MANAGEMENT GUIDELINES FOR NURSE PRACTITIONERS WORKING WITH OLDER ADULTS

Second Edition

Laurie Kennedy-Malone, *PhD, APRN-BC, GNP*
Associate Professor
Director of the Adult/Gerontological Nurse Practitioner Program
School of Nursing
The University of North Carolina at Greensboro
Greensboro, North Carolina

Kathleen Ryan Fletcher, *RN, MSN, APRN-BC,*
GNP, FAAN
Gerontological Nurse Practitioner
Administrator, Senior Services
Assistant Professor of Nursing
University of Virginia Health System
Charlottesville, Virginia

Lori Martin Plank, *PhD(c), MSPH, MSN, RN,*
APRN, BC
Assistant Professor, School of Nursing
College of Allied Health Sciences
Temple University
Family and Gerontological Nurse Practitioner, Temple Health Connection,
a member of the National Nursing Centers Consortium
Philadelphia, Pennsylvania

F. A. DAVIS COMPANY | Philadelphia

F. A. Davis Company
1915 Arch Street
Philadelphia, PA 19103

Printed in Canada

Last digit indicates print number: 10 9 8 7 6 5 4 3 2 1

Acquisitions Editor: Joanne Patzek DaCunha, RN, MSN
Developmental Editor: Diane Blodgett
Cover Designer: Louis J. Forgione

As new scientific information becomes available through basic and clinical research, recommended treatments and drug therapies undergo changes. The authors and publisher have done everything possible to make this book accurate, up to date, and in accord with accepted standards at the time of publication. The authors, editors, and publisher are not responsible for errors or omissions or for consequences from application of the book, and make no warranty, expressed or implied, with regard to the contents of the book. Any practice described in this book should be applied by the reader in accordance with professional standards of care used with regard to the unique circumstances that may apply in each situation. The reader is advised always to check product information (package inserts) for changes and new information regarding dose and contraindications before administering any drug. Caution is especially urged when using new or infrequently ordered drugs.

Library of Congress Cataloging-in-Publication Data

Management guidelines for nurse practitioners working with older adults / [edited by] Laurie Kennedy-Malone, Kathleen Ryan Fletcher, Lori Martin Plank.—2nd ed.
  p. ; cm.
  Rev. ed. of: Management guidelines for gerontological nurse practitioners / [edited by] Laurie Kennedy-Malone, Kathleen Ryan Fletcher, Lori Martin Plank.©2000.
  Includes bibliographical references and index.
  ISBN 0-8036-1120-X
  1. Geriatric nursing. 2. Geriatrics. 3. Nurse practitioners. 4. Aged—Diseases—Treatment. I. Kennedy-Malone, Laurie, 1957– II. Fletcher, Kathleen Ryan, 1951– III. Plank, Lori Martin. IV. Management guidelines for gerontological nurse practitioners.
  [DNLM: 1. Geriatric Nursing—methods. WY 152 M2657 2003]
RC954.M356 2003
610.73′65—dc21
                                                                    2003053078

I dedicate this book to my husband Chris, young son Brendan,
and my parents Edward and Nancy Kennedy, for their years of support,
encouragement, and understanding throughout this endeavor.

L.K.-M.

I dedicate this book to my husband Steve, my son Ian, and my mother
Eleanor, who understand my professional commitments and provide
unfailing support and encouragement.

K.R.F.

I dedicate this book to my husband Rick and daughter Erin
and to my dear aunt, Madeleine Plank, for sharing her
end-of-life experience with us.

L.M.P.

PREFACE

Because of the continuing rapid growth of the older adult population, there will be an increased need for primary care providers to deliver age-specific care and direct disease management. This second edition of *Management Guidelines for Nurse Practitioners Working with Older Adults* serves as a clinical resource for advanced practice nurses and students who are privileged to provide primary care to older adults. This helpful guide is a useful resource for clinical nurse specialists, nurse case managers, and registered nurses caring for older adults in ambulatory care settings.

Unit I, "The Healthy Older Adult," covers updated information pertaining to health promotion and disease prevention strategies for older adults, including an immunization schedule, components of nutritional assessment, and recommendations for a healthy diet for older adults. Because older adults are often at risk for nutritional deficiencies, the unit covers unique signs and symptoms of this condition in older adults.

Unit II, "Managing Illness: Symptom-Based Problems," provides the clinician with a concise description of more than 20 symptoms prevalent in older adults. In the next 11 chapters, updated information pertaining to the disease management of illnesses common in older adults is presented. Clinical pearls highlighting the atypical presentation of illness in older adults are featured throughout the chapters. Each disease presentation includes updated ICD-9 codes. Rapid access to diagnostic test interpretation accompanied by CPT codes for each disease condition is included for each disease. The unit concludes with appendices that contain valuable information for the busy practitioner to have readily available for reference.

ACKNOWLEDGMENTS

This book would not have become a reality if not for the kind assistance of some wonderful people whom we would like to thank. To Joanne DaCunha, our editor, who continued to encourage us to complete this task, and to Karen Yandell and Mary Flemming, for assistance with literature review and information retrieval.

L.K.-M.

CONTRIBUTORS

Susan J. Appel, PhD RN, ACNP-BC, FNP-BC, CCRN
Assistant Professor of Nursing
The University of North Carolina at Greensboro
Greensboro, North Carolina
Chapter 11—Hyperlipidemia; Obesity

Kathleen M. Pelletier Brown, MSN, CRNP, PhD
University of Pennsylvania
School of Nursing
Philadelphia, Pennsylvania
Chapter 7—Breast Cancer; Endometrial Cancer; Ovarian Cancer

Karen Beard Byrd, MSN, RN, C-GNP, OCN
The Comprehensive Cancer Center of Wake Forest University
Winston Salem, North Carolina
Chapter 10—Brain Tumor

Robert B. Davis, RN/FNP, MSN
Family Nurse Practitioner
Department of Nephrology and Renal Services
University of Virginia Health System
Charlottesville, Virginia
Chapter 2—Cough; Hemoptysis

Sheree L. Loftus Fader, MSN, CRRN, RNC
Coordinator/Nurse Practitioner
National Parkinson Foundation
Beth Israel Phillips Ambulatory Care Center
New York, New York
Chapter 10—Parkinson's Disease

Kathleen Ryan Fletcher, RN, MSN, APRN-BC, GNP, FAAN
Gerontological Nurse Practitioner
Administrator Senior Services
Assistant Professor of Nursing
University of Virginia Health System
Charlottesville, Virginia
Chapter 2—Symptom-Based Problems; Appendices

Stacey Hamilton, MSN, RN, CS, GGNP
Austin Geriatric Specialists, P.A.
Austin, Texas
Chapter 2—Tremor

Gretchen Hope Miller Heery, APRN, BC
Occupational Health Nurse Practitioner
WorkForce Wellness Program
Family Nurse Practitioner
Gnaden Huetten Memorial Hospital
Lehighton, Pennsylvania
Chapter 3—Pressure Ulcers

Ellen Jones, ND, FNP, RNC
Assistant Professor of Nursing
School of Nursing
The University of North Carolina at Greensboro
Greensboro, North Carolina
Chapter 11—Diabetes Mellitus

Laurie Kennedy-Malone, PhD, APRN-BC, GNP
Associate Professor
Director of the Adult/Gerontological Nurse Practitioner Program
School of Nursing
The University of North Carolina at Greensboro
Greensboro, North Carolina

Virginia Lee, RN, APRN-BC, MSN
Adult Nurse Practitioner
Senior Services
University of Virginia Health System
Charlottesville, Virginia
Chapter 2—Confusion; Involuntary Weight Loss

Terri L. Moore, RN, BSN
Vascular Care Coordinator
TCV Services
University of Virginia Health System
Charlottesville, Virginia
Chapter 9—Abdominal Aortic Aneurysm; Peripheral Vascular Disease

Margo Packheiser, MSN, RN, APRN-BC, ANP/GNP
Clinical Associate Professor
School of Nursing
The University of North Carolina at Greensboro
Greensboro, North Carolina
Chapter 11—Malnutrition

Lori Martin Plank, PhD(c), MSPH, MSN, RN, APRN, BC
Assistant Professor, School of Nursing
College of Allied Health Sciences
Temple University
Family and Gerontological Nurse Practitioner, Temple Health Connection,
a member of the National Nursing Centers Consortium
Philadelphia, Pennsylvania
Chapter 1—Health Promotion; Chapter 3—Chronic Bronchitis; Lung
Cancer; Pneumonia; Pulmonary Embolism; Pulmonary Tuberculosis;
Restrictive Lung Disease; Upper Respiratory Tract Infection; Chapter 4—
Head, Neck, and Face Disorders; Chapter 7—Reproductive Disorders;
Chapter 12—Hematological and Immune System Disorders; Chapter
13—Psychosocial Disorders

Catherine Ratliff, PhD, GNP, CWOCN, CS
Enterostomal Therapy
University of Virginia Health System
Charlottesville, Virginia
Chapter 2—Dehydration; Nausea and Vomiting

Marianne Shaughnessy, PhD, CRNP
Associate Director Education/Evaluation
Baltimore VA Geriatrics Research, Education and Clinical Center
Assistant Professor
University of Maryland, Baltimore
School of Nursing
Baltimore, Maryland
Chapter 10—Cerebrovascular Accident (Stroke); Transient Ischemic
Attack

Lois L. VonCannon, MSN, RN, APRN, BC
Clinical Associate Professor
School of Nursing
The University of North Carolina at Greensboro
Greensboro, North Carolina
Chapter 11—Chronic Pancreatitis; Pancreatic Cancer

CONTENTS

Unit 1
THE HEALTHY OLDER ADULT

Chapter *1*
HEALTH
PROMOTION

Health Promotion   ICD-9-CM: V70.0

The concept of health promotion includes activities to which an individual is committed and performs proactively to further his or her health and well-being. This includes not only preventive and health-protective measures, but also actualization of one's health potential. The broadest definition, identified by the World Health Organization, includes healthy lifestyle promotion, creation of supportive environments for health, community action, redirection of health services, and healthy public policy formulation. All these measures are within the scope of the nurse practitioner and enhance the visibility of his or her role while advancing the needs of patients.

Nurse practitioners are in a unique and pivotal position to guide and encourage health promotion programs and individual efforts. From our nursing background, we bring a holistic orientation to health and wellness, knowledge of developmental tasks, and of the wellness-illness continuum. Our advanced practice education helps us to diagnose and treat patients in a way that supports their return to optimal levels of function and maximizes their coping abilities within the limits of their existing function.

This particular blend of competencies is especially valuable in working with older patients. Heterogeneity increases with aging, presenting the gerontological nurse practitioner with the challenge of individualizing health promotion recommendations for each patient. Given that average life expectancy in developed countries is approximately 80 years, with a potential to live to 120 years, it behooves us to focus on prevention and health promotion in older patients to maximize the quality of these years.

The guidelines of the United States Preventive Services Task Force (USPSTF) and other authorities can be used to provide a framework and timeline for health promotion and preventive activities. These guidelines represent the best effort to date to identify screenings and interventions that have scientific merit and efficacy. Many of these items do not target specifically the older age group, but they may be adapted as clinical judgment permits. Primary and secondary prevention in the areas of immunizations, screening, and counseling is addressed; the active roles of the primary health-care provider and patient are emphasized. As the science of evidence-based practice evolves, the USPSTF is continually re-evaluating and updating recommendations. The Agency for Healthcare Research and Quality has also developed a clearinghouse for evidence-based practice guidelines addressing prevention and disease management. With the cost of medical interventions rising astronomically, mandated cost controls limit treatment options and make prevention economically desirable. Despite these advances in the science of evidence-based health care, a survey of adults in several U.S. cities revealed that most are uninformed and cling to the myth of the annual physical examination without recommended screenings (Oboler et al, 2002).

Healthy People 2010, the U.S. Surgeon General's prevention agenda for a healthy population, is a statement of national health objectives designed to identify the most significant preventable threats to health and to establish national goals to reduce these threats. Ten leading health indicators representing these preventable threats include physical activity, overweight and obesity, tobacco use, substance abuse, responsible sexual behavior, mental health, injury and violence, environmental quality, immunization, and access to health care(contact: http://web.health.gov/healthypeople/LHI/lhiwhat.htm). On a global level, similar prerequisites for healthy aging were unveiled at the Second World Assembly on Aging of the World Health Organization (contact: http://www.who.int/inf/en/pr-2002-24.html).

The message is clear that individual lifestyle interventions are the key to health promotion and healthy aging. The USPSTF confirms the need to individualize preventive services. The USPSTF has identified personal counseling and patient education as being more effective than diagnostic testing in health promotion and health protection and found that the most effective interventions are focused on patients' personal health practices. For optimal outcomes, health promotion and preventive counseling should be addressed at each encounter including goal setting and scheduled follow-up if indicated. Use of a reminder system or flow sheet may be helpful in implementing and tracking progress. Other tools include writing a wellness prescription or designing an individual contract for the patient to sign.

The USPSTF has presented a comprehensive plan for implementing and evaluating behavioral interventions in the primary care setting. The Five A's Organizational Construct for Clinical Counseling from this plan are summarized as follows:

Assess: Ask about/assess behavioral health risks and factors affecting choice of behavior change goals and methods. For older adults, consider present and anticipated level of function and barriers to implementation.

Advise: Give clear, specific, and personalized behavior change advice, including information about personal health harms and benefits and effectiveness of specific preventive interventions for older adults.

Agree: Collaboratively select appropriate treatment goals and methods based on the patient's interest in and willingness to change the behavior.

Assist: Using behavior change techniques (self-help or counseling or both), aid the patient in achieving agreed-on goals by acquiring the skills, confidence, and social and environmental supports for behavior change, supplemented with adjunctive medical treatments when appropriate (e.g., pharmacotherapy for tobacco dependence).

Arrange: Schedule follow-up contacts (in person or by telephone) to provide ongoing assistance and support and to adjust the treatment plan as needed, including referral to more intensive or specialized treatment (contact: http://www.ahrq.gov/clinic/uspstfix.htm).

The USPSTF research found that brief interventions incorporated into everyday practice can produce meaningful changes in behavioral risk factors. Specific areas for health promotion counseling of the older adult are addressed next.

EXERCISE

The health benefits of regular physical activity are well documented and include flexibility, increased muscle mass, maintenance of desirable weight, decreased insulin resistance, decreased peripheral vascular resistance, lower blood pressure, and a sense of well-being. Two thirds of older adults are sedentary, however, or only sporadically active. Some common barriers to regular physical activity identified in a study of older men included pain, fatigue, mobility impairment, and sensory impairment. Adaptation of the exercise program to surmount these and other perceived barriers is challenging but key to success. For most healthy older adults and adults with stable chronic health problems, a regular exercise program is achievable and desirable. It should incorporate stretching for flexibility, strengthening and resistive training, and a cardiovascular fitness component of moderate intensity over a 30-minute period daily or on most days. For many older adults, brisk walking can achieve the desired aerobic benefit. Active hobbies, such as gardening, golfing, tennis, dancing, bowling, hiking, and swimming, are also beneficial. Tai chi and yoga are helpful for stretching and balance. Frail elderly or older adults with impaired mobility can benefit from armchair exercises and modified ambulation. It may take 20 weeks for measurable results to occur, so ongoing encouragement is essential to success.

To avoid musculoskeletal complications that may sabotage the program, a gradual stepwise approach is advised. Before embarking on an exercise program, all patients should have an evaluation of health history, including medications, present physical activity and functional level, potential barriers to exercise, and physical examination (Table 1–1). Older adults with known or suspected cardiac risk factors should have a stress test before engaging in vigorous exercise. All participants should be reminded of the need for adequate hydration and caution during extreme weather conditions.

NUTRITION

The heterogeneity of older adults is evident in the wide range of nutritional issues affecting them. Before initiating counseling on diet, obtain

Table 1–1   Initial Evaluation of the Elderly Patient for Physical Activity Prescription

Objectives/Principles	Interventions	Tips to Suggest to Patients
Identify chronic disease or physical limitations that could affect exercise capabilities. Modified exercise is generally safe and will help maintain independence and quality of life.	Individualize the exercise program within the safety guidelines or physical limitations.	Monitor blood pressure and heart rate before, during, and after exercise. Exercise only when feeling well. Exercise 2 hours after eating a meal.
Modify physical activities to provide enjoyable and practical exercises so that exercise is more likely to be maintained.	Help the patient choose low- to moderate-impact exercises such as walking or swimming. Incorporate a variety of activities into the routine.	Begin slowly and increase duration gradually. Adjust exercise to the weather. Dress in confortable clothes.
Set realistic program goals that the patient is likely to attain and continue.	Determine the elder's willingness to include exercise.	Walk with the Senior Citizens group three times a week.
Evaluate dietary history with emphasis on dietary inadequacies. Dietary inadequacies are common and may be compounded by modest increases in caloric expenditure due to increased activity.	Encourage patient to eat a regular balanced diet high in protein, minerals, and vitamins.	Stop exercising if faintness, upper body discomfort, and/or bone/joint pain occur.
Evaluate for potential injury. Degenerative joint disease is common in this age group. Neuropathy, gait disturbance, impaired equilibrium, orthostatic hypotension, and cardiovascular symptoms may be present.	Use assistive devices such as walkers with wheels to provide stability. Include range of motion and resistance training to increase stability.	

Table 1–1   Initial Evaluation of the Elderly Patient for Physical Activity Prescription *(continued)*

Objectives/Principles	Interventions	Tips to Suggest to Patients
Review medications to avoid adverse interactions with activity program, in particular, note whether patient is taking: diuretics (can cause hyper-calcemia, hypokalemia, arrhythmias, and volume depletion) beta blockers (can reduce exercise tolerance) tranquilizers (can cause orthostatic hypotension and dizziness and can impair thermoregulation) insulin (may require dose adjustment).	Teach the patient self-monitoring of heart rate, blood pressure, respirations.	Monitor heart rate, blood pressure, respirations. Drink enough water before and after exercise. Eat foods high in calcium and potassium. Take prescribed calcium and potassium supplements. Reduce the intensity of exercise. Take extra time for warming up and cooling down. Get up and down slowly. Eat high-carbohydrate snacks before exercising. Keep hard candy readily available.

Used with permission from Allison, M, and Keller, C: Physical activity in the elderly: Benefits and intervention strategies. Nurse Practitioner 22:53–69, 1997. © Springhouse Corporation.

baseline information on current dietary intake and activity pattern and combine this with height and weight data and other health status information. For patients in the long-term care setting, this information is obtained easily from chart documentation. For community-dwelling older adults, the Nutrition Screening Initiative tools are most specific and easily administered (Table 1–2). The initial, self-administered questionnaire can be given to patients waiting to see the health-care provider. After scoring the questionnaire, at-risk patients are referred for additional screening, using the mnemonic *DETERMINE* to identify risk for nutritional deficiencies:

Disease
Eating poorly
Tooth loss or mouth pain
Economic hardship
Reduced social contact and interaction
Multiple medications
Involuntary weight loss or gain
Need for assistance with self-care
Elder at an advanced age

Additional screening using the mnemonic *ABCDEF* gathers more information to complete the assessment and pinpoint interventions:

Anthropometric: Height and weight
Biochemical: Serum albumin <3.5 mg/dL is a nonspecific indicator of poor nutrition; hemoglobin determination for anemia,

Table 1–2   Determine Your Nutritional Health (NSI)

	Yes
I have an illness or condition that made me change the kind and/or amount of food I eat.	2
I eat fewer than 2 meals per day.	3
I eat few fruits or vegetables, or milk products.	2
I have 3 or more drinks of beer, liquor, or wine almost every day.	2
I have tooth or mouth problems that make it hard for me to eat.	2
I don't always have enough money to buy the food I need.	4
I eat alone most of the time.	1
I take 3 or more different prescribed or over-the-counter drugs a day.	1
Without wanting to, I have lost or gained 10 pounds in the last 6 months.	2
I am not always physically able to shop, cook, and/or feed myself.	2
TOTAL	

Total Your Nutritional Score. If it's—		*These materials developed and distributed by the Nutrition Screening Initiative, a project of:*
0–2	**Good!** Recheck you nutritional score in 6 months.	AMERICAN ACADEMY OF FAMILY PHYSICIANS
		THE AMERICAN DIETETIC ASSOCIATION
		NATIONAL COUNCIL ON THE AGING, INC.
3–5	**You are at moderate nutritional risk.** See what can be done to improve your eating habits and lifestyle. Your office on aging, senior nutrition program, senior citizens center, or health department can help. Recheck your nutritional score in 3 months.	
6 or more	**You are at high nutritional risk.** Bring this checklist the next time you see your doctor, dietitian, or other qualified health or social service professional. Talk with them about any problems you may have. Ask for help to improve your nutritional health.	**Remember that warning signs suggest risk, but do not represent diagnosis of any condition.**

Reprinted with permission from the Nutrition Screening Initiative, a project of the American Academy of Family Physicians, the American Dietetic Association, and the National Council on the Aging, Inc., and funded in part by a grant from Ross Products Division, Abbott Laboratories.

hematocrit for hemoconcentration with dehydration, serum cholesterol for cholesterol elevation, and serum vitamin B_{12} to rule out deficiencies complete the screen.

Clinical: Physical and medical history (self-explanatory)

Dietary history: Food diary of a normal 24- to 48-hour period, listing all food and drink, supplements, food sources, storage, and cooking facilities as well as any cultural and religious preferences and taboos

Empathy: Active listening, inquiring about diet, and giving the patient time to share any problems

Functional assessment: Assessment of activities of daily living and instrumental activities of daily living abilities related to meal planning, shopping, preparation, and storage

Although this approach may seem redundant, it yields more specific information for designing individualized interventions and is more likely to be successful.

General guidelines for dietary counseling include:

- Limiting fat and cholesterol
- Maintaining a balanced caloric intake
- Emphasizing the inclusion of grains, fruits, and vegetables daily
- Ensuring an adequate calcium intake, especially for women
- Limiting alcohol, if used, to one drink daily for women and two drinks daily for men: one drink $=$ 12 oz. beer, 5 oz. wine, or 1.5 oz. of 80-proof distilled spirits

More than half of U.S. adults are overweight or obese. Overweight and obesity are associated with heart disease, certain types of cancer, type 2 diabetes, breathing difficulties, stroke, arthritis, and psychological problems. Although there is a decline in the prevalence of overweight and obesity after age 60 years, it remains a problem for many older adults. It is a major risk factor for decreased mobility and functional impairment as well as a cardiovascular risk. The National Heart, Lung, and Blood Institute has an Obesity Education Initiative, complete with provider training and patient education materials (contact: http://www.nhlbi. nih.gov/about/oei/index.htm). The Obesity Education Initiative endorses treatment of obesity up to age 80 years with precautions to preserve bone health and nutritional status. The National Cholesterol Education Program's Adult Treatment Panel III Guidelines provide health-care professionals and patients with a comprehensive plan for lowering cholesterol to prevent heart disease and for patients who already have heart disease. The Adult Treatment Panel III Guidelines At-A-Glance Quick Desk Reference (contact: http://www.nhlbi.nih.gov/guidelines/cholesterol/index.htm) offers clinicians an abbreviated step-by-step guide to evaluation and management of high cholesterol.

SAFETY

Prevention of injury in the older adult is of paramount importance to continuing functionality and quality of life. Part of this counseling involves reinforcement of extant recommendations, including wearing lap and shoulder seatbelts in a motor vehicle, avoiding drinking and driving, having working smoke detectors in the residence, and keeping hot water set at $<120°F$. For older adults who drive a motor vehicle, periodic assessment of their ongoing ability to drive safely is vital to the older adult and the public at large. Most motor vehicle accidents involve young drivers and older drivers.

Two other recommendations are especially important for the older adult. The first involves the safe storage and removal of firearms. Possession of a firearm combined with depression, caregiver stress, irreversible illness, or decline in functional abilities can invite self-inflicted injury, suicide pacts, or other acts of violence. Counsel patients to avoid firearms in the home and to use alternative means for self-protection, such as alarm systems and pepper mace spray. Falls are the leading cause of nonfatal injuries and unintentional death from injury in older persons. Certain combinations of physiological and environmental factors place some patients at increased risk. About 85% of falls occur at home, in the later part of the day. Table 1–3 lists the known risk factors.

Evaluation of risk factors and a home safety assessment by a home health nurse or a geriatric assessment team can provide direction for preventive intervention and education (Table 1–4). Potential recommendations include exercise programs to build strength, modification of environmental hazards, monitoring and adjusting of medications, external protection against falling on hard surfaces, and measures to increase bone density. If urinary incontinence is a contributing factor, a urological workup may be indicated. Falls are often alarming to patients and families; in some cases, family members may desire nursing home placement for the patient because of a fall. In other cases, patients may be fearful of ambulation as a result of a fall. Falls also pose a challenge in the long-term care environment. The use of active restraining devices does not prevent falls; some patients are injured further because of the restraints. Families may insist on restraining the patient for safety, however. Education and counseling combined with an assessment of the patient's environment are helpful. Keeping water, call bell, telephone, and other necessities available and toileting regularly can minimize the potential for falling.

Health promotion in older adults can be expanded to include presence or absence of social and financial support systems, completion of an advanced directive, and evaluation of spiritual needs. The last-men-

Table 1–3   Risk Factors for Falls in the Elderly

Physiological	Environmental
Gait disturbances	Stairs
Poor vision	Pavement irregularities
Decreased muscle strength	Slippery surfaces (loose rugs)
Postural instability	Incorrect footwear
Cognitive impairment	Low chairs
Number of medications	Inadequate lighting
Psychoactive drugs	Unexpected objects
Antihypertensive drugs	
Multiple physiological problems	

Table 1–4 Home Safety Checklist

Place a check mark next to each question if the answer is yes. Use this checklist to correct all hazards in the home.

Housekeeping

—— Do you clean up spills as soon as they occur?
—— Do you keep floors and stairways clear and free of clutter?
—— Do you put away books, magazines, sewing supplies, and other objects as soon as you are through with them and never leave them on floors or stairways?
—— Do you store frequently used items on shelves that are within easy reach?

Floors

—— Do you keep everyone from walking on freshly washed floors before they are dry?
—— If you wax floors, do you apply 2 thin coats and buff each thoroughly or use self-polishing wax?
—— Do all area rugs have nonslip backings?
—— Have you eliminated small rugs at the tops and bottoms of stairways?
—— Are all carpet edges tacked down?
—— Are rugs and carpets free of curled edges, worn spots, and rips?
—— Have you chosen rugs and carpets with short, dense pile?
—— Are rugs and carpets installed over good quality, medium-thick pads?

Lighting

—— Do you have light switches near every doorway?
—— Do you have enough good lighting to eliminate shadowy areas?
—— Do you have a lamp or light switch within easy reach of every bed?
—— Do you have night lights in your bathrooms and in hallways leading from bedrooms to bathrooms?
—— Are all stairways well lit, with light switches at both top and bottom?

Bathrooms

—— Do you use a rubber mat or nonslip decals in tubs and showers?
—— Do you have a grab bar securely anchored over each tub and shower?
—— Do you have a nonslip rug on all bathroom floors?
—— Do you keep soap in easy-to-reach receptacles?

Traffic Lanes

—— Can you walk across every room in your home, and from one room to another, without detouring around furniture?
—— Is the traffic lane from your bedroom to the bathroom free of obstacles?
—— Are telephone and appliance cords kept away from areas where people walk?

Stairways

—— Do securely fastened handrails extend the full length of the stairs on each side of the stairways?
—— Do the handrails stand out from the walls so you can get a good grip?
—— Are handrails distinctly shaped so you are alerted when you reach the end of a stairway?
—— Are all stairway in good condition, with no broken, sagging, or sloping steps?
—— Are all stairway carpeting and metal edges securely fastened and in good condition?
—— Have you replaced any single-level steps with gradually rising ramps or made sure such steps are well lighted?

Ladders and Step Stools

—— Do you always use a step stool or ladder that is tall enough for the job?
—— Do you always set up your ladder or step stool on a firm, level base that is free of clutter?
—— Before you climb a ladder or step stool, do you always make sure it is fully open and that the stepladder spreaders are locked?
—— When you use a ladder or step stool, do you face the steps and keep your body between the side rails?
—— Do you avoid standing on the top step of a step stool or climbing beyond the second step from the top on a stepladder?

(Continued on the following page)

Table 1–4 **Home Safety Checklist** *(Cont'd)*

Outdoor Areas

——— Are walks and driveways in your yard and other areas free of breaks?
——— Are lawns and gardens free of holes?
——— Do you put away garden tools and hoses when they are not in use?
——— Are outdoor areas kept free of rocks, loose boards, and other tripping hazards?
——— Do you keep outdoor walkways, steps, and porches free of wet leaves and snow?
——— Do you sprinkle icy outdoor areas with de-icers as soon as possible after a snowfall or freeze?
——— Do you have mats at doorways for people to wipe their feet on?
——— Do you know the safest way of walking when you can't avoid walking on a slippery surface?

Footwear

——— Do your shoes have soles and heels that provide good traction?
——— Do you avoid walking in stocking feet and wear house slippers that fit well and don't fall off?
——— Do you wear low-heeled oxfords, loafers, or good-quality sneakers when you work in your house or yard?
——— Do you replace boots or galoshes when their soles or heels are worn too smooth to keep you from slipping on wet or ice surface?

Personal Precautions

——— Are you always alert for unexpected hazards, such as out-of-place furniture?
——— If young children visit or live in your home, are you alert for children playing on the floor and toys left in your path?
——— If you have pets, are you alert for sudden movements across your path and pets getting underfoot?
——— When you carry packages, do you divide them into smaller loads and make sure they do not obstruct your vision?
——— When you reach or bend, do you hold onto a firm support and avoid throwing your head back or turning it too far?
——— Do you always move deliberately and avoid rushing to answer the phone or doorbell?
——— Do you take time to get your balance when you change position from lying down to sitting and from sitting to standing?
——— Do you keep yourself in good condition with moderate exercise, good diet, adequate rest, and regular medical checkups?
——— If you wear glasses, is your prescription up to date?
——— Do you know how to reduce injury in a fall?
——— If you live alone, do you have daily contact with a friend or neighbor?

Adapted from National Safety Council, Falling—The Unexpected Trip: A Safety Program for Older Adults (Program Leader's Guide). National Safety Council, Chicago, 1982. Used with permission of the National Safety Council; copyright © 1982.

tioned area, wellness spirituality, has been discussed in detail by Leetun (1996), who identified four key domains for assessment: self-actualization activities, connectedness activities, healing and new life activities, and religious and humanistic orientation activities. Spiritual health promotion also may benefit older adults dealing with the loss of significant others or losses secondary to chronic health problems and functional decline. Referral to a support group or congregational health ministry team can be initiated.

SEXUAL BEHAVIOR

Assumptions regarding lack of sexual expression in the healthy older adult are unfounded. With the possibility of pregnancy eliminated, many mature adults feel less restraint. Because of divorce or widowhood, they may seek satisfaction with new partners, yet lack the knowledge to protect themselves from sexually transmitted diseases, especially human immunodeficiency virus (HIV). More than 10% of HIV cases diagnosed in the United States are in people >50 years old. Older adults need to be taught about methods for safe sex with use of a barrier to avoid sexually transmitted diseases, including HIV and hepatitis B. Using the patient's sexual history, explore patient needs, preferences, and medical or psychological obstacles to sexual expression. This exploration facilitates counseling and interventions to promote healthy sexuality.

DENTAL HEALTH

Counseling regarding dental health in the older adult includes the need for regular visits to the dental-care provider, daily flossing, and brushing with a fluoride toothpaste. Many elders have dentures or dental implants and assume that dental checkups are no longer necessary. Oral screening for cancer is still indicated, as is periodic assessment of denture fit and functionality. Another concern is for the condition of the remaining teeth of some older adults. Periodontal disease, erosion of dentin, or other problems may render the teeth nonfunctional for chewing and a potential source for infection. Dependence on others for transportation or lack of availability of dental resources for patients in long-term care settings further complicate the problem. Caregivers simply may overlook this aspect of preventive health, or financial considerations may preclude treatment. Patient and family education regarding dental health is essential.

SUBSTANCE USE

Counseling about substance use (tobacco, alcohol, and drugs) and injury prevention can be combined naturally within the issue of safety. Smoking is the leading preventable cause of death in the United States. Smoking cessation yields many benefits to former smokers in terms of reduction of risk for several chronic illnesses and stabilization of pulmonary status. Clear and specific guidelines are available to help health-care providers advise tobacco users to quit and to provide them with follow-up encouragement and relapse prevention management. Quitting smoking may not be a choice for the institutionalized older adult but rather dictated by the policy of the institution. Health-care providers can offer support and encouragement, emphasizing the positive health changes that will result.

Counseling regarding alcohol or other drug use can be preventive or interventional, depending on the initial assessment. Use the Michigan Alcohol Screening Test (MAST), CAGE, or Alcohol Use Disorders Identification Test (AUDIT) to assess risk. Emphasize the dangers of drinking and driving and the increased risk of falling while under the influence of alcohol or any drug that acts on the central nervous system. Teach patients about the coincidental interactions between alcohol and many prescription drugs, over-the-counter preparations such as acetaminophen, and herbal remedies. The contribution of alcohol abuse to problems such as insomnia, depression, aggressive behaviors, and deteriorating social relationships should be addressed. Likewise, the problem of dependence on prescription drugs, such as analgesics, hypnotics, tranquilizers, and anxiolytics, should be assessed and addressed. Counseling in the form of individual follow-up sessions, group support, or outpatient or inpatient rehabilitation may be indicated. In a group-living situation, the governing body (i.e., resident council) may become involved if the patient's behavior threatens the safety or well-being of the other group members.

IMMUNIZATIONS

Influenza vaccine is now recommended annually for all adults >50 years old, unless contraindicated. Residents of long-term care facilities that house persons with chronic medical conditions are at especially high risk for developing the disease. Health-care workers also should receive the vaccine. Patients with a severe egg allergy or severe reaction to the influenza vaccine in the past and patients with a prior history of Guillain-Barré syndrome should talk with their health-care provider before getting the vaccine.

Tetanus-diphtheria (Td) vaccine is administered as a booster every 10 years or at least once in later adulthood. For acute, traumatic wound management, a booster may be given if >5 years have elapsed since the previous tetanus immunization. If a primary series was not given during childhood, administer three doses. The second dose is given 4 to 6 weeks after initial dose, the third dose is given 6 to 12 months after the second dose, then revert to booster schedule. Adults >60 years old account for 60% of tetanus cases.

Pneumococcal vaccine usually is administered once to adults ≥65 years old. Younger persons with severe chronic health conditions, including hemoglobinopathies, renal disease, diabetes, heart disease, lung disease, or immunodeficiency or immunosuppressive disorders also should receive the vaccine. A repeat dose may be given 5 years after the initial dose for adults at highest risk or adults vaccinated before 65 years of age.

Hepatitis A vaccine is recommended for persons traveling to countries where the disease is common. It is given in two doses; the initial dose should be administered at least 4 weeks before departure. The second dose should be given 6 to 12 months later.

Hepatitis B vaccine is recommended for high-risk persons, such as intravenous drug users or persons who are sexually active with multiple partners. The initial dose is given, followed 1 month later by the second dose, then the third dose given 4 to 6 months after the second dose.

Table 1–5 presents recommended adult immunization schedules. Table 1–6 summarizes preventive services to consider for older adults.

Table 1–5 Recommended Adult Immunization Schedule, United States, 2002–2003, and Recommended Immunizations for Adults with Medical Conditions, United States, 2002–2003

Recommended Adult Immunization Schedule, United States, 2002–2003

Legend:
- For all persons in this group
- Catch-up on childhood vaccinations
- For persons with medical/ exposure indications

Vaccine ▼	19–49 Years	50–64 Years	65 Years and Older
		Age Group	
Tetanus, Diphtheria (Td)*	1 dose booster every 10 years[1]		
Influenza	1 dose annually for persons with medical or occupational indications, or household contacts of persons with indications[2]	1 annual dose	
Pneumococcal (polysaccharide)	1 dose for persons with medical or other indications. (1 dose revaccination for immunosuppressive conditions)[3,4]		1 dose for unvaccinated persons[3] / 1 dose revaccination[4]
Hepatitis B*	3 doses (0, 1–2, 4–6 months) for persons with medical, behavioral, occupational, or other indications[5]		
Hepatitis A	2 doses (0, 6–12 months) for persons with medical, behavioral, occupational, or other indications[6]		

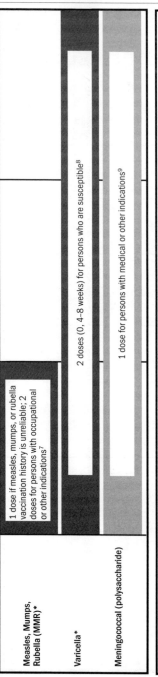

Measles, Mumps, Rubella (MMR)*	1 dose if measles, mumps, or rubella vaccination history is unreliable; 2 doses for persons with occupational or other indications[7]
Varicella*	2 doses (0, 4–8 weeks) for persons who are susceptible[8]
Meningococcal (polysaccharide)	1 dose for persons with medical or other indications[9]

* Covered by the Vaccine Injury Compensation Program. For information on how to file a claim call 800-338-2382. Please also visit www.*hrsa.asp.gov/osp/vicp*. To file a claim for vaccine injury write: U.S. Court of Federal Claims, 717 Madison Place, N.W., Washington D.C. 20005.

This schedule indicates the recommended age groups for routine administration of currently licensed vaccines for persons 19 years of age and older. Licensed combination vaccines may be used whenever any components of the combination are indicated and the vaccine's other components are not contraindicated. Providers should consult the manufacturers' package inserts for detailed recommendations.

Report all clinically significant post-vaccination reactions to the Vaccine Adverse Event Reporting System (VAERS). Reporting forms and instructions on filing a VAERS report are available by calling 800-822-7967 or from the VAERS website at www.*vaers.org*.

For additional information about the vaccines listed above and contraindications for immunization, visit the National Immunization Program Website at www.*cdc.gov/nip/* or call the National Immunization Hotline at 800-232-2522 (English) or 800-232-0233 (Spanish).

Approved by the Advisory Committee on Immunization Practices (ACIP), and accepted by the American College of Obstetricians and Gynecologists (ACOG) and the American Academy of Family Physicians (AAFP)

(continued on the following page)

Table 1-5 Recommended Adult Immunization Schedule, United States, 2002–2003, and Recommended Immunizations for Adults with Medical Conditions, United States, 2002–2003 (continued)

Recommended Adult Immunization Schedule, United States, 2002–2003

Legend: ■ For all persons in this group | Catch-up on childhood vaccinations | For persons with medical/exposure indications | ■ Contraindicated

Medical Conditions	Tetanus-Diphtheria (Td)*	Influenza	Pneumococcal (polysaccharide)	Hepatitis B*	Hepatitis A	Measles, Mumps, Rubella (MMR)*	Varicella*
Pregnancy		A				Contraindicated	Contraindicated
Diabetes, heart disease, chronic pulmonary disease, chronic liver disease, including chronic alcoholism		B	C		D		
Congenital immunodeficiency, leukemia, lymphoma, generalized malignancy, therapy with alkylating agents, antimetabolites, radiation or large amounts of corticosteroids			E				Contraindicated F
Renal failure/end stage renal disease, recipients of hemodialysis or clotting factor concentrates			E	G			
Asplenia including elective splenectomy and terminal complement component deficiencies			E, H, I				
HIV infection			E, J			K	Contraindicated

A. If pregnancy is at 2nd or 3rd trimester during influenza season.

B. Although chronic liver disease and alcoholism are not indicator conditions for influenza vaccination, give 1 dose annually if the patient is ≥ 50 years, has other indications for influenza vaccine, or if the patient requests vaccination.

C. Asthma is an indicator condition for influenza but not for pneumococcal vaccination.

D. For all persons with chronic liver disease.

E. Revaccinate once after 5 years or more have elapsed since initial vaccination.

F. Persons with impaired humoral but not cellular immunity may be vaccinated. *MMWR* 1999; 48 (RR-06): 1–5.

G. Hemodialysis patients: Use special formulation of vaccine (40 μg/mL) or two 1.0 mL 20 μg doses given at one site. Vaccinate early in the course of renal disease. Assess antibody titers to hep B surface antigen (anti-HBs) levels annually. Administer additional doses if anti-HBs levels decline to <10 milliinternational units (mIU)/mL.

H. Also administer meningococcal vaccine.

I. Elective splenectomy: vaccinate at least 2 weeks before surgery.

J. Vaccinate as close to diagnosis as possible when CD4 cell counts are highest.

K. Withhold MMR or other measles containing vaccines from HIV-infected persons with evidence of severe immunosuppression. *MMWR* 1996; 45:603–606, *MMWR* 1992; 41 (RR-17):1–19.

Footnotes for Recommended Adult Immunization Schedule, United States, 2002–2003

1. **Tetanus and diphtheria (Td)**—A primary series for adults is 3 doses: the first 2 doses given at least 4 weeks apart and the 3rd dose, 6–12 months after the second. Administer 1 dose if the person had received the primary series and the last vaccination was 10 years ago or longer. *MMWR* 1991; 40 (RR-10): 1–21. The ACP Task Force on Adult Immunization supports a second option: a single Td booster at age 50 years for persons who have completed the full pediatric series, including the teenage/young adult booster. *Guide for Adult Immunization.* 3rd ed. ACP 1994:20.

2. **Influenza vaccination**—Medical indications: chronic disorders of the cardiovascular or pulmonary systems including asthma; chronic metabolic diseases including diabetes mellitus, renal dysfunction, hemoglobinopathies, immunosuppression (including immunosuppression caused by medications or by human immunodeficiency virus [HIV], requiring regular medical follow-up or hospitalization during the preceding year; women who will be in the second or third trimester or pregnancy during the influenza season. Occupational indications: health-care workers. Other indications: residents of nursing homes and other long-term care facilities; persons likely to transmit influenza to persons at high-risk (in-home care givers to persons with medical indications, household contacts and out-of-home caregivers of children birth to 23 months of age, or children with asthma or other indicator conditions for influenza vaccination, household members and care givers of elderly and adults with high-risk conditions); and anyone who wishes to be vaccinated. *MMWR* 2002; 51 (RR-3):1–31.

3. **Pneumococcal polysaccharide vaccination**—Medical indications: chronic disorders of the pulmonary system (excluding asthma), cardiovascular diseases, diabetes mellitus, chronic liver diseases including liver disease as a result of alcohol abuse (e.g., cirrhosis), chronic renal failure or nephrotic syndrome, functional or anatomic asplenia (e.g., sickle cell disease or splenectomy), immunosuppressive conditions (e.g., congenital immunodeficiency, HIV infection, leukemia, lymphoma, multiple myeloma, Hodgkin's disease, generalized malignancy, organ or bone marrow transplantation), chemotherapy with alkylating agents, anti-metabolites, or long-term systemic corticosteroids. Geographic/other indications: Alaskan natives and certain American Indian populations. Other indications: residents of nursing homes and other long-term care facilities. *MMWR* 1997; 47 (RR-8);1–24.

(continued on page 18)

4. **Revaccination with pneumococcal polysaccharide vaccine**—One time revaccination after 5 years for persons with chronic renal failure or nephrotic syndrome, functional or anatomic asplenia (e.g., sickle cell disease or splenectomy), immunosuppressive conditions (e.g., congenital immunodeficiency, HIV infection, leukemia, lymphoma, multiple myeloma, Hodgkin's disease, generalized malignancy, organ or bone marrow transplantation), chemotherapy with alkylating agents, antimetabolites, or long-term systemic corticosteroids. For persons 65 and older, one-time revaccination if they were vaccinated 5 or more years previously and were aged less than 65 years at the time of primary vaccination. *MMWR* 1997; 47 (RR-8):1-24.

5. **Hepatitis B vaccination**—Medical indications: hemodialysis patients, patients who receive clotting-factor concentrates. Occupational indications: health-care workers and public-safety workers who have exposure to blood in the workplace, persons in training in schools of medicine, dentistry, nursing, laboratory technology, and other allied health professions. Behavioral indications: injecting drug users, persons with more than one sex partner in the previous 6 months, persons with a recently acquired sexually-transmitted disease (STD), all clients in STD clinics, men who have sex with men. Other indications: household contacts and sex partners of persons with chronic HBV infection, clients and staff of institutions for the developmentally disabled, international travelers who will be in countries with high or intermediate prevalence of chronic HBV infection for more than 6 months, inmates of correctional facilities. *MMWR* 1991; 40 (RR-13):1-25. (*www.cdc.gov/travel/diseases/hbv.htm*)

6. **Hepatitis A vaccination**—For the combined HepA-HepB vaccine use 3 doses at 0, 1, 6 months). Medical indications: persons with clotting-factor disorders or chronic liver disease. Behavioral indications: men who have sex with men, users of injecting and noninjecting illegal drugs. Occupational indications: persons working with HAV-infected primates or with HAV in a research laboratory setting. Other indications: persons traveling to or working in countries that have high or intermediate endemicity of hepatitis A. *MMWR* 1999; 48 (RR-12):1-37. (*www.cdc.gov/travel/diseases/hav.htm*)

7. **Measles, Mumps, Rubella vaccination (MMR)**—Measles component: Adults born before 1957 may be considered immune to measles. Adults born in or after 1957 should receive at least one dose of MMR unless they have a medical contraindication, documentation of at least one dose or other acceptable evidence of immunity. A second dose of MMR is recommended for adults who:

   - are recently exposed to measles or in an outbreak setting
   - were previously vaccinated with killed measles vaccine
   - were vaccinated with an unknown vaccine between 1963 and 1967
   - are students in post-secondary educational institutions
   - work in health care facilities
   - plan to travel internationally

   Mumps component: 1 dose of MMR should be adequate for protection. Rubella component: Give 1 dose of MMR to women whose rubella vaccination history is unreliable and counsel women to avoid becoming pregnant for 4 weeks after vaccination. For women of child-bearing age, regardless of birth year, routinely determine rubella immunity and counsel women regarding congenital rubella syndrome. Do not vaccinate pregnant women or those planning to become pregnant in the next 4 weeks. If pregnant and susceptible, vaccinate as early in postpartum period as possible. *MMWR* 1998; 47 (RR-8):1-57.

8. **Varicella vaccination**—Recommended for all persons who do not have reliable clinical history of varicella infection, or serological evidence of varicella zoster virus (VZV) infection; health-care workers and family contacts of immunocompromised persons, those who live or work in environments where transmission is likely (e.g., teachers of young children, day care employees, and residents and staff members in institutional settings), persons who live or work in environments where VZV transmission can occur (e.g., college students, inmates and staff members of correctional institutions, and military personnel), adolescents and adults living in households with children, women who are not pregnant but who may become pregnant in the future, international travelers who are not immune to infection. Note: Greater than 90% of U.S. born adults are immune to VZV. Do not vaccinate pregnant women or those planning to become pregnant in the next 4 weeks. If pregnant and susceptible, vaccinate as early in postpartum period as possible. *MMWR* 1996; 45 (RR-11):1–36, *MMWR* 1999; 48 (RR-6):1–5.

9. **Meningococcal vaccine (quadrivalent polysaccharide for serogroups A, C, Y, and W-135)**—Consider vaccination for persons with medical indications: adults with terminal complement component deficiencies, with anatomic or functional asplenia. Other indications: travelers to countries in which disease is hyperendemic or epidemic ("meningitis belt" of sub-Saharan Africa, Mecca, Saudi Arabia for Hajj). Revaccination at 3–5 years may be indicated for persons at high risk for infection (e.g., persons residing in areas in which disease is epidemic). Counsel college freshmen, especially those who live in dormitories, regarding meningococcal disease and the vaccine so that they can make an educated decision about receiving the vaccination. *MMWR* 2000; 49 (RR-7):1–20. Note: The AAFP recommends that colleges should take the lead on providing education on meningococcal infection and vaccination and offer it to those who are interested. Physicians need not initiate discussion of the meningococcal quadravalent polysaccharide vaccine as part of routine medical care.

Recommended Adult Immunization Schedule United States, 2002-2003 and Recommended Immunizations for Adults with Medical Conditions United States, 2002-2003
Summary of Recommendations Published by The Advisory Committee on Immunization Practices
Department of Health and Human Services Centers for Disease Control and Prevention

Table 1–6 Summary of Preventive Services to Consider

Immunizations and Chemoprophylaxis

Tetanus-diphtheria booster
Influenza vaccine
Pneumococcal vaccine
Hepatitis A, hepatitis B (high-risk)

Discussion of aspirin prophylaxis in high-risk group

Conditions and Factors to Remain Alert for

Depression symptoms
Suicide risk factors
Abnormal bereavement
Medications that increase risk for falls
Change in functional status

Signs of physical abuse or neglect
Malignant skin lesions
Peripheral arterial disease
Tooth decay, gingivitis, loose teeth
Change in mental or cognitive status

Screening/Counseling

History
Dietary intake
Physical activity
Tobacco, alcohol, or drug use
Functional status in normal environment
Social supports
Financial supports
Spiritual supports
Physical Examination
Clinical breast examination
Blood pressure
Height and weight
Visual acuity
Hearing screening
Multisystem examination
  Skin: premalignant/malignant changes, dietary fiber and sodium, lymphadenopathy
  Cardiovascular: arrhythmias, murmurs, bruits, peripheral vascular disease, ulcers
  Pulmonary: adventitious sounds
  Oral/dental: denture fit, lesions (examination by dental professional every 6 months)
  Abdomen: organomegaly, masses
  Genitourinary/rectal: prostate, incontinence, cystocele, rectocele, atrophic vaginitis, lesions or masses
  Neuromuscular: gait, balance, strength, mobility

Laboratory/Diagnostic Tests
Cholesterol
Mammogram
Fecal occult blood test and/or sigmoidoscopy
Papanicolaou smear
High-Risk Groups
Human immunodeficiency virus screen
Prior history of transient ischemic attacks
Tuberculin skin test (purified protein derivative)
Electrocardiogram
Complete blood count
Cholesterol profile
Ophthalmoscopic examination
Thyroid-stimulating hormone level
Counseling
Diet: Fat, cholesterol, calcium (women), caloric balance
Substance use: smoking cessation, alcohol, other drugs including prescription, drinking and driving, treatment for substance abuse
Injury prevention: falls, seatbelts, smoke detectors, hot water heater
Dental health: daily brushing with fluoridated toothpaste, flossing, regular checkups, denture fit
Skin: protection from ultraviolet light
Physical activity: exercise prescription

REFERENCES

Agency for Healthcare Research and Quality: What's new in preventive services. Contact: http://www.ahrq.gov/clinic/prevnew.htm. Accessed May 2, 2002.

Allison, M, and Keller, C: Physical activity in the elderly: Benefits and intervention strategies. Nurse Practitioner 22:53, 1997.

American Heart Association: Dietary guidelines for healthy Americans. Contact: http://www.americanheart.org/presenter.jhtml?identifier=1330. Accessed May 5, 2002.

American Heart Association: Exercise tips for older Americans. Contact: http://www.americanheart.org/presenter.jhtml?identifier=814. Accessed May 5, 2002.

American Heart Association: Older Americans and physical activity. Contact: http://www.americanheart.org/presenter.jhtml?identifier=811. Accessed May 5, 2002.

Balducci, L, and Kennedy, BJ: Cancer screening in older patients. Patient Care Nurse Practitioner 4:41, 2001.

Burke, MM, and Laramie, JA: Primary Care of the Older Adult: A Multidisciplinary Approach. Mosby, St. Louis, 2000.

Chen, K, et al: Clinical use of Tai Chi in elderly populations. Geriatr Nurs 22:198, 2001.

Cooper, KM, et al: Health barriers to walking for exercise in elderly primary care. Geriatr Nurs 22:258, 2001.

Cotter, VT, and Strumpf, NE (eds): Advanced Practice Nursing with Older Adults. McGraw-Hill, New York, 2002.

Davidhizar, R, et al: Health promotion for aging adults. Geriatr Nurs 23:28, 2002.

Dunphy, LM, and Winland-Brown, JE: Primary Care: The Art and Science of Advanced Practice Nursing. FA Davis, Philadelphia, 2001.

Elder, BM: Measuring physical fitness of adults in the primary care setting. Am J Nurse Practitioners 6:9, 2002.

Evans, WJ: Aging and malnutrition: Treatment guidelines. Contact: http://www.medscape.com/viewprogram/715_pnt. Accessed March 22, 2002.

Hill, C: Caring for the aging athlete. Geriatr Nurs 22:43, 2001.

Houde, AC, and Melillo, KD: Physical activity and exercise counseling in primary care. Nurse Practitioner 25:11, 2000.

Leetun, M: Wellness spirituality in the older adult: Assessment and intervention protocol. Nurse Practitioner 21:60, 1996.

Loeb, SJ, et al: Health motivation: A determinant of older adults' attendance at health promotion programs. J Commun Health Nurs 18:151, 2001.

Martin, AC: It's never too late to start: Seven steps towards good health. Topics in Advanced Practice Nursing eJournal 2(1), 2002.

Miller, J, et al: Postmenopausal estrogen replacement and risk for venous thromboembolism: A systematic review and meta-analysis for the U.S. Preventive Services Task Force. Ann Intern Med 36:680, 2002.

Molony, SL, et al: Gerontological Nursing: An Advanced Practice Approach. Appleton & Lange, Stamford, Conn., 1999.

National Heart, Lung, and Blood Institute: Aim for a healthy weight. Contact: http://www.nhlbi.nih.gov/health/public/heart/obesity/lose_wt/index.htm. Accessed May 10, 2002.

National Heart, Lung, and Blood Institute: Clinical guidelines on the identification, evaluation, and treatment of overweight and obesity in adults. Contact: http://www.nhlbi.nih.gov/guidelines/obesity/ob_home.htm and http://www.nhlbi.nih.gov/about/oei/index.htm. Accessed May 10, 2002.

National Heart, Lung, and Blood Institute: Third report of the expert panel on detection, evaluation, and treatment of high blood cholesterol in adults (adult treatment panel III). Contact: http://www.nhlbi.nih.gov/guidelines/cholesterol/index.htm. Accessed May 11, 2002.

National Immunization Program: Adult immunization schedule. Contact: http://www.cdc.gov/nip/recs/adult-schedule.html. Accessed May 2, 2002.

Nied, RJ, and Franklin, B: Promoting and prescribing exercise for the elderly. Am Fam Physician 65:419, 2002.

Oboler, SK, et al: Public expectations and attitudes for annual physical examinations and testing. Ann Intern Med 36:652, 2002.

Padden, DL: The role of the advanced practice nurse in the promotion of exercise and physical activity. Topics in Advanced Practice Nursing eJournal 2(1), 2002. Contact: http://www.medscape.com/viewarticle/421475. Accessed May 2, 2002.

Pizzi, ER, and Wolf, ZR: Health risks and health promotion for older women: Utility of a health promotion diary. Holistic Nursing Practice 12:62, 1998.

Resnick, B: Geriatric health promotion. Topics in Advanced Practice Nursing eJournal 1(3), 2001. Contact: http://www.medscape.com/viewarticle/408406. Accessed May 2, 2002.

Ruffing-Rahal, M, and Wallace, J: Successful aging in a wellness group for older women. Health Care Women Int 21:267, 2000.

Siccardi, A: Healthcare needs of the older adult and competencies of the advanced practice nurse. Topics in Advanced Practice Nursing eJournal 1(3), 2001. Contact: http://www.medscape.com/viewarticle/408415. Accessed May 2, 2002.

Stanley, M, and Beare, PG: Gerontological Nursing: A Health Promotion/Protection Approach, ed 2. FA Davis, Philadelphia, 1999.

Stevenson, JS: Health promotion for chronically ill elders. In Swanson, EA, and Tripp-Reimer, T (eds): Chronic Illness and the Older Adult. New York: Springer Publishing Company, New York, 1999.

Stone, EG, et al: Interventions that increase use of adult immunization and cancer screening services: A meta-analysis. Ann Intern Med 36:641, 2002.

U.S. Department of Health and Human Services: Healthy people 2010: Lifestyle health indicators. 2000. Contact: http://web.health.gov/healthypeople/LHI/lhiwhat.htm. Accessed May 5, 2002.

U.S. Preventive Services Task Force: Evaluating primary care behavioral counseling interventions: An evidence-based approach. Am J Prev Med 22:267, 2002. Contact: http://www.ahcpr.gov/clinic/3rduspstf/behavior/behsum1.htm and http://www.ahcpr.gov/clinic/3rduspstf/behavior/behsum2.htm#RationaleFive A. Accessed May 2, 2002.

U.S. Preventive Services Task Force: Guide to Preventive Services, ed 2. 1996. Contact: http://odphp.osophs.dhhs.gov/pubs/guidecps. Accessed March 22, 2002.

U.S. Public Health Service: Put Prevention into Practice: Clinician's Handbook of Preventive Services, ed 2. International Medical Publishers, McLean, Va., 1997.

van der Bij, AK, et al: Effectiveness of physical activity interventions for older adults: A review. Am J Prev Med 22:120, 2002.

Wenger, NK, et al: Exercise and elderly persons. Am J Geriatr Cardiol 10:241, 2001.

World Health Organization: (2002). Active ageing: a policy framework. Contact: http://www.who.int/hpr/ageing. Accessed May 10, 2002.

Unit 2
MANAGING ILLNESS

Chapter 2

SYMPTOM-BASED PROBLEMS

BOWEL INCONTINENCE

Feces/anal sphincter	ICD-9-CM: 787.6
Without sensory awareness	ICD-9-CM: 788.34
Continuous leakage I	ICD-9-CM: 788.37

Description: Fecal or bowel incontinence, the inability to control evacuation of stool or flatus from the rectum, can be episodic and self-limiting or a chronic problem in the older adult. In either scenario, this socially and emotionally devastating situation interferes with quality of life and self-esteem.

Etiology: The most common cause of significant fecal incontinence is denervation of the puborectalis muscles and the external sphincters that is associated with rectal prolapse, habitual straining with defecation, pelvic floor dysfunction, diabetes mellitus, and spinal cord injuries. Distention of the rectum by the impacted stool can lead to overflow incontinence as the liquid stools pass around the impaction through an inhibited sphincter.

Occurrence: Among community-dwelling older adults, approximately 3% to 4% have a problem with bowel incontinence. In older adults in hospitals and long-term care facilities, the incidence is 30% to 50%.

Age: Bowel incontinence is found more frequently in older adults than in the general population.

Ethnicity: Not significant.

Gender: Bowel incontinence occurs equally in men and women.

Contributing factors: Diarrhea from gastrointestinal (GI) disease, irritable bowel syndrome, infectious causes, or medication side effects can contribute to acute, short-term bowel incontinence. Constipation and fecal impaction from inadequate dietary fiber, insufficient fluid intake, or the effects of certain medications are also implicated. Protracted laxative abuse can damage the myenteric plexus, leading to retention of feces and soiling. Altered cognitive functioning related to delirium, dementia, or depression also can contribute to inability to respond appropriately to the urge to defecate. Impaired mobility from acute musculoskeletal conditions, chronic degenerative changes, or neurological problems is also a risk factor. Traumatic injury to the anal sphincter muscles can occur even during minor surgery (hemorrhoidectomy, episiotomies, and anal fissure procedures).

 Clinical Pearl: Functional fecal incontinence occurs when the physiological mechanisms to control evacuation are intact but persons to assist the dependent older adult with toileting are unavailable.

Signs and symptoms: Initially, patients may deny the problem or use incontinence pads because of the embarrassment associated with the problem. Family members or caregivers may notice and report fecal smearing, soiling, or accidents. A history of abrupt onset and short course suggests an acute or self-limiting process. A more insidious and progressive course warrants a different workup. Inquiring about the frequency, duration, severity, and character of the incontinence (gas, liquid, solid) is essential. Presence or absence of associated symptoms, such as pain, urinary incontinence, diarrhea, constipation, bleeding, or vomiting, should be ascertained.

A history of medications that can produce diarrhea or constipation should be elicited along with a diet history. Past medical history for gastroenterological and neurological diseases and diabetes as well as surgical and obstetrical history is reviewed. Physical examination should include a thorough abdominal assessment, looking for rigidity, distention, hyperactive or absent bowel sounds, and pain. A rectal examination, including a digital examination to check for hemorrhoids, impaction, and sphincter control, is indicated. The patient's weight should be measured and compared with previous measurements to determine any significant change.

Diagnostic tests: There is no routine testing for fecal incontinence; the tests are determined by the history and physical examination findings. Possible tests include abdominal ultrasound, radiograph of the abdomen, and computed tomography (CT) scan if an acute surgical abdomen or partial obstruction is suspected. Barium contrast studies, particularly a barium enema, may be helpful. Fecal hemoccult testing, sigmoidoscopy, or colonoscopy also may be indicated. If an infectious or food-borne cause is suspected, collection of stools for culture, ova, and parasites is appropriate. Anorectal manometry and defecography may help establish a cause. Proctosigmoidoscopy might identify the presence of inflammation.

Differential diagnosis: Fecal incontinence is a symptom. Differential diagnosis is broad and includes gastroenteritis, food-borne illness, ruptured diverticulum, colon cancer, fecal impaction, anal fistula, diabetic neuropathy, and rectal prolapse; upper motor neuron lesions secondary to cerebrovascular accident, multiple sclerosis, spinal cord compression, degenerative processes, dementia, and trauma; inflammatory bowel disease, irritable bowel syndrome, and functional bowel disease; and depression with self-care deficits.

Treatment: Treatment is aimed at alleviating the cause of bowel incontinence, when possible, or at minimizing its consequences, restoring self-esteem, maintaining function, and improving quality of life. For depression and functional bowel disease, treatment is individualized. Reviewing and adjusting a patient's medications is needed when the incontinence results from prescribed drugs. If chronic laxative abuse is involved, intervention and design of a successful bowel management program are needed. When fecal impaction is the cause, disimpaction (manual/mechanical or pharmacological removal of impaction) and preventive bowel hygiene measures should be instituted. Dietary modifications and the addition of a bulk-forming agent, such as bran or fiber supplements, may be considered. Other treatment options include biofeedback, bowel training, and toileting. Toileting is a treatment because frail elderly persons who are dependent for activities of daily living (ADLs) need to be given the opportunity to evacuate at regular intervals. Surgery is rarely indicated except for ruptured diverticulum, rectal prolapse, some fistulas, and possibly colon cancer. For acute gastroenteritis and food-borne illnesses, treatment includes maintaining hydration, monitoring for life-threatening consequences, and possibly antimicrobial therapy.

Follow-up: Follow-up is indicated by cause. Ongoing monitoring is needed in all cases.

Sequelae: Possible complications depend on the cause of the symptom. Complications of bowel incontinence may include peritonitis, septic shock, dehydration, electrolyte imbalance, skin breakdown, and depression. If the patient is functionally dependent or cognitively impaired, bowel incontinence may result in placement in a long-term care facility.

Prevention/prophylaxis: Prevention strategies depend on the cause of incontinence. Eating a balanced diet with adequate fiber and fluid intake, maintaining regular physical activity, avoiding use of laxatives and cathartics, making time for bowel evacuation, and avoiding unnecessary over-the-counter (OTC) drug use are good general preventive measures. Proper food preparation and storage can prevent food-borne illness.

Referral: Refer the patient to (or consult with) appropriate specialist, as indicated by cause of incontinence symptom or if the cause is not known, onset is rapid, or there is weight or blood loss.

Education: Educate the patient and caregivers in rationale for and implementation of preventive strategies as indicated, focusing especially on the need to avoid regular laxative use and to appreciate that a normal bowel evacuation pattern may not require a bowel movement every day.

Explain the cause of the incontinence, the rationale for any diagnostic tests, and the appropriate treatment plan. Advise the patient when to seek medical care.

CHEST PAIN

Central	ICD-9-CM: 786.50
Atypical	ICD-9-CM: 786.59
Midsternal/substernal	ICD-9-CM: 786.51
Musculoskeletal/noncardiac	ICD-9-CM: 786.59
Anterior wall	ICD-9-CM: 786.52

Description: Acute nontraumatic chest discomfort, perceived as pain or as a sensation of tightness, pressure, or squeezing in the chest, is associated with actual or potential tissue damage.

Etiology: The many different pathophysiologies of major chest pain syndromes may be attributed to segmental overlap of the neurons of cardiopulmonary and noncardiopulmonary origin. Chest pain may originate from organs within or outside the thorax. Causes associated with the highest mortality and morbidity include acute myocardial infarction, pulmonary embolism, aortic aneurysm or dissection, pericarditis, myocarditis, pneumothorax, and pneumonia.

 Clinical Pearl: Herpes zoster is common in the elderly and can affect a chest wall dermatological root. The chest pain often is described as shooting or as paresthesias and often is experienced before the lesions appear.

Occurrence: Chest pain is one of the most common presenting symptoms, accounting for 7% of all visits to the emergency department or outpatient clinic.

Age: In elderly persons, the most common causes of chest pain are ischemia (angina), gastroesophageal reflux disease (GERD), and panic disorder. The older adult is more likely to describe a symptom of chest discomfort rather than chest pain.

Ethnicity: African-Americans have a high prevalence of hypertensive heart disease, which is a cause of ischemic pain. The symptoms of coronary heart disease may differ between African-Americans and whites in that African-Americans report less typical anginal features. African-Americans are also less likely to attribute their symptoms to underlying coronary heart disease and tend to delay longer before going to the emergency department.

Gender: Coronary artery disease is the leading cause of death in women, and it is more difficult to diagnose in women because of a greater prevalence of atypical symptoms, variant angina, and microvascular angina. Silent ischemia and infarction also occur more frequently in women.

Contributing factors: Differentiating the etiology of chest pain in elderly persons is problematic owing to the more common atypical presentation and comorbidity. In elderly individuals, esophageal disease coexists with myocardial infarction in 50% of patients with coronary artery disease. Hyperventilation, a frequent symptom in patients with panic attacks, has been shown to cause coronary artery and esophageal spasm. Heartburn can reduce blood flow to the heart causing cardiac ischemia. Medications, including sildenafil (Viagra), which can cause a drop in the blood pressure, and sumatriptan (Imitrex), which can cause coronary vasoconstriction, can trigger chest pain.

Signs and symptoms: Ask the patient to describe generally the severity of the discomfort and to characterize the feeling. The older adult is more likely to describe a symptom of chest discomfort rather than chest pain. If there is radiation or discomfort, have the patient point to the exact location, then trace any radiation with the finger. Some significant parameters of symptom assessment of chest pain are listed in Table 2–1. The presentation may be different in the aged or diabetic patient with altered pain perception or altered ability to localize the discomfort or altered cognition impairing the ability to describe the pain. An absence of chest pain with myocardial infarction in elderly persons is common. Dyspnea, not chest pain, is the most common presenting symptom of acute myocardial infarction in patients >85 years old. Obtain information relative to coronary artery disease risk factors.

Table 2–1   Chest Pain: Symptom Assessment

Descriptors
Onset and Duration: Trauma relationship, predictable. **Precipratating and Aggravating Factors:** Emotional upset; swallowing; cold weather; sexual intercourse; deep breathing; coughing; neck, arm, or chest movement; position change. **Relieving Factors:** Food, antacid, nitroglycerine, resting, change in position, massage. **Associated Symptoms:** Anxiety, depression, faintness, palpitation, numbness or tingling in hands or around mouth, fever, chills, sweating, syncope, cough, sputum production, hemoptysis, dyspnea, tenderness, trouble swallowing, nausea, vomiting, leg swelling or pain, weight change, confusion, fatigue. **Past Treatment or Evaluation:** Electrocardiogram; upper gastrointestinal x-ray; chest x-ray.

Medical History
Lung disease, chest surgery, chest injury, cardiovascular disease, hypertension, diabetes, elevated cholesterol or triglyceride, angina, phlebitis, emotional problems, recent immobilization.

Medications
Hormones, diuretics, digitalis, bronchodilators, nitroglycerine, tranquilizers, sedatives, antacids, sildenafil, sumatriptan, illicit drug use.

Family History
Cardiovascular disease, diabetes, hypertension, elevated blood lipids.

Environmental History
Smoking, alcohol use, diet history, cocaine use.

Focus the physical examination on the general appearance of the patient, including the level of distress. For vital signs, concentrate on the regularity and symmetry of the pulse, blood pressure in both arms, and temperature. Assess the skin for moisture, color, and capillary refill. Evaluate the lower extremities for temperature, tenderness, and edema. Conduct a complete cardiac examination, assessing for extra heart sounds and checking carotid arteries for bruit, murmurs, and pericardial rubs.

 Clinical Pearl: The most common physical finding in the setting of acute ischemia is the presence of a fourth heart sound, which reflects decreased ventricular compliance.

The pulmonary examination consists of palpation for tenderness of the chest wall and auscultation for crackles, wheezes, or pleural rubs. You also might examine the abdomen, spine, and musculoskeletal or neurological systems, as guided by the history. A normal physical examination can never be used to rule out myocardial ischemia or infarction.

Diagnostic tests: Order diagnostic tests based on the history and physical examination findings. Generally, the following are indicated in evaluating a patient with chest pain:

Test	Results Indicating Disorder	CPT Code
12-lead ECG	ST segment depression or elevation, T wave inversion, new left bundle-branch block, or Q wave development supports myocardial ischemia.	93000
Chest x-ray	Pulmonary finding of tumors, effusion, pulmonary edema, pneumonia, or vasculature changes Left ventricular hypertrophy or dissecting aortic aneurysm may be identified.	71010, 71030
CK-MB; troponin T and I	Elevations 4–24 hours after the onset of chest pain indicate myocardial cell damage. Troponin may elevate within one hour after myocardial cell injury	82553; 84484, 84512

ECG, electrocardiogram.

Additional tests may be indicated, including:

- Cardiac: complete blood count, thyroid function, lipids, exercise ECG, echocardiogram, perfusion studies, coronary arteriography, cardiac catheterization
- Pulmonary: D-dimer, arterial blood gases, lung scan, pulmonary arteriography, sputum culture or cytology, bronchoscopy, biopsy
- Aortic: echocardiogram, aortic angiography, CT scan, magnetic resonance imaging (MRI), transesophageal echocardiogram

- GI: esophageal manometry, acid perfusion testing, 24-hour pH monitoring
- Psychogenic: neuropsychiatric consultation and testing, electroencephalogram.

Differential diagnosis: The differential diagnosis for individuals presenting with chest pain is broad, including cardiopulmonary and noncardiopulmonary possibilities. The greatest challenge is differentiating ischemic chest pain from chest pain of another etiology. Many conditions can present with pain similar to that of myocardial ischemia, and the broad differential diagnosis includes pulmonary, musculoskeletal, GI, and anxiety disorders.

Treatment: Therapeutic management of chest pain is always based on the specific cause of the symptom. For cardiac pain, it may include nitrates, β-blockers, calcium channel blockers, aspirin, analgesics, oxygen, and thrombolytics. Pulmonary embolism is treated with anticoagulation, herpes zoster is treated with antivirals, and esophageal pain is treated with an H_2-receptor antagonist. If a psychogenic cause is determined, selected patients may benefit from antidepressants or anxiolytics.

Follow-up: Monitor patients with acute chest pain closely and appropriately as the diagnosis and response to treatment dictate. Follow regularly patients with chronic chest pain caused by known chronic disease. Instruct the patient to report immediately to the health-care professional any changes in the characteristics of the symptom.

Sequelae: The significance of an episode of chest pain is evidenced by the fact that 50% of patients presenting with a myocardial infarction had an episode of prior angina. Silent ischemia is equally significant; 25% of all myocardial infarctions are discovered only by new ECG changes without clinically recognizable associated events. Older adults have higher frequencies of unrecognized infarcts than other groups (approximately 68%). For adults >70 years old with known infarction, the in-hospital mortality rate is 37.5% compared with 17% for adults <70 years old.

Prevention/prophylaxis: Maintaining a healthy lifestyle, including maintaining appropriate weight, eating a balanced nutritional diet, and getting adequate exercise, is the best way to prevent the development of disease. Individuals with major cardiac risk factors, including diabetes, smoking, hypertension, hypercholesteremia, and a positive family history for coronary artery disease, need specific instructions and ongoing support in risk reduction.

Referral: Chest pain that is acute, is of recent onset, or has increased recently in frequency or severity should always be considered unstable and evaluated immediately in the hospital. Patients who have a history of coronary artery disease, who have ST segment changes on ECG, who have rest or variant angina, or whose vital signs are unstable also should be evaluated immediately in the hospital.

Education: Teach patients and families to call the emergency response system without delay when an acute new onset of chest pain or a change in chronic chest pain is experienced. Teach individuals with coronary artery disease and known ischemia to avoid precipitants, including stress, heavy meals, and strenuous exercise. Patients with GERD are taught about prudent lifestyle changes, including stopping smoking, avoiding alcohol and coffee, and weight reduction. Because pain often occurs after meals in a supine position, teach the patient to avoid late night feedings and to keep the head of the bed elevated.

CONFUSION

Confusion	ICD-9-CM: 298.9
Acute	ICD-9-CM: 293.0
Acute confusion with arteriosclerotic dementia	ICD-9-CM: 290.41
Acute confusion with presenile brain disease	ICD-9-CM: 290.11
Acute confusion with senility	ICD-9-CM: 290.3
Alcoholic	ICD-9-CM: 291.0
Delirium (delirious)	ICD-9-CM: 780.09
Epileptic	ICD-9-CM: 293.0
Postoperative	ICD-9-CM: 293.9
Psychogenic	ICD-9-CM: 298.2
Reactive	ICD-9-CM: 298.2
Subacute	ICD-9-CM: 293.1

Description: Acute confusion or delirium is a transient condition characterized by an abrupt onset (hours or days), a fluctuating course, and disturbances of cognition and consciousness. The presentation may vary. Some individuals are loud, agitated, hyperactive, and obviously confused, whereas others may be quiet and lethargic or present with a mixture of these behaviors. Particularly if patients have a quiet or mixed presentation or if they have an underlying diagnosis of dementia or other cognitive impairment, the delirium is often not identified by clinicians. Increased mortality is associated with delirium; when delirium is suspected, there should be an aggressive workup, and the underlying cause should be identified and treated.

Etiology: Acute confusion is a common response to a myriad of factors and problems in the elderly. Its causes may be physiological, psychological, sociological, or environmental in nature; however, the usual cause is often a combination of several factors. Delirium develops more often in individuals with cognitive impairments, advanced age, severe illness, and sensory deficits. The more vulnerable the patient, the less noxious the precipitant or combination of precipitants needed to result in delirium. Despite this variability in etiology, the major physiological causes have been identified. The most common is medications, particularly drugs with anticholinergic properties or drugs with potent central nervous system effects. Infection is the second most common cause, especially urinary and respiratory infections. Fluid and electrolyte imbalances, nutrition problems, and extremes in the patient's environment, such as sensory overload or deprivation, are also commonly associated with acute confusion.

 Clinical Pearl: Assume medical illness in cases of delirium, and work aggressively to identify a cause. It is important to name the confusion as delirium. In patients with dementia or other underlying cognitive impairment, it is easy to attribute the current delirium to the underlying condition.

Occurrence: Estimates are that delirium affects 2.3 million elderly each year and is responsible for >17.5 million hospital days. Of elderly patients, 10% to 16% are delirious on admission to hospitals, and during hospitalization delirium is the most frequent complication of older patients. The attributed costs are >$4 billion. These costs rise if in-home care, rehabilitation, and nursing home placement costs are added for patients whose cognitive dysfunction does not resolve.

Age: Individuals of any age can become delirious, but individuals >70 years old are at particular risk.

Ethnicity: Not available.

Gender: No significance.

Contributing factors: Generally, individuals who are older, who are sicker, or who have a preexisting cognitive or functional impairment are more vulnerable to acute confusion. Elements contributing to this increased vulnerability include a variety of aging changes, such as decreased sensory awareness, slower cognitive function, less physiologic reserve and ability to respond to stress, and increased sensitivity to medications. Additionally, poor nutrition, the presence of multiple chronic diseases, and polypharmacy are common factors. The use of alcohol and other intoxicating substances and previous episodes of confusion add to an individual's risk of developing delirium.

Signs and symptoms:

- Acute onset and fluctuating course
- Inattention
- Altered level of consciousness
- Disorganized thinking

Additional signs or symptoms that are often present but not necessary for the diagnosis include abnormal psychomotor activity, acute changes in function, sleep/wake cycle disturbances, hallucinations, delusions, and tremor.

Diagnostic tests: There are two necessary steps in establishing a diagnosis of delirium: first, to verify specifically the existence of delirium and, second, to identify the cause. Evaluation of the first four above-listed signs is essential to distinguish the presence of delirium using the confusion assessment method (CAM). The diagnosis of delirium using CAM requires the presence of the first two features and either the third or the fourth feature. Using CAM, it is possible to detect delirium even in the presence of dementia. If delirium exists or is suspected, it is essential to establish the underlying cause. A thorough history is required to determine the frequency and duration of the mental status changes and other clinical features. A drug review, including OTC medications and alcohol, is essential. Look particularly at recent changes in dosage or the recent addition or discontinuation of drugs. The patient's history, drug review, and physical examination guide the laboratory evaluation. CBC, serum electrolytes, urinalysis, and cultures are the most useful screening tools. An ECG or a chest x-ray or both can be obtained if an underlying cardiac or pulmonary disorder is suspected.

Tests	Results Indicating Disorder	CPT Code
Urinalysis	Positive nitrates indicate bacteria present WBCs and leukocyte esterase are usually present with bacteria	81000, 81005
Urine culture	One organism with $>10^5$ highly indicative of infection	87088
CBC	Results are of little value unless related to the clinical presentation. Elevated WBCs indicate severity of disease process, bacterial and viral infections, and tissue necrosis. This response may be suppressed in the elderly	85025, 85027
Basic metabolic panel	Significant deviations from normal in a variety of elements may affect cognition—electrolytes (sodium, calcium), glucose, blood urea nitrogen	80048
Oxygen saturation, blood gases	Insufficient oxygen or increased levels of carbon dioxide can lead to confusion	82805–82810

WBC, white blood cell.

Treatment: The most important aspect of the management of delirium is treatment of the underlying cause. In addition, address contributing factors, manage safety and behavioral problems related to the delirium episode, avoid iatrogenic complications, and support the patient and family. Psychoactive drug treatment may be required to treat the associated agitation that is sometimes present. For most patients, low doses of high-potency antipsychotics are preferred (e.g., haloperidol, 0.25–1 mg orally, intramuscularly, or intravenously). Risperidone also has been used (0.25–1 mg) and is gaining popularity because it produces less sedation and fewer extrapyramidal symptoms and anticholinergic effects. Benzodiazepines with short half-lives, such as lorazepam, may be more useful for treating delirium related to drug or sedative withdrawal.

Follow-up: Adequately treat the underlying cause. Because several contributing factors frequently are involved, an interdisciplinary team approach is often helpful to ensure the best care. Failure to provide sufficient care may lead to life-threatening complications and long-term loss of function.

Sequelae: If delirium is promptly identified and the underlying cause adequately treated, individuals usually return to their baseline cognitive function within a few days or weeks. Delirium increases the risk of falls, however, and other untoward events that may start the older adult on a downward spiral of decreasing function, additional complications, and frailty. About one third of patients with delirium in the hospital remain confused at the time of discharge.

Prevention/prophylaxis: Preventive measures that have been helpful include:

Compensate for sensory deficits by providing glasses, magnification, and hearing aids.

Institute mobility or range of motion programs three times a day.

Periodically review medications for continued need and the development of associated side effects.

Avoid the addition of medications unless there is a clear medical cause.

Minimize the use of devices that contribute to immobility, such as indwelling catheters or physical restraints.

Maintain adequate hydration.

Use nonpharmacological means, such as music, massage, herbal tea, and relaxation tapes, to help induce sleep and relieve anxiety.

Referral: Refer to a specialist for sophisticated diagnostic workup or management of a patient condition beyond your current scope of practice. Referral to other members of the interdisciplinary team also may be helpful in addressing contributing factors.

Education: Patients and families should be taught the signs of delirium so that they know the importance of reporting signs and symptoms early. Families or significant others should be supported to advocate for the prompt identification of causative or contributing factors that should be addressed. Frail elderly and elderly with dementia, depression, significant hearing loss, or prior episodes of delirium are particularly at risk.

CONSTIPATION

Constipation	ICD-9-CM: 564.00
Atonic	ICD-9-CM: 564.09
Drug induced, correct substance properly administered	ICD-9-CM: 564.09
Overdose or wrong substance given or taken	ICD-9-CM: 977.9
Neurogenic	ICD-9-CM: 564.09
Other specified	ICD-9-CM: 564.09
Outlet dysfunction	ICD-9-CM: 564.02
Psychogenic	ICD-9-CM: 306.4

Simple	ICD-9-CM: 564.00
Slow transit	ICD-9-CM: 564.01
Spastic	ICD-9-CM: 564.09

Description: Constipation is subjectively defined as infrequent elimination of no more than three bowel movements per week or straining at stool 25% of the time. In true clinical constipation, a large amount of stool is objectively found by the digital examination, or fecal loading is revealed by x-ray examination.

Etiology: Colonic motility depends on the integrity of the nervous system impulses and circular smooth muscle tone and motor complexes stimulated by increasing intraluminal pressure generated by bulk. Any pathophysiologic process that interferes with this process can cause constipation. Common causes for constipation may be organic or functional (Table 2–2).

Occurrence: Constipation rates in the general public are not known, but constipation is reported more frequently among children, pregnant women, and older adults.

Age: Constipation is a frequent complaint of elderly persons; 30% to 50% of individuals report taking laxatives on a regular basis; an estimated $400 million are spent on laxatives annually.

Ethnicity: Not significant.

Gender: At all ages, constipation is reported more frequently in women than in men.

Contributing factors: The functional factors described earlier contribute to constipation if they are not the primary etiology. Additional contributing factors include anxiety, depression, and dementia. Medications that may contribute to constipation include calcium channel blockers, narcotics, iron supplements, aluminum-containing antacids, nonsteroidal anti-inflammatory drugs (NSAIDs), and any drug that has anticholinergic side effects. Certain types of laxatives also may be constipating, such as stimulant laxatives, which may cause cathartic colon and laxative dependency, and bulk laxatives taken with insufficient fluids. Immobility and reduced fluid intake also can contribute to constipation.

Signs and symptoms: Patients may describe constipation as an inability to pass or difficulty in passing stool, hard or dry stool, a feeling of abdominal or rectal fullness, and less than normal frequency or less than normal amount of passing stool. Ask the patient to describe specifically the frequency, character, and amount of stool. Determine the patient's fluid and fiber intake and exercise level. Conduct a through medication review to determine use of constipating drugs and laxatives. For cognitively impaired or communication-impaired individuals who are unable to self-report bowel frequency or elimination of discomfort, encourage the caregiver to maintain a record of the frequency and character of

Table 2–2 Etiologies of Constipation

Organic	Functional
Anatomical: tumors (benign or malignant), Hirschsprung's disease	Poor eating habits
Metabolic: hypothyroidism, hypercalcemia, diabetes	Inadequate fiber intake
Neurological: multiple sclerosis, Parkinson's disease, cord lesion depression, dementia, stroke	Inadequate fluid intake
Gastrointestinal idiopathic megarectum, idiopathic megacolon, diverticular disease, Chagas' disease	Lack of exercise
Medications: analgesics, iron, calcium, antacids, anticholinergics	Failure to respond to normal defecation impulses

bowel elimination. The physical examination of the constipated patient should focus on a general assessment for signs of dehydration, such as inadequate skin turgor or dry mucous membranes. Perform an abdominal examination to check for distention and visible peristalsis. Auscultate bowel sounds, and check the patient for abdominal masses. Do a rectal examination, assessing for fissures and external hemorrhoids and checking for anal stricture and sensation. Do a digital examination to assess for the presence of rectal masses and stool. The absence of stool found on examination does not exclude the possibility of constipation or fecal impaction.

Diagnostic tests:

Test	Results Indicating Disorder	CPT Code
CBC	Presence of anemia	85004
Fasting blood glucose	Increased fasting glucose level warrants further testing for diabetes	82947
Thyroid-stimulating hormone	Presence of hypothyroidism	84443

CBC, complete blood count.

An abdominal radiograph may help to determine the extent and distribution of feces. Sigmoidoscopy or barium enema or both may be indicated in patients with a recent onset of constipation when a lesion is suspected. Checking colonic transit times may be indicated in patients who have a normal number of bowel movements but still complain of constipation. Colonic motility testing may be useful in identifying patterns of colonic activity.

Differential diagnosis: The differential diagnosis involved in evaluating a patient with a complaint of constipation involves first determining what the patient perception is of normal bowel frequency. The clinician then evaluates the etiology and contributing causes.

Treatment: After the specific etiology is established and factors contributing to constipation are identified, the appropriate pharmacological and nonpharmacological interventions are initiated. Nonpharmacological measures to treat constipation include encouraging fluids (1500–2000 mL/day minimum), increasing fiber intake (approximately 20 g/day), and prescribing exercise (20–30 minutes of walking daily when appropriate). Modify existing medication therapies if they are contributing to the constipation. Laxatives typically prescribed and their mechanism of action are listed in Table 2–3.

If nonpharmacological measures are unsuccessful, consider bulk laxatives as the first line of pharmacological laxative therapy. Start bulk laxatives slowly, increasing the dose as the patient tolerates. Avoid bulk-forming laxatives in patients who cannot take adequate fluids and patients with swallowing difficulties. If these agents are unsuccessful or not suitable, saline or osmotic laxatives might be added on a scheduled basis. Avoid long-term use of stimulant laxatives in older adults because these can cause malabsorption, electrolyte imbalance, dehydration, and cathartic colon. Mineral oil is always avoided in older adults, owing to the risk of aspiration and the depletion of fat-soluble vitamins. Natural laxatives, mixtures of fruits and fruit juices, have been successful in treating and preventing constipation.

 Clinical Pearl: Fecal softeners (docusate sodium) do not act as laxatives and are not useful in constipation, although they may reduce the strain associated with bowel elimination.

The prokinetic misoprostol can increase bowel movement frequency. Enemas work through lavage and can cause fluid and electrolyte imbalance and can increase the risk of bowel perforation, particularly if the patient is not manually disimpacted first.

Follow-up: Chronically constipated individuals often need to have combined nonpharmacological with periodic pharmacological intervention. When laxatives are prescribed, these individuals need regular monitoring for the side effects and the responses to treatment.

Sequelae: Constipation, although uncomfortable, is rarely life-threatening. When associated with pain, distention, or vomiting, constipation may

Table 2–3   Laxatives and Mode of Action

Laxative	Action
Stimulant: senna, biscadyl, cascara	Stimulates myenteric plexus, increases intra-luminal fluid
Bulk: bran, psyllium, methylcellulose	Increases water absorption, resists bacterial degradation
Saline: magnesium hydroxide, magnesium citrate	Osmotically draws fluid into the small bowel lumen
Hyperosmolar: sorbitol, lactolose, glycerine, polyethylene glycol	Nonabsorbable dissacharrades metabolized by cecal lactobacilli

be a sign of a life-threatening mesenteric infarction or a partial or complete bowel obstruction. Straining in elderly persons may have serious effects on the cerebral, coronary, and peripheral arterial circulation. If stool is not eliminated from the colon and the patient becomes dehydrated, stool may harden, resulting in fecal impaction. Hardened stool may back up farther into the colon and become difficult to remove with either cathartics or enemas. Some individuals have needed surgical intervention to remove hard stool that is obstructing the bowel.

Prevention/prophylaxis: Adequate dietary fluid and fiber and regular exercise habits help to promote colonic mobility. Bowel elimination patterns should be monitored regularly in individuals who are unable to report bowel habits or bowel discomfort.

Referral: Patients with recent-onset constipation associated with bleeding, anemia, or family history of colon cancer; patients with chronic constipation with anemia, abdominal pain, and weight loss; and patients with recent-onset fecal incontinence should be referred to a gastroenterologist. Referral to a specialist also should be considered when there is a failure to alleviate constipation despite escalating attempts.

Education: In addition to giving instruction in the dietary measures appropriate in preventing constipation, encourage older patients to maintain regular bowel habits and respond to the urge to defecate rather than suppress it. Patients should be taught to take advantage of the gastrocolic reflex, which is strongest about 30 minutes after meal consumption. All individuals should avoid the use of laxatives and OTC medications known to have constipating side effects.

COUGH

Cough	ICD-9-CM: 786.2
With hemorrhage	ICD-9-CM: 786.3
Affected	ICD-9-CM: 786.2
Bronchial	ICD-9-CM: 786.2
Chronic	ICD-9-CM: 786.2
Epidemic	ICD-9-CM: 786.2
Functional	ICD-9-CM: 306.1
Hemorrhagic	ICD-9-CM: 786.3
Hysterical	ICD-9-CM: 300.11
Laryngeal spasmodic	ICD-9-CM: 786.2
Nervous	ICD-9-CM: 786.2
Psychogenic	ICD-9-CM: 306.1
Smoker's	ICD-9-CM: 491.0
Tea taster's	ICD-9-CM: 112.89

Description: Cough is the forceful expelling of air from the lungs involving the use of accessory muscles of the chest and constriction of the glottis.

Etiology: Cough is the voluntary or involuntary mechanism used to eject aspirants or noxious substances, including fluids, solid, dust, and gases from the body's upper and lower airways. Cough is also the body's mechanism to remove mucus from the upper or lower respiratory tracts.

Occurrence: Cough is the most common respiratory symptom. It is most often a transient symptom associated with infections, allergies, and postnasal drip.

Age: Occurs at any age.

Ethnicity: No direct ties to ethnicity have been documented, but immigrants and individuals living in poverty are at higher risk for tuberculosis (TB) and other pulmonary infections.

Gender: No gender-specific differences.

Contributing factors: Knowing a history of the following activities is crucial to the assessment of cough:

Smoking is almost the exclusive cause of throat and lung cancer. Smoking as well as second-hand smoke is the primary cause of chronic cough.

Bronchogenic cancers are often associated with cough, but metastatic cancers to the lungs seldom result in cough until late in the course of the disease.

Trauma that can contribute to cough includes assault, motor vehicle accidents, or falls leading to contusion of the lungs.

Living environment can have exposure to infectious agents or poorly ventilated heating.

Work environment can have exposure to chemicals and dust.

Comorbid conditions include immune compromise leading to fungal pneumonitis, hypertension, and GERD.

Medications can contribute to cough. Angiotensin-converting enzyme (ACE) inhibitors cause cough as a side effect in 20% of users.

Signs and symptoms: A thorough history of the disease, the patient's risk factors, and the work and home environments is the first step in narrowing the cause of cough. Risk factors for cough include smoking, stroke, immigrant status, use of ACE inhibitors, human immunodeficiency virus (HIV)–positive status, and heart disease. The cough may be productive or nonproductive, and the sputum may be tinged with blood. Identify if the onset is acute or chronic; the duration and character of the cough; and if it is associated with other symptoms, including fever and dyspnea.

Vital signs should include temperature, heart rate, respirations, and oxygen saturation. Next, the physical examination begins with a thorough examination of the nose and orophyaryngeal mucosa. Tenderness to percussion of the facial and maxillary sinuses and swollen, mucus-covered, boggy turbinates indicate allergic rhinitis. A "cobblestone" appearance (from chronic stimulation of submucosal lymphoid follicles) to the posterior pharynx and swollen eyelids are other indicators of an allergic origin.

The chest must be assessed for adventitious breath sounds. Wheezes indicate bronchitis or asthma caused by mucus in or constriction of the airways. Rhonchi or crackles are suspicions for pneumonia or infiltrates. Diminished or absent lung sounds by auscultation and dullness to percussion are highly suggestive of pneumonia's consolidation. Rhonchi or crackles with cardiomegaly on x-ray or ECG indicate congestive heart failure and may not be accompanied by edema.

Diagnostic tests: No specific tests are indicated when the patient has a cough. The selection and extent of testing depend on the findings on history and physical examination and whether these services are available on-site. The following tests are listed with their efficacy, specificity, and expense:

- Oxygen saturation test—to assess pulmonary status; if low, consider pneumonia (inexpensive, quick, nonspecific)
- TB skin testing—if at risk (moderately specific and may show false-negatives on immunocompromised patients, requires 48–72 hours, moderately invasive, moderate cost)
- Sputum sampling—is difficult to obtain without contamination with oral flora (nonspecific if contaminated, time-consuming, moderately expensive)
- CBC—increased WBC count indicates infection (moderately expensive, nonspecific, moderately invasive)
- Chest x-ray—to evaluate for pneumonia, congestive heart failure, or cancer; chest x-rays are usually negative in bronchitis and may not detect lung cancer until the late stages of the disease (requisite assessment tool for the evaluation of cough, limited specificity, expensive, minimally invasive)
- ECG—for initial evaluation of cardiomegaly, heart failure, and mitral valve stenosis (minimally invasive, practically specific, moderately expensive)
- Bronchoscopy—to determine the specific pathogen or type of cancer (specific, expensive, invasive)

Differential diagnosis: Distinguish acute from chronic cough. Consider potential causes, including chronic obstructive pulmonary disease (COPD), chronic bronchitis, acute bronchitis, allergic rhinitis, aspiration, asthma, congestive heart failure, drug reaction, flu, GERD, lung cancer, pertussis, pneumonia, sinusitis, tuberculosis, and viral syndrome.

 Clinical Pearl: A nocturnal cough associated with shortness of breath suggests heart failure and without shortness of breath is more indicative of an allergy.

Treatment: If the source of the cough has been reasonably isolated to the respiratory system and the condition is not life-threatening, the following treatments are recommended:

Acute bronchitis: Most acute bronchitis is viral, and the use of antibiotics does not shorten the course of the disease. If the patient smokes, he or she should be counseled to quit or cut back significantly. Albuterol helps open the airways, but expectorants such as guaifenesin mobilize secretions, as does drinking two additional glasses of water per day. Cough suppressants should be avoided except to help the patient sleep. A cool mist humidifier in the bedroom is helpful.

Chronic bronchitis: A combination bronchodilator as an inhaler or as a nebulizer is needed. Because chronic bronchitis is usually a result of smoking, the patient should be counseled to stop. Antibiotics and oral steroids should be reserved for acute exacerbations heralded by increasing shortness of breath, change in the color of the sputum to dark yellow or green, or fever. Inhaled steroids may be of benefit but there are few data to guide use.

Bacterial pneumonia: Pneumonia most often is caused by *Staphylococcus, Klebsiella,* or *Pseudomonas* in the otherwise healthy individual. If pneumonia is suspected, broad-spectrum antibiotic therapy should be initiated empirically. Immuno-compromised patients, patients with any respiratory distress, and elderly patients with significantly elevated WBC counts may need to be hospitalized.

Fungal infection: A fungal infection should be suspected if the pneumonia does not respond to conventional antibiotic therapy. Amphotericin should be considered and the patient referred to a pulmonologist.

TB: Antituberculosis drugs should be begun with a positive Mantoux test and the patient referred to a health department.

Drug reaction: A reaction that is due to ACE inhibitors can be tested with a trial of another antihypertensive medication.

Follow-up: The tenacity of follow-up depends on the severity of the illness. For pneumonia or bronchitis with minimal dyspnea, a call to check on the patient is appropriate. Rising temperature or increasing difficulty breathing requires immediate attention or emergency department evaluation. Patients with resolving pneumonia should be evaluated in 2 to 3 weeks; a repeat chest x-ray may be taken.

Sequelae: If the cough is caused by lung cancer, the prognosis is ominous. Cigarette smoking is the most significant preventable cause of disease in the United States. Deaths from lung cancer peaked for men in the early 1990s as smokers from the 1940s and 1950s reached the crest of their mortality. Mortality rates from lung cancer continue to be three times higher than the next most significant cause of cancer death (prostate). Lung cancer has surpassed breast cancer as the leading cause of cancer in women. Death rates from lung cancer continue to rise among women in the United States. Cough from COPD worsens in intensity and duration if the patient continues to smoke.

Prevention/prophylaxis: Preventive measures include smoking avoidance or cessation intervention, evaluation of the work and home environment, and humidification of the sleeping area with a cool mist humidifier. Stress the need for flu shots for all patients and Pneumovax for older and immunocompromised patients.

Referral: If cough persists or increases despite treatment, the patient needs to be referred to a pulmonologist for possible bronchoscopy. If lesions suspicious for cancer are found on x-ray, the radiologist likely will request a chest CT scan with contrast dye followed by referral to an oncologist or a surgeon.

Education: Recommend smoking cessation classes and allergen avoidance training.

DEHYDRATION

Dehydration	ICD-9-CM: 286.5
With hypernatremia	ICD-9-CM: 276.0
With hyponatremia	ICD-9-CM: 276.1

Description: Dehydration or fluid volume depletion is a common condition in older patients whether they live in the community or in long-term care facilities. Most adults rely on thirst to drink more, but this signal is not always reliable in the elderly.

Etiology: Total body water decreases with age. The total body water of an adult age 61 to 74 is approximately 43% for women and 51% for men compared with 80% for children. Even small decreases in fluid intake can cause more dehydration in an older adult. The ability of the kidneys to concentrate urine declines with age, so that even when deprived of water, urination is not significantly reduced. Also, thirst decreases as a person ages, which is an important self-regulation against dehydration.

Dehydration can be defined as a fluid and electrolyte disturbance arising from either a water depletion or a sodium depletion in which there is accompanying water loss. It can be classified into three different types based on the possible causes (Table 2–4): isotonic, hypotonic, and hypertonic.

Occurrence: Dehydration has been reported to be the most common fluid and electrolyte imbalance in older adults. Every year, 1 million elderly individuals are admitted to U.S. hospitals with isotonic dehydration as a major component. Individuals >85 years old are particularly susceptible.

Table 2–4   Classification of Dehydration

Types	Description	Causes
Isotonic	Sodium loss = water loss	Fasting Vomiting Diarrhea
Hypotonic	Sodium loss > water loss Serum sodium < 135 mmol/L	Diuretics
Hypertonic	Sodium loss < water loss Serum sodium > 145 mmol/L	Fever Decreased fluid intake Fluid deprivation Neglect

Adapted from The Joanna Briggs Institute for Evidenced Based Nursing and Midwifery: Maintaining oral hydration in older people. Best Practice 5:1–6, 2001. Contact: http://www.joannabriggs.edu.au/BPISHyd.pdf.

Age: Older people are particularly susceptible to dehydration because of age-related changes. Renal perfusion and sensitivity to antidiuretic hormone decrease. Sense of thirst is reduced, and total body water is decreased.

Ethnicity: Not significant.

Gender: Female nursing home residents have been suggested to be dehydrated more often than males, having a lower percentage of water intake than males. Male residents (68–90 years old) in a long-term care unit and a geriatric admission unit received less fluid; however, these differences were not significant, and more research is needed.

Contributing factors: Decreased mobility, confusion, depression, dementia, and the presence of chronic diseases such as diabetes and cardiovascular and renal disease make older adults more sensitive to fluid and electrolyte imbalance. Other risk factors for dehydration in the elderly include the following: needs help to eat or drink, eats less than half of meals/snacks, mouth pain, dentures do not fit, and hard time chewing or swallowing. Vomiting, diarrhea, hemorrhage, and increased metabolic states (fever, infection) that result in excess loss of fluids are also contributing factors. The use of certain medications, such as diuretics, anticholinergics, and tricyclic antidepressants, also may increase the risk.

 Clinical Pearl: Inadequate fluid intake is the most common cause of dehydration in long-term care facilities.

Signs and symptoms: A dry, furrowed tongue and mucous membranes, sunken eyes, confusion, and upper body muscle weakness may indicate dehydration. Clinical signs may not appear, however, until dehydration is far advanced. In addition, the usual signs of constipation, disorientation, dry mucous membranes, orthostatic hypotension, and weight loss may be caused by other factors. If one or more of these are present or are a change from baseline, dehydration may be the cause.

Clinical Pearl: The most reliable sign of general dehydration is dry tongue with longitudinal furrows, and this typically occurs when the fluid deficit is >3 L. Dry tongue without furrows may be due to mouth breathing or a lack of saliva.

Diagnostic test:

Test	Results Indicating Disorder	CPT Code
Basic metabolic panel	Serum osmolarity >300 mOsm/kg, serum sodium >145 mEq/L, blood urea nitrogen >20 mg/dL, serum creatinine >1.2 mg/dL	80048

Differential diagnosis: When dehydration is identified, it is important to identify the cause and contributing factors and address these.

Treatment: Individualize treatment, depending on the underlying cause of the dehydration (see Table 2–4). The recommended daily intake of fluids should be ≥1600 mL/24 hours to ensure adequate hydration. Regular presentation of fluids to bedridden individuals can maintain adequate hydration status. Fluids given with medication can be an important source of fluids, and so fluids should be encouraged at this time.

Follow-up: See patient as indicated by cause and response to treatment.

Sequelae: Dehydration has severe consequences for the elderly. Inadequate fluid intake can have serious medical consequences, such as urinary tract infections, bowel obstructions, delirium, cardiovascular symptoms, and death.

Prevention/prophylaxis: Educate patients, families, and caregivers that to prevent dehydration one needs to ensure adequate fluid intake. All liquids are not the same in maintaining fluid balance. Water is the best and should be at least half of the daily intake of fluid. Add milk, fruit and vegetable juices, and nonsalty soups for variety. Decrease coffee, tea, alcohol, colas, and liquid diet supplements because they may cause dehydration.

Referral: Refer as indicated by source of symptom.

Education: Explain causes of symptoms and measures taken to determine cause and treatment. Aim for 1500 mL of oral liquids per day unless contraindicated by certain medical conditions, such as congestive heart failure. Allow adequate time for eating at mealtimes. Meals can provide two thirds of daily fluids. Offer fluids regularly during the day. Encourage consumption of fluids with medications.

DIARRHEA

Diarrhea	ICD-9-CM: 787.91

Description: Diarrhea is an increase in the frequency, volume, or fluidity of stools. It can be acute (<3–5 days' duration) or chronic (>2 weeks' duration). Diarrhea is defined as a frequency of more than three

bowel movements per day or a volume >200 g/day. Regardless of its etiology, diarrhea in the frail older adult is a significant cause for concern.
Etiology: Acute diarrhea is usually a result of infection or a drug
effect. Viral infection secondary to rotavirus is the most common cause
of acute diarrhea. Bacterial pathogens include *Shigella, Campylobacter,
Salmonella,* and less commonly *Escherichia coli. Clostridium difficile*
is a significant cause of diarrhea in institutionalized older adults receiving antibiotic therapy. Other causes of diarrhea are traveler's diarrhea (often rotavirus) and protozoal infections with *Giardia lamblia,
Cryptosporidium,* or *Entamoeba histolytica.* Several drugs have significant side-effect profiles for diarrhea, including antibiotics, anticancer
drugs, cardiovascular and central nervous system drugs, and GI drugs.
Inflammatory bowel disease, irritable bowel syndrome, colitis, lactase
deficiency, fecal impaction, malabsorption, and bowel ischemia are other
causes of diarrhea in older adults. Diarrhea is also a common occurrence in individuals with diabetes mellitus, although the pathogenesis is
unclear. In many patients, no explanation for diarrhea is identified, and
the symptoms subside spontaneously.
Occurrence: Diarrhea is common, second only to respiratory infections
in frequency in the United States.
Age: Diarrhea may occur at any age; however, the most serious effects
are found in the very young and very old. Of deaths from diarrheal illness,
>50% occur in people >74 years old, accounting for approximately
1600 deaths annually.
Ethnicity: Not significant.
Gender: Diarrhea occurs equally in men and women.
Contributing factors: Foreign travel, contaminated food or water, laxative abuse, immunocompromise, and alcohol use are contributing factors. A group living situation, such as in long-term care, presents an
environmental factor favoring the spread of certain types of diarrhea,
particularly if good hand washing is not enforced. Medications, particularly those listed previously, can be causative as well as contributing factors to diarrhea. Nutritional factors include foods containing sorbitol,
lactulose, fructose, and caffeine.
Signs and symptoms: The history should include symptom assessment
parameters, including onset, frequency, amount and character of the
stool (including the presence of blood, mucus, or atypical color), and
any associated symptoms. The patient's baseline bowel pattern, usual
dietary intake, food intolerance history, exposure to others with illness,
and any recent dining out need to be identified. A thorough medication
review, including the use of OTC herbal remedies and laxatives, needs to
be conducted. A dietary history of the 2 days before symptom onset is
helpful, with particular attention to ingestion of meat, dairy products, and
seafood. Exploration of associated signs and symptoms is key in targeting
the source of the problem. Associated symptoms including fever, abdom-

inal pain and distention, vomiting, myalgia, and headache and abrupt onset suggest acute diarrhea etiologies. Fatigue, muscle weakness, weight loss, alternating diarrhea and constipation, incomplete evacuation, abdominal pain, and protracted or recurring symptoms suggest chronic diarrhea etiologies.

Physical examination should include vital signs and weight. Assess the skin for turgor and the condition of the tongue and mucous membranes. Check for evidence of jaundice, rashes, or lesions. Examine the thyroid for lesions. Perform a thorough examination of the abdomen for distention, rigidity, tenderness, bowel sounds, masses, hepatomegaly, or splenomegaly. Perform a rectal examination, including Hemoccult testing, to assess for bleeding, hemorrhoids, polyps, fissures, fistulas, or evidence of malignancy. Include a general inspection for arthritis or lymphadenopathy. Stool should be examined for blood or mucus.

Diagnostic tests:

Test	Results Indicating Disorder	CPT Code
Stool check for leukocytes, blood, ova, and parasites	Positive findings indicate underlying cause. If positive for leukocytes, the stool should be cultured to identify any bacterial etiology	82274, 87177

Concurrent use of tetracycline, sulfonamides, magnesium hydroxide, castor oil, kaolin, bismuth, antiprotozoals, or enemas with barium, soap, hypertonic saline, or tap water interferes with ova and parasite collection. Abuse of the laxative phenolphthalein also interferes with some stool testing. If you suspect laxative abuse, order a stool laxative screen.

Additional diagnostic tests are indicated as guided by the history and physical examination. Complete CBC, electrolytes, and renal function identify infections and imbalances caused by diarrhea and dehydration. If obstruction or ischemia is suspected, an abdominal x-ray helps to confirm this or may point to the need for more sophisticated testing. A barium enema can reveal malignancies, polyps, or abnormalities of the mucosal pattern. Colonoscopy or sigmoidoscopy may be useful when symptoms are persistent and unexplained. D-xylose testing and serum iron, vitamin B_{12}, and folate levels may be needed if malabsorption is suspected in patients with chronic diarrhea. Plasma protein levels may highlight loss of protein stores in patients with chronic diarrhea.

Differential diagnosis: Distinguish first between acute diarrhea and chronic diarrhea. In acute diarrhea, consider inflammatory bowel disease, fecal impaction, irritable bowel syndrome, diverticulitis, antibiotic-associated pseudomembranous colitis, bowel ischemia, drug side effects, food-borne pathogens, and viral gastroenteritis. In chronic diarrhea, possibilities include malabsorption, occult neoplasm, postradiation enterocolitis, irritable bowel syndrome, and factitious and functional problems.

Treatment: Treatment depends on the cause. Frail elderly persons are at risk for dehydration and multisystem failure from diarrhea. If diarrhea is severe, refer the patient for emergent evaluation and treatment. In the hospital, the elderly patient should be treated aggressively with intravenous fluid therapy with close monitoring of the patient's cardiopulmonary status. In cases of acute-onset diarrhea in which a viral cause is likely, provide symptomatic treatment to maintain hydration and electrolyte balance. If the patient is not vomiting, encourage frequent fluids with carbohydrates and electrolytes. Tea, juice, flat carbonated beverages, Gatorade, or oral rehydration products such as Pedialyte can be given. Advance the diet to include rice, bananas, applesauce, crackers, soup, and toast. High-fiber foods including raw fruits and cruciferous vegetables, dairy products, caffeine, alcohol, and spicy or stimulant foods should be avoided until the diarrhea subsides and normal bowel function returns. If diarrhea persists for >3 days on this regimen, re-evaluate the patient. Use of antidiarrheals is controversial owing to side effects, particularly if the patient is taking other medications. Bismuth subsalicylate (Pepto-Bismol), two tablets four times daily, is effective in treatment of traveler's diarrhea. *C. difficile* may be treated with metronidazole 250 mg orally four times daily; no alcohol is permitted with this medication. Because any antibiotic has the ability to disrupt normal bowel flora and precipitate further episodes of diarrhea, watchful waiting may be useful before prescribing.

For patients with chronic diarrhea, treat as indicated by cause. The addition of a bulk-forming agent such as psyllium may be helpful in giving stools a solid consistency; however, patients must take adequate fluids to prevent impaction or obstruction from use of this substance. Dietary counseling to promote adequate fiber in the diet is helpful, if this is not contraindicated.

Follow-up: Schedule follow-up visits as indicated by cause of the diarrhea. In the case of acute diarrhea, re-evaluate the patient after 3 days of following the initial treatment plan. If diarrhea persists, diagnostic studies are indicated, and the patient's state of hydration must be addressed.

Sequelae: Depending on the cause and extent of the diarrhea, complications may include dehydration, sepsis, shock, anemia, fluid and electrolyte imbalances, malnutrition, and peritonitis.

Prevention/prophylaxis: Prevention depends on the cause. For community-dwelling older adults, especially adults who live alone, the following guidelines are helpful:

Careful cooking and storage of food is important to avoid spoilage. Date leftover food and discard after 5 days. Check expiration dates on dairy and meat products before using. Clean cutting boards and utensils. All patients not on a medically prescribed diet should be taught about the food pyramid and the need for adequate fluid and fiber in the diet.

For individuals planning travel to a foreign country, prophylactic treatment with Pepto-Bismol may be prescribed, or the individual may be given a 3- to 5-day course of an antimicrobial such as ofloxacin (Floxin) to take if diarrhea develops. This is particularly recommended for individuals with underlying chronic disease. Caution travelers to avoid uncooked or undercooked foods, raw fruits and vegetables, buffet foods, unpasteurized dairy products, tap water, and ice. Carbonated drinks, bottled water, and boiled water are considered safe for drinking and to use for oral hygiene.

Prevention of transmission of diarrhea in hospitals and long-term care facilities is extremely important. Frequent hand washing by patients and health-care workers in long-term care facilities and hospitals is the key to preventing transmission of infectious diarrhea. Avoidance of long-term laxative use and prudent use of antimicrobial agents are also important in preventing diarrhea.

Referral: Consult with or refer the patient to the appropriate specialist, as the cause of diarrhea indicates.

Education: Explain to the patient, family, and caregivers the cause of symptoms, diagnostic and treatment measures, follow-up, and preventive strategies. Emphasize the need for early intervention to prevent dehydration.

DIZZINESS

Dizziness	ICD-9-CM: 780.4
Hysterical	ICD-9-CM: 300.11
Psychogenic	ICD-9-CM: 306.9

Description: *Dizziness* is an imprecise term commonly used to describe various subjective symptoms. The practitioner must understand the patient's personal meaning of dizziness to classify the symptom and determine its cause. The most frequently used categories of dizziness are vertigo, presyncopal lightheadedness, disequilibrium, other (psychiatric or organic disease), and mixed (more that one type exists in >40% of cases).

Etiology: Dizziness may be caused by neurological, systemic, psychiatric, or mixed pathologies. Causes seen most often in primary care practice are anxiety, benign positional vertigo, vestibular, cerumen-impacted ears, medication, cardiovascular disease, systemic or viral infections, multiple neurosensory impairments, transient vertebrobasilar ischemia, and vasovagal conditions.

Occurrence: Dizziness is the 13th leading reason for visits to general internists and accounts for approximately 6 million visits per year.

Age: A common complaint in individuals >75 years old; an estimated 30% of this age group are seen in primary care with this symptom.

Ethnicity: Not significant.

Gender: Dizziness occurs equally in men and women.

Contributing factors: Factors contributing to dizziness in older adults include use of medications, particularly antihypertensives, anticonvulsants, psychotropic drugs, and ototoxic drugs. Changes in body systems with age can affect coordination and equilibrium and cause delays in recovery of balance. Altered sensitivity of the baroreceptors over time increases the vulnerability to presyncope, and the sensory receptors are diminished with aging.

Signs and symptoms: The patient's description of the symptom should help determine the type of dizziness experienced. What does the patient mean by the word *dizzy*? The parameters of symptom assessment include the onset and trigger for the symptom, relieving or aggravating factors, symptom pattern, and associated symptoms. A careful medication review needs to be completed.

Vertigo: Patients describe the environment or themselves as spinning; an illusion of movement, continuous or positional; or the sensation of being pushed. Associated symptoms include nausea, vomiting, unsteadiness, hearing loss, visual disturbances, and tinnitus.

Presyncopal lightheadedness: Patients have the sensation one feels when about to faint. Associated symptoms include perspiration, pallor, palpitations, and syncope.

Disequilibrium: Patients describe a sense of imbalance. It may be a sensation localized to the body and relieved by bracing oneself, sitting, or lying down. Associated symptoms are numbness, poor coordination, and general weakness. When patients give a vague description of dizziness, assess further for anxiety and depression.

The physical exam should be comprehensive and include the following components.

General: Observe how the patient moves around in the physician's office. Does he or she hold onto the furniture or walls? Check vital signs, especially postural blood pressure. A drop in systolic blood pressure of ≥ 20 mm Hg without normalization after 2 minutes is significant. It is important to determine whether the test of abruptly going from a lying to a sitting or standing position reproduces the patient's sensation. Check for an irregular heart rate and presence of fever.

HEENT examination: Test for extraocular movement, watching for nystagmus. Rotatory nystagmus suggests a peripheral cause of dizziness; vertical nystagmus suggests a central lesion. Check the patient's visual acuity and corneal reflexes. Perform a funduscopic examination, looking for papilledema. Inspect the ears for accumulation of fluid, bulging tympanic membrane, inflamed tympanic membrane, presence of cerumen impaction, or pus accumulation and discharge. Perform Weber's and Rinne's hearing tests if gross hearing is diminished. Acute hearing loss is associated with Ménière's disease, acoustic neuroma, and vestibular neuronitis.

Cardiovascular examination: Assessment should include central and peripheral function. Auscultate for heart sounds and check the carotid artery for bruit.

Neurologic examination: Assessment includes cerebellar testing. If the patient points past the examiner's finger, suspect a vestibular lesion. Intentional tremor or abnormal alternating movements suggest cerebellar dysfunction (point-to-point). Perform sensory testing, position sense, and Romberg's test. Patients with cerebellar disease have difficulty standing with their feet together. Patients with decreased position sense are able to compensate with eyes open but sway with eyes closed. Perform gait assessment; patients with cerebellar disease perform this maneuver poorly. Check deep tendon reflexes.

Special diagnostic and screening tests:

Have the patient breathe 20 to 30 times/minute for 2 to 3 minutes (forced hyperventilation). This normally causes dizziness and finger and perioral numbness. Determine whether these are the same sensations the patient has been feeling; if so, the dizziness may be related to anxiety.

Have the patient march in place for 30 seconds with the eyes closed and arms extended in front. Be careful not to orient the patient with any sounds (e.g., your voice or a ticking clock). Patients with absent or reduced vestibular function (from prior vestibular damage) rotate $>30°$ to $45°$ while marching.

For the Hallpike maneuver, assist the patient quickly to lay down on the examination table with the head hanging over the back of the table at about a $30°$ angle and the face turned $45°$ to the right. While holding the patient's head in place for 1 minute, observe the patient for nystagmus and ask whether this reproduces the dizziness (vertigo) symptoms. Bring the patient back to a sitting position and observe for 1 minute. Repeat the test with the head turned $45°$ to the left. If vertigo is reproduced, the test should be repeated two or three times on the side that caused the most severe symptoms to determine if the nystagmus and symptoms begin to disappear. Patients with benign postural vertigo experience severe vertigo 5 to 15 seconds after the head is turned and nystagmus is induced. Position change must be completed in 2 seconds, the signs typically fade in <1 minute, and repeated testing causes the symptoms to disappear.

Perform the minicalorie test to screen for vestibular dysfunction. Position the patient supine with the head turned 30°. Instill 0.2 mL of ice water from a tuberculin syringe into the ear canal. Then turn the patient's head to midline and observe the eyes for nystagmus. With repetition, failure to induce nystagmus indicates peripheral disease on that side.

Diagnostic tests: There are no routine tests to evaluate the complaint of dizziness. If indicated by history, selected testing might be done: CBC for anemia, serum glucose for hypoglycemia, ECG or Holter monitoring for arrhythmia, audiometry if hearing loss is present. Neuroimaging (CT or MRI) may be ordered if neurological symptoms are present.

Differential diagnosis: Differentiate between vertigo (a sensation of movement), lightheadedness (a sensation of being about to faint), and syncope (an actual loss of consciousness).

 Clinical Pearl: If dizziness has a predictable pattern associated with it (e.g., mid to late morning, mid to late afternoon, 2–4 hours after eating), suspect hypoglycemia.

Treatment: Patients are treated according to the cause of the dizziness. Patients with benign positional vertigo can perform therapeutic exercises, such as the Epley maneuver, which loosens particles out of the posterior semicircular canal and back into the utricle. If the cause of lightheadedness is medication side effects or volume deficiencies, adjustments are indicated. Support stockings may help to reduce pooling in the lower extremities. Medications for dizziness (e.g., meclizine), although they are commonly prescribed, have not been rigorously tested and can worsen the symptoms of dizziness and have anticholinergic side effects.

Follow-up: Patients should return for follow-up visits if symptoms worsen, change from one type of dizziness to another, or do not resolve within 2 weeks.

Sequelae: Sequelae depend on the underlying cause of the dizziness.

Prevention/prophylaxis: Teach older adults to move extremities before rising from positions held for any length of time to compensate for age-related changes in vascularity. Try to determine if dizziness is from medication side effects before adding additional medications to combat the dizziness.

Referral: If the etiology remains unclear, refer the patient to a specialist. Consider neurology, cardiology, ENT, or psychiatry as appropriate if the symptom persists and is disabling or a new abnormality is detected.

Education: Explain the underlying cause, rationale for treatment, and importance of exercises. Teach the patient the exercises and ask him or her to demonstrate. Explain that this condition may return intermittently for several years. Encourage the use of assistive devices for safety until the condition resolves. Placement of handrails in the bathroom and halls may assist with safe ambulation. If the condition worsens (e.g., the patient develops a fever, increased dizziness, or tinnitus), advise the patient to seek medical attention.

DYSPHAGIA

Dysphagia	ICD-9-CM: 787.2
Functional/hysterical/nervous	ICD-9-CM: 300.11
Sideropenic	ICD-9-CM: 280.8
Psychogenic	ICD-9-CM: 306.4
Spastica	ICD-9-CM: 478.79

Description: Dysphagia is a swallowing disorder involving the inability to get the food from the mouth to the stomach. The problem is commonly divided into oropharyngeal (the inability to initiate deglutition successfully) and esophageal (the sensation of impeded transit through the esophagus).

Etiology: The causes of dysphagia are multiple and diverse, and the diagnosis of dysphagia is abnormal at any age. Aging does not cause clinical dysphagia; however, some normal changes of aging can aggravate any swallowing problems. Oropharyngeal dysphagia is usually related to neuromuscular impairments of the tongue, pharynx, and upper esophageal sphincter. Afferent stimulation triggers saliva production, and inadequate saliva can impede swallowing and digestion. Stroke is the most common cause of oropharyngeal dysphagia in the elderly. Esophageal dysphagia is usually a result of a motor, motility, or neurological disorder or an obstruction from either an intrinsic (carcinoma, stricture, web, diverticula) or an extrinsic (mediastinal tumors, vascular anomalies) source. Muscle diseases that may result in motor disorders of the esophagus include muscular dystrophy, myasthenia gravis, and scleroderma. Neurological disorders that may result in motor disorders of the esophagus include achalasia, multiple sclerosis, and amyotrophic lateral sclerosis. Esophagitis is another etiology, usually secondary to GERD, herpesvirus, or a retained pill (primary offenders include NSAIDs, quinidine, potassium, ferrous sulfate, tetracycline, and alendronate).

Occurrence: Swallowing disorders occur in about 20% of individuals >50 years old and 60% of nursing home patients.

Age: Dysphagia occurs predominantly in older adults because the causes for this problem primarily affect the elderly.

Ethnicity: Not significant.

Gender: Dysphagia occurs equally in males and females, although this varies based on the etiology of the disorder.

Contributing factors: Factors that contribute to dysphagia include changes in swallowing with aging, such as decreased facial muscle and masticatory strength, delay in pharyngeal swallow, delay in emptying of the esophagus, and decreased lower esophageal sphincter relaxation.

Medications with anticholinergic side effects (e.g., antidepressants, opiates, sedatives, antipsychotics, antispasmodics, antihistamines, and some antihypertensives) may produce slowing or disruption of the oral phase of swallowing and affect salivation. Other drugs can increase the likelihood of reflux (i.e., calcium channel blockers, β-adrenergic agents, aspirin, theophylline, nitrates, vitamin C, and NSAIDs), particularly if the patient has inadequate fluid intake. Inadequate fluid intake with medication or meals may contribute to dysphagia.

Signs and symptoms: Symptoms typically associated with oropharyngeal dysphagia include difficulty initiating swallowing, food sticking in the throat, nasal regurgitation, and coughing during the swallow. Voice changes (wet vocal quality) may be associated with swallowing incompetence. Patients with esophageal dysphagia most commonly present with a complaint that food is stuck in chest (sternum or suprasternal area) and may report choking or a feeling of pressure sensation. Reflux symptoms may be present. If total obstruction occurs, salivation increases, and vomiting may result. Weight loss and aspiration pneumonia may occur.

Clinical Pearl: Weight gain may be a sign of dysphagia if the patient consumes significant amounts of processed foods such as milkshakes that have a higher calorie count.

It is important for the clinician to distinguish between difficulty swallowing solids, liquids, or both. In general, patients with obstructions (strictures, webs) complain of solid rather than liquid dysphagia. The time of the presentation of signs and symptoms is important because a rapid onset may indicate infection, irritation, or a food impaction, whereas a more insidious onset suggests a motor disorder. Physical examination consists of checking the oral cavity in conjunction with a neuromuscular examination. The mouth should be assessed for signs of irritation, ill-fitting dentures, and any pharyngeal masses. The head and neck should be examined, checking for lymph node or thyroid enlargement.

Clinical Pearl: Dentures may block palatal mechanoreceptors, which can lead to poor bolus control, oral transit delays, and longer feeding times.

Neurological evaluation must be comprehensive and include a mental status evaluation, cranial nerve examination, and muscle weakness. A bedside swallow assessment to determine aspiration risk is often inadequate and misleading.

Diagnostic tests:

Test	Results Indicating Disorder	CPT Code
Modified barium swallow with videofluoroscopy	Aspiration, pooling, abnormal bolus transit or motor function	74230

Other tests that may be indicated based on the history and physical examination include testing the stool for occult blood and a CBC with indices if associated esophagitis is suspected. Ambulatory 24-hour pH testing of intraesophageal pH and pressures has been found to be useful when evaluating for GERD. If malnutrition is suspected, a serum albumin level is appropriate. Fiberoptic endoscopic evaluation is an option when the patient cannot be transported to the radiology department for the modified barium swallow. Additional swallowing studies include radiography, and manometry may be indicated to identify specific abnormalities.

Differential diagnosis: It is important to differentiate whether the patient has a feeding problem (inability to present food to the mouth) or a swallowing problem (inability to get food from the mouth to the stomach) or both. Cognitive impairments frequently are associated with feeding problems. Determination of specific motor, neurological, or obstructive cause needs to be accomplished. For the patient complaining of burning associated with swallowing, reflux esophagitis, esophageal infection, and tablet-induced esophagitis need to be explored.

Treatment: Treatment always targets the specific cause. Management of dysphagia after a stroke is directed toward increasing the sensory awareness of food and improving bolus movement by the chin-tuck and double-swallow technique. A nutritionist works to ensure appropriate consistency and nutritional content. Stable patients can be treated as outpatients. Hospitalization may be required when dysphagia is associated with total or near-total obstruction of the esophageal lumen. Esophageal dilation (pneumatic or bougie), surgical intervention for an esophageal stent, or laser therapy for late cancer also may be part of the treatment plan, depending on the etiology of the dysphagia. Patients with esophageal spasms can be given calcium channel blockers (nifedipine, 10–30 mg three times daily). Patients with associated esophagitis may receive antacids; H_2 blockers, adjusting the dosage for the creatinine clearance (ranitidine, 150 mg orally twice daily; nizatidine, 150 mg twice daily; or famotidine, 20 mg twice daily); or, in cases of severe esophagitis, a proton-pump inhibitor, such as omeprazole, 20 mg once a day for 4 to 8 weeks.

Follow-up: Patient monitoring depends on the specific etiology of the dysphagia.

Sequelae: Complications from dysphagia depend on its cause. The most common complications are malnutrition and aspiration.

Prevention/prophylaxis: People with dysphagia should remain upright with the head midline and slightly flexed when eating or drinking. Extremely hot or cold foods may worsen symptoms of dysphagia. Aspiration precautions include modifying food and fluid consistencies, giving verbal and physical prompts, and allowing additional time for feeding to encourage double swallows and small amounts taken per mouthful.

Referral: A gastroenterologist should be consulted for the endoscopy and for possible hospitalization of patients with severe dysphagia. Other referrals may include a speech therapist, radiologist, and dentist.

Education: Patients and caregivers should be encouraged to provide foods and fluids at appropriate consistency. All foods, especially meat products, should be chewed thoroughly. Patients also should be informed that it is important to swallow all medications with plenty of fluid while in an upright position.

FATIGUE

Fatigue	ICD-9-CM: 780.79
Chronic	ICD-9-CM: 780.7
Chronic fatigue syndrome	ICD-9-CM: 780.71
Combat	ICD-9-CM: 308.9
Psychogenic	ICD-9-CM: 300.5
Heat	ICD-9-CM: 992.6

Description: Fatigue is a subjective state often described as a feeling of tiredness, weariness, or exhaustion that is unrelieved or only partially relieved by rest and often results in a decreased capacity for physical or mental work.

Etiology: Physiological fatigue occurs normally with inadequate rest, excess exertion, or insufficient diet. Fatigue that interrupts the patient's ADLs may have a physical or psychological cause and be either acute or chronic. Acute fatigue lasts <6 months, and chronic fatigue lasts >6 months. Fatigue is a commonly reported symptom in patients with cancer.

Clinical Pearl: Chronic fatigue syndrome is determined when on clinical evaluation the fatigue is persistent, unexplained, unrelieved, and accompanied by four or more of the following: impairment in short-term memory or concentration, sore throat, tender cervical or axillary nodes, muscle pain, multiple joint pain without redness or swelling, headaches of a new pattern or severity, unrefreshing sleep, and postexertional malaise lasting >24 hours.

Occurrence: Fatigue is the seventh most common complaint in primary care and accounts for 1% to 7% of all office visits.

Age: Fatigue is common among the elderly. It is problematic for 70% of older adults; 59% report experiencing it often.

Ethnicity: Not significant.

Gender: Fatigue occurs equally in males and females.

Contributing factors: Poor dietary habits, alcohol abuse, smoking, stress, chronic illness, drug interactions, misuse of drugs, and sleep apnea may contribute to fatigue.

Signs and symptoms: Obtain a complete medical history and perform a physical examination because fatigue may indicate various psychological or physiological illnesses. Conduct a complete symptom assessment, including the onset and precipitating, aggravating, and relieving factors. Identify other indicators or associated symptoms of fatigue, which may include decreased energy expenditure, decreased endurance, sleep disturbance, attention deficits, somatic complaints (aching body, tired eyes), and weakness. Carefully review the adequacy of the diet, any medication side effects, and potential causes or contributing factors. Identify the impact fatigue is having on the person's ADLs and quality of life. A complete physical examination is indicated. Distinguish between generalized fatigue and actual weakness by testing for muscle strength and presence of localized tenderness. A mental status examination should be included as part of the physical examination to screen for dementia. Using a geriatric depression scale, establish a baseline diagnosis.

Diagnostic tests: Consider the following diagnostic tests on all patients with persistent unresolved fatigue because these are low cost and offer significant screening capacity.

Test	Results Indicating Disorder	CPT Code
CBC with differential	Anemia or infection	85025
ESR	Nonspecific but elevations may indicate an inflammatory or infectious process	85651
Urinalysis	Renal disorder or systemic disease	81002

ESR, erythrocyte sedimentation rate.

Additional tests may be indicated by history and physical examination and might include a metabolic panel, electrolytes, thyroid function, renal function, and liver panel. An ECG may reveal cardiac arrhythmias, enlargement of the heart, myocardial infarction, or abnormalities in the conduction system. Monitor drug levels carefully in appropriate patients. Digoxin toxicity is especially common in older adults, and the signs and symptoms are similar to that of anemia.

 Clinical Pearl: Masked hyperthyroidism may present with a chief complaint of fatigue.

Differential diagnosis: Fatigue can be related to many psychological and physiological etiologies. Psychiatric disorders including depression and generalized anxiety disorder account for 70% of cases of fatigue. In approximately 25% of cases, the cause remains undetermined.

Treatment: Treatment depends on the etiology identified in the comprehensive workup. Symptom management includes regular exercise, attention-restoring activities, psychosocial techniques, energy conservation measures, and good sleep hygiene. Pharmacological management is directed at the cause of the fatigue.

Follow-up: Follow-up depends on the findings. Monitor the patient periodically as indicated by diagnosis or symptoms, symptom persistence, and disability associated with the symptom.

Sequelae: The potential for complications relates to the cause of fatigue and the impact the symptom has on the person's function.

Prevention/prophylaxis: Optimal health maintenance, including maintaining a healthy diet and regular exercise, may prevent or enable early recognition of signs and symptoms of systemic or psychological illness.

Referral: Referral to a specialist may be indicated based on the results of the workup.

Education: If the fatigue has a physiological cause, teaching should be related to the findings; psychological counseling, changes in the environment, behavior modification, and stress reduction may be needed. The goal of fatigue management is to provide the patient with self-help tools to eliminate or alleviate fatigue.

HEADACHE

Headache	ICD-9-CM: 784.0
Allergic	ICD-9-CM: 346.2
Cluster	ICD-9-CM: 346.2
Due to spinal fluid loss/lumbar puncture/saddle block	ICD-9-CM: 349.0
Emotional/psychogenic	ICD-9-CM: 307.81
Histamine	ICD-9-CM: 346.2
Menopausal	ICD-9-CM: 627.2
Migraine	ICD-9-CM: 346.9
Nonorganic origin	ICD-9-CM: 307.81
Sick	ICD-9-CM: 346.1
Tension	ICD-9-CM: 307.81
Vascular	ICD-9-CM: 784.0
Vasomotor	ICD-9-CM: 346.9

Description: Headache describes many entities in which the primary symptom is pain in the head, neck, or face. Headache is one of the most commonly encountered problems in primary care of adults. Most headaches are benign; however, some are life-threatening. The risk of organic pathology is greater in the elderly. Symptoms of headache often interfere with optimal functioning and quality of life.

Etiology: Principal pain structures are extracranial (vascular, muscle contraction), although intracranial causes (tumor, hemorrhage, inflammation, infection) are also responsible for some head pain. The most common type of headache, the tension headache, is caused by stress and muscle contraction. Vascular headaches (migraine and cluster) are also common, although less so in older adults than the general population. Many people with chronic or recurrent headaches have a combination of vascular and tension causes. The International Headache Society has a classification system that provides operational definitions for all headache types.

Occurrence: Headache is one of the 10 most common symptoms seen in primary care. Of the population, 90% have had headaches, with 45 million individuals reporting recurring headache. About 5% of individuals experiencing headaches seek medical attention for them.

Age: Approximately 10% of women and 5% of men report severe headache at age 70. Tension headaches often increase in frequency with age. Migraine headaches are less common, although approximately 2% of individuals >65 years old experience new onset of migraines. New or sudden onset of headache after age 50 must be investigated because it may indicate new disease.

 Clinical Pearl: Migraines presenting without headache can be difficult to distinguish from a transient ischemic attack. A visual or sensory disturbance may be the only presenting symptom. Scintillating scotoma with the classic zigzag edge or fortification spectra is characteristic of the migraine aura.

Ethnicity: Not significant.

Gender: Women are affected more often than men; 76% of women and 57% of men report one headache per month. Migraine headaches are more common in women than in men, tending to begin in early adulthood. Cluster headaches are more common in men than in women, with a mean age of onset at 30 years.

Contributing factors: Stress, depression, anxiety, sleep disorders, and joint disorders and pain may contribute to or complicate the symptoms of headaches. Medications commonly taken by older adults, such as steroids, estrogen, calcium channel blockers, nitrates, anti-Parkinson drugs, indomethacin, and theophylline can cause or contribute to headaches. Migraine triggers include dietary factors (aged or smoked cheese, chocolate, caffeine, MSG), changes in sleep pattern, weather changes, and smoking. Alcohol may trigger vascular headaches.

Signs and symptoms: Diagnosis frequently is made on the basis of history because the physical examination is often normal. The symptom is characterized by manifestations including onset, location, duration, frequency, severity, character, triggering or aggravating factors, and alleviating factors. Associated symptoms are elicited and might include nausea and vomiting, eye tearing, nasal congestion, teeth grinding, and neck pain. For recurrent headaches, having the patient keep a headache diary is helpful in identifying patterns and identifying the impact the symptom has on function.

Past history should be explored for a history of migraine or head trauma, and family history should be explored for migraine and tension headache. Medications should be reviewed thoroughly. Alcohol and smoking consumption should be examined.

The physical examination should include observation of general appearance, including facies, and evaluation of mental status. Assess vital signs for extremes in blood pressure, which suggest a neurological event. Examine the head and palpate for tenderness, signs of trauma, pain over the temporal artery, and strength of the temporal arterial pulse. Test the cranial nerves. Perform a funduscopic examination to assess for papilledema, hemorrhages, exudates, and venous pulsations, and check extraocular movements and position of the eyelids. Evaluate gross and fine motor and sensory functions, including gait, balance, and tactile sense. Test deep tendon reflexes for presence and symmetry; measure muscle strength for grading and equality.

Conduct an examination of the head and neck for lymphadenopathy, thyroid enlargement, carotid bruits, trigger points, meningeal irritation, or limitation in normal range of motion. Check the temporomandibular joint for alignment, mobility, and clicking. Examine the ears, nose, throat, and teeth for contributing problems.

Evaluate the patient for postural alignment problems, muscle spasms, or trigger points in the back or shoulders.

Diagnostic tests: Individualize diagnostic tests according to the suspected cause of the symptom. Neuroimaging sometimes is indicated for emergency evaluation of suspected vascular, neoplastic, or infectious disease. Generally, MRI is preferred to CT scan. MRI is considered if the headache is of sudden onset, severe, worsening, unresponsive to treatment, and associated with neurological or constitutional symptoms. Blood tests are generally not helpful, unless anemia, infection, or electrolyte imbalance is suspected. ESR or C-reactive protein may be indicated if an inflammatory condition, such as giant cell arteritis, is under consideration. An elevated ESR warrants referral of the patient for temporal artery biopsy to confirm diagnosis. If thyroid abnormalities are a possibility, perform thyroid function studies. A lumbar puncture should be done for cerebrospinal fluid analysis if a diagnosis of subarachnoid hemorrhage or meningeal infection is being considered, although about 30% of lumbar punctures result in a low cerebrospinal fluid headache. Sinus or cervical spine x-rays may be indicated.

Differential diagnosis: Symptoms of headaches of various types and etiologies can mimic each other. Potentially serious causes include temporal arteritis, stroke, brain lesions, and hemorrhage. Severe or persistent pain, sudden onset, headaches that worsen over time, and early morning head pain suggest an organic etiology. Migraines are often unilateral, throbbing in quality, and associated with nausea and vomiting and visual symptoms, including light sensitivity. A prodrome or aura is often present, and head pain is aggravated by exertion and lasts 4 to 72 hours. Tension headaches are bilateral and pressing in quality, are not aggravated by exertion, and may last minutes to days. The cluster headache is usually periorbital, unilateral, and associated at times with eye tearing and nasal congestion. The cluster is worse in the supine position and occurs two to six times daily, lasting 15 to 90 minutes.

 Clinical Pearl: Temporal arteritis occurs generally in older adults and often in patients with polymyalgia rheumatica. These headaches are fixed in location, high in severity, and increase in frequency over time. Accompanied by systemic symptoms, such as malaise and aches, the scalp vessels may be found to be tender and thickened to the touch.

Treatment: Treatment of headache depends on its cause. Analgesics such as acetaminophen, aspirin, and NSAIDs in appropriate doses may be used cautiously along with nonpharmacological modalities, and this is often effective for pain relief. Nonpharmacological treatment, including biofeedback, imagery, progressive relaxation techniques, and other stress management strategies, should be tried initially for muscle tension, migraine, and mixed (tension and migraine) headaches. Additional treatments that may be effective include acupuncture, acupressure, transcutaneous electrical nerve stimulation, massage, intermittent use of a cervical collar, heat or cold application, and resting in a darkened room.

For frequent migraine headaches, prophylactic therapy may be instituted to prevent development of symptoms. Medication is taken daily for a trial period (usually 1–2 months) to evaluate the effect on headache frequency, and all categories of drugs should be started at low doses and incrementally increased to therapeutic dosing. Although β-blockers (propranolol [Inderal LA], 80 mg orally daily; atenolol [Tenormin], 50–100 mg orally daily; or nadolol [Corgard], 40 mg orally daily) have been used prophylactically for migraine and cluster headaches, they are contraindicated in patients with a history of bronchospastic disease, asthma, diabetes, or congestive heart failure.

Calcium channel blockers (verapamil, 240 mg orally daily in divided doses, or nifedipine, 30–180 mg orally daily) also have been used prophylactically to prevent migraines. Contraindications include congestive heart failure, heart block, hypotension, sick sinus syndrome, and atrial fibrillation. Low doses of tricyclic antidepressants (amitriptyline [Elavil], 25–50 mg orally daily, or desipramine [Norpramin], 50 mg orally daily) have been prescribed prophylactically, although these agents may be contraindicated because of adverse effects on the cardiovascular system or anticholinergic effects. Anticonvulsants (carbamazepine, 600 mg twice daily, or valproic acid, 250–500 mg in daily divided doses) are newer drugs being used.

For abortive treatment of migraine or cluster headache, if nonprescription analgesics such as aspirin and acetaminophen are ineffective, ergotrate preparations (Midrin, Cafergot) or a selective serotonin agonist (sumatriptan) have been used with some success in adults; however, all are contraindicated in patients with coronary artery disease or peripheral vascular disease, limiting their use in older patients. In cluster headaches, the same drugs may work in some cases, and if not contraindicated, prednisone, 40 to 60 mg orally daily for 1 week, then tapered off for another week, also may be prescribed. Intranasal lidocaine 4% topical solution, 1 mL in the nostril corresponding to the location of the headache, also has been effective in relieving migraine or cluster headaches. Cluster headaches may be treated with lithium.

For giant cell arteritis, patients may take prednisone, 40 to 60 mg daily for several weeks, then tapered gradually to 10 to 20 mg daily and continued for 18 months. Long-term steroid therapy of this nature has important implications related to immune system function, GI bleeding, and bone deterioration.

 Clinical Pearl: Feverfew is a medicinal herb used in self-treatment of migraine with mixed results shown in clinical trials. The side effects include mouth ulcerations and a loss of sense of taste.

Follow-up: Monitoring depends on cause and treatment strategies. Patients should be monitored for effectiveness of treatment.

Sequelae: Sequelae depend on cause. Missed diagnosis of acute, life-threatening symptoms can prove fatal. Most common causes have recurrence or chronicity, which affects quality of life.

Prevention/prophylaxis: Preventive measures include avoidance of triggers, early intervention with medication as soon as symptoms present, and stress reduction techniques as appropriate.

Referral: Refer patients to collaborating physician or neurologist whenever red flags are noted to be present.

Education: Teach patients how to live with a chronic or recurrent problem, to avoid triggers, to reduce stress, and to promote self-care. If medications are prescribed, ensure that the patient understands proper use and safety considerations.

HEMOPTYSIS

Hemoptysis	ICD-9-CM: 786.3

Description: Coughing or spitting blood from the respiratory tract.
Etiology: Determining the source of the blood that the patient coughs up can be a difficult task. Potential locations and causes of blood loss from the respiratory tract include:

- Oronasopharyngeal area—nosebleed, rhinitis, irritation, dental disease
- Larynx—trauma, cancer
- Cardiopulmonary—trauma, bronchitis, pneumonia, tuberculosis, cancer, abscess, congestive heart failure, pulmonary hypertension, mitral stenosis

Rarer causes of hemoptysis include:

- Bleeding disorders

- Pulmonary infarction, thrombus, and emboli

Occurrence: Upper respiratory infections are the most common cause of blood-streaked sputum. In >15% of patients, the source of minor hemorrhage is often never identified and disappears after a few days. Of all patients with hemoptysis, >50% have a normal x-ray. At some time in the course of their disease, 50% of lung cancer patients have hemoptysis. Of all patients, 20% have hemoptysis with mitral stenosis from capillary rupture caused by pulmonary hypertension.

Age: May occur at any age.

Ethnicity: No direct ties to ethnicity have been documented, but immigrants and persons living in poverty are at higher risk for TB and other pulmonary infections.

Gender: No gender-specific differences.

Contributing factors: Knowing a history of the following activities is crucial to the assessment of hemoptysis:

- Smoking (including second-hand smoke)—leading to cancer of the throat and lungs.
- Alcohol use—leading to liver cirrhosis and varices as well as raising the risk of stomach cancer
- Trauma—assault, motor vehicle accidents, or falls leading to contusion of the lungs
- Living environment—exposure to infectious agents, poorly ventilated heating in the home
- Work environment—exposure to chemicals and dust
- Hypertension—may be heralded by persistent nosebleeds
- Comorbidity—immune compromise leading to fungal pneumonitis or clotting disorders
- Medications—aspirin, acetaminophen, and anticoagulant ingestion

Signs and symptoms: The quantity of blood and the length of time the symptoms have been occurring are the first points to determine in assessing the patient. Hemoptysis >100 mL ($^1/_2$ cup) in <24 hours is potentially life-threatening and requires treatment in an emergency department. Likewise, sudden onset of hemoptysis without other mitigating circumstances usually is caused by pulmonary thrombus and needs emergent treatment.

A comprehensive history of the disease, the patient's risk factors, and the work and home environment is the first step in narrowing the cause of the hemoptysis. Risk factors include smoking, long-term alcohol abuse, stroke, older age, emigrant status, HIV-positive status, and heart disease. Use of tobacco with long-standing or increasingly severe hoarseness may indicate cancer of the mouth or throat. A history of persistent "heartburn" may be a clue to consider esophageal erosion as the source of the bleeding.

Vital signs should include oxygen saturation, temperature, heart rate, and respirations. The physical examination begins with a thorough examination of the nose and oropharyngeal mucosa. The lymphatic chains of the neck and supraclavicular nodes must be palpated carefully to assess for infection, lymphoma, and other cancers.

The chest must be assessed for adventitious breath sounds. Wheezes indicate bronchitis or asthma caused by mucus in the larger airways. Rhonchi or crackles are suspicious for pneumonia or infiltrates. Diminished or absent lung sounds by auscultation and dullness to percussion are highly suggestive of consolidation of pneumonia. Rhonchi or crackles with cardiomegaly on x-ray or ECG indicate congestive heart failure and may or may not be accompanied by edema. A prominent first heart sound, early diastolic snap, and rumbling diastolic murmur are signs of mitral valve stenosis. A patient's abdomen distended owing to ascites is likely to be accompanied by esophageal varices from cirrhosis of the liver.

 Clinical Pearl: A prodrome of a tingling sensation at the back of the throat may be experienced before blood is coughed up.

Diagnostic tests: No routine testing is indicated for hemoptysis; however, if the amount of blood loss is substantial, a CBC is in order. The extent of testing depends on whether these services are available on-site. Following are tests along with their efficacy, specificity, and expense:

- pH testing—blood from the respiratory tract being more alkaline than acidic blood from the GI tract (optional, noninvasive, limited specificity, quick, low cost)
- Oxygen saturation test—to assess pulmonary status; if low, consider pneumonia (inexpensive, quick, nonspecific)
- TB skin testing—if at risk (moderately specific, requires 48–72 hours, moderately invasive, moderate cost)
- Sputum sampling—difficult to obtain without contamination with oral flora (nonspecific if contaminated, time-consuming, moderately expensive)
- CBC—increased WBC count indicates infection, low hemoglobin, low hematocrit (moderately expensive, nonspecific, moderately invasive)
- Chest x-ray—to evaluate for pneumonia, congestive heart failure, or cancer; usually negative in bronchitis (obligatory assessment tool for hemoptysis, limited specificity, expensive, minimally invasive)
- ECG—for initial evaluation of cardiomegaly, heart failure, and mitral valve stenosis (minimally invasive, practically specific, moderately expensive)
- Bronchoscopy/laryngoscopy—to determine the specific source of the hemorrhage if the bleeding is increasingly severe or lasts >1 week (specific, expensive, invasive)

Differential diagnosis: Determine first if the blood is coming from the respiratory tract (hemoptysis) or the GI tract (hematemesis).

- Aspiration
- Coagulopathy
- Flu
- Goodpasture's syndrome
- Leukemia
- Lupus pneumonitis
- Mitral valve stenosis
- Pulmonary embolus
- Thrombocytopenia
- Wegener's granulomatosis

Treatment: If the source of the bleeding has been reasonably isolated to the respiratory system and the condition is not life-threatening, the following treatments are recommended:

Acute bronchitis: Acute bronchitis is predominantly viral, and antibiotics do not shorten the course of the disease. If the patient smokes, he or she should be counseled to quit or cut back significantly. Bronchodilators help open the airways; expectorants such as guaifenesin used to mobilize secretions is about as effective as drinking two additional glasses of water per day. Cough suppressants should be avoided except to help the patient sleep. A cool mist humidifier in the bedroom is useful in loosening secretions.

Chronic bronchitis: Chronic bronchitis needs a combination bronchodilator as an inhaler or as a nebulizer. Because chronic bronchitis is usually a result of smoking, the patient should be counseled to stop. Antibiotics or oral steroids should be reserved for acute exacerbations heralded by increasing shortness of breath, change in the color of the sputum to dark yellow or green, or fever.

Bacterial pneumonia: Pneumonia is most often caused by *Staphylococcus, Klebsiella,* or *Pseudomonas* in the otherwise healthy individual. If pneumonia is suspected, broad-spectrum antibiotic therapy should be initiated empirically. Immuno-compromised patients, patients with any respiratory distress, and elderly patients with significantly low or elevated WBC counts may need to be hospitalized.

Fungal infection: A fungal infection should be suspected if the pneumonia does not respond to conventional antibiotic therapy. Amphotericin may be initiated, and the patient should be referred to a pulmonologist.

Tuberculosis: Antituberculosis drugs should be begun with a positive Mantoux test and the patient referred to a health department.

Follow-up: The tenacity of follow-up depends on the severity of the illness. For pneumonia or bronchitis with minimal dyspnea, a call to check on the patient is appropriate. Worsening temperature, bleeding, or difficulty breathing requires immediate attention or emergency department evaluation. Patients with resolving pneumonia should be evaluated in 2 to 3 weeks and a repeat chest x-ray considered.

Sequelae: Death can occur if the etiology is not identified quickly and treated, particularly if it causes cardiovascular collapse or acute respiratory insufficiency.

Prevention/prophylaxis: Smoking cessation intervention is always indicated. The work and home environment should be evaluated. Humidification of the sleeping area with a cool mist humidifier is recommended. Stress the need for flu shots for all patients and Pneumovax for older and immunocompromised patients.

Referral: If hemoptysis persists or increases, the patient needs to be referred for bronchoscopy or laryngoscopy. If lesions suspicious for cancer are found on x-ray, the radiologist may request a chest CT scan with contrast dye, followed by referral to an oncologist or surgeon.

Education: Patient education includes smoking cessation classes. Recommend Alcoholics Anonymous if alcoholism is suspected.

INVOLUNTARY WEIGHT LOSS

| Involuntary weight loss | ICD-9-CM: 783.21 |

Description: Involuntary weight loss occurs when the number of calories available are less than the patient's daily needs. Recent, marked weight loss is a more ominous sign than gradual loss over many months or years; the rapidity of weight loss is an important clue. Recent loss is usually defined as a substantial loss of ≥ 10 lb occurring over the past 3 to 6 months. In the older adult, a loss of at least 10% of body weight over 2 months is cause for concern.

Etiology: Involuntary weight loss can be classified in three ways:

- Inadequate nutrient intake
- Excessive energy expenditure that occurs in catabolism
- A combination of inadequate intake and excessive energy expenditure

Organic causes of inadequate nutrient intake include alcoholism, mechanical causes such as poor dentition, and dysphagia. Psychogenic causes of unexplainable weight loss include depression, anxiety, and dementia. Patients who have hyperthyroidism, diabetes mellitus, pheochromocytoma, malignancy, or fever lose weight because of excessive energy expenditure. For patients with neoplasms, infection, liver disease, renal disease, endocrine disorder, and GI disease, weight loss results from the anorexia that often occurs with these diseases and the excessive energy expended.

Occurrence: The occurrence of involuntary weight loss completely depends on the etiology and underlying disease (e.g., 71% of patients with COPD commonly lose weight). A high incidence of involuntary weight loss occurs with metastatic disease, alcoholism, dementia, depression, and acquired immunodeficiency syndrome.

Age: Age as an isolated factor has no documented significance; however, age-related changes (e.g., smell, taste) and chronic diseases common in the elderly predispose this age group to weight loss. About half of Americans >65 years old have lost all their teeth. This tooth loss and teeth in poor repair may affect significantly the ability to eat a nutritious diet in adequate amounts.

Ethnicity: Not significant.

Gender: No documented significance; however, gender data are affected if the specific underlying disease causing the weight loss is more common in men or in women.

Contributing factors: Pulmonary and cardiac diseases, cancer, dementia, alcoholism, depression, medications, GI tract dysmotility, sensory changes, decreased functional status, lack of transportation, financial problems, malnutrition, hyperthyroidism, chronic infection, dentition, smoking, family history of involuntary weight loss, and history of exposure to hepatitis have been known to contribute to involuntary weight loss.

Signs and symptoms: Patients may report depression, poor dentition, dysphagia, alcohol and drug use, persistent localized pain, sore tongue, paresthesia, anorexia, nausea, vomiting, change in stools, and diarrhea. Patients with accelerated metabolism may describe episodes of fatigue, fever, melena, heat intolerance, polydipsia, polyphagia, and polyuria. On physical examination, patients with significant weight loss appear pale and cachectic, with a malnourished appearance (hair loss, muscle wasting, loss of subcutaneous fat, especially around the face). Look for evidence of loose skin, petechiae, cyanosis, clubbing of the fingers, and edema. There may be temporal wasting, icterus, dry mucous membranes, and flattened papillae of the tongue. The oral examination also should note denture fit; tooth and gum disease; and oral lesions such as ulcers, stomatitis, and candidiasis. Examination of the cardiorespiratory system may reveal loud or palpable murmurs and diminished breath sounds. Liver or spleen may be palpable. Check for masses in the abdomen, breasts, and rectum. Muscle wasting may be apparent on the extremities, and deep tendon reflexes may have a prolonged relaxation phase. Patients may have diminished position and vibratory sense. Check women for ovarian masses, cervical lesions, and any obvious neoplasia. In men, examine the prostate gland for enlargement. An early focus of the assessment should be screening for a functional cause of weight loss (i.e., is the patient able to prepare and eat an appropriate diet; if functional limitations are present, is adequate help consistently available to assist with ADLs).

Diagnostic tests: Physical findings and history indicate most organic causes of weight loss and guide the choice of diagnostic tests. A nutritional or diet history and calorie counts add objective data to evaluate the amount and quality of food intake. A complete review of medications is always a good idea, looking for medication effects on appetite, taste, mouth dryness, nutrient absorption, or increased indigestion or reflux. Standard screening tests are as follows:

Test	Results Indicating Disorder	CPT Code
Albumin (has a half-life of about 21 days and reflects level about 3 weeks in past).	2.9–3.5 g/dL, mild nutritional deficiency 2.1–3 g/dL, moderate nutritional deficiency <2.1 g/dL, severe nutritional deficiency	82040
Prealbumin	10.7–16 g/dL, moderate deficiency <10.7 g/dL, severe deficiency	84134
Serum cholesterol	≤160 mg/dL, consider protein-calorie malnutrition if signs/symptoms of poor nutrition present	82480
CBC with differential	Low total lymphocyte count or an unexplained normocytic anemia may indicate malnutrition. A blood loss anemia should raise concern of malignancy	85025
TSH	1.9–5.4 μIU /mL, normal reference range Decreased levels in hyperthyroidism, often associated with weight loss Increased levels in hypothyroidism, associated with weight change (usually gain, but loss also occurs in elderly)	84443
Transferrin	150–200 mg/dL, mild depletion 100–150 mg/dL, moderate depletion <200 mg/dL, severe visceral protein depletion Limited use in monitoring response to therapy, but better than albumin. Not specific to nutritional issues	84466

TSH, thyroid-stimulating hormone.

 Clinical Pearl: For patients whose nutrition is being monitored closely, an increase in the prealbumin of 1 mg/day indicates a good response to nutritional supplementation. A response of <2 mg/week signifies an inadequate response or an inadequate level of nutritional support.

In the absence of localized symptoms, routine cancer screening is indicated in certain patients. Consider a neoplastic origin when benign causes of weight loss appear unlikely. Evidence of blood loss anemia on the CBC or one positive fecal occult blood result is a reason to perform GI imaging. In general, imaging studies performed in the hope that they will show something are expensive, are as likely to yield false-positive results as true-positive results, and are overused for general screenings. These methods have a higher diagnostic yield if directed at a specific organ, system, or region of the body. With frail older persons, however, before this kind of invasive and expensive workup is begun, it is important to address the question of treatment options with the patient and family. There is no need to proceed further if surgery, radiation, or other treatment options are not feasible or if the patient or family is not interested. If the cause of weight loss is not clear from these results, watchful waiting is recommended; watch for further weight loss or specific symptoms, and reconsider a functional cause of weight loss. If no abnormalities are detected from the standard tests, history, and physical examination, an organic cause is unlikely (<5%). When the findings from the initial workup are negative, psychological problems, particularly depression and anxiety, are among the most common reasons for weight loss. For gradual weight loss, the workup can take 6 months.

 Clinical Pearl: In elderly patients with multiple or nonspecific complaints (often including weight loss), a high index of suspicion for depression is warranted. An adequate trial of an antidepressant is almost always appropriate.

Differential diagnosis: For weight loss that occurs with increased food intake, consider diabetes, thyrotoxicosis, malabsorption, leukemia, lymphoma, and adrenal insufficiency. For weight loss that occurs with normal or decreased food intake, consider alcoholism; malignancy; infection; gastrointestinal, hepatic, renal, dental, endocrine, respiratory, cardiac, or psychological causes; anorexia nervosa; malnutrition; or a functional origin.

Treatment: Watchful waiting is recommended if no organic cause is determined immediately. Otherwise, treat or manage the identified underlying cause. Drugs that stimulate the appetite are not a first-line therapy in those with weight loss since few studies show efficacy.

Follow-up: If results of the standard tests listed earlier are negative, and the history and physical examination are negative, the recommended approach is to watch for further weight loss and to reconsider functional causes. Have the patient or caregiver keep a daily record of food intake, activity levels, and symptoms, and schedule a return visit in 2 to 4 weeks.

Sequelae: Malnutrition is the first complication to consider in involuntary weight loss. Long-term unexplained weight loss may indicate failure to thrive and the beginning of a downward spiral in health and function.

 Clinical Pearl: Many patients in acute and long-term care have unrecognized protein-calorie malnutrition. Protein-calorie malnutrition is a common iatrogenic complication of hospitalization.

Prevention/prophylaxis: Discuss proper nutrition and the need for dental care, if appropriate. Address functional, financial, and social issues that may affect nutrition (i.e., address depression, arrange for socialization at mealtime if feasible, arrange Meals on Wheels).

Referral: Refer to a specialist for rapid or acute decline; for positive diagnostic test results indicating malignancy, thyrotoxicosis, or other acute organic illnesses requiring sophisticated diagnostic workup or management; or for a patient condition beyond your current scope of practice. Refer patients for assistance if social or functional issues may be contributing to weight loss. Refer to an appropriate specialist or perform additional assessments to confirm patient's denial of problems (e.g., nutritional, psychological, in-home, functional).

Education: Instruct patients about proper nutrition and hydration. Encourage exercise to improve strength or function and to stimulate appetite. Teach patients about medication side effects that may affect nutrition and about signs or symptoms of overmedication or undermedication.

JOINT PAIN

Joint pain	ICD-9-CM: 719.40
Ankle	ICD-9-CM: 719.47
Elbow	ICD-9-CM: 719.42
Foot	ICD-9-CM: 719.47
Hand	ICD-9-CM: 719.44
Hip	ICD-9-CM: 719.45
Knee	ICD-9-CM: 719.46
Multiple sites	ICD-9-CM: 719.49
Pelvic region	ICD-9-CM: 719.45
Psychogenic	ICD-9-CM: 307.89
Shoulder	ICD-9-CM: 719.41
Specified site	ICD-9-CM: 719.48
Wrist	ICD-9-CM: 719.43

Description: Joint pain is discomfort or pain arising from one of the various joints in the body (neck, spine, shoulder, hand, wrist, distal interphalangeal, proximal interphalangeal, elbow, hip, knee, ankle, or metatarsophalangeal). Joint pain can arise from muscular, bone, or systemic disease. The knee is the most commonly affected joint in older adults.

Etiology: The description, location, onset, and associated symptoms are crucial to diagnosing the etiology of joint pain. The cause can be as varied as the type of pain with which the patient presents. Narrowing down or clarifying the etiology of the pain depends on the clinical presentation, complete history, and findings from physical examination and appropriate diagnostic testing. The pain can be mild (from strained muscles or ligaments that support the joint), chronic (lasting >6 months, from degenerative joint disease arthritis, osteoarthritis), inflammatory (from joint effusion, rheumatoid arthritis [RA]), or severe and acute (from fracture, cartilage injury, avascular septic necrosis). The following should be considered as causes of joint pain:

- Chronic infection (TB, fungal)

- Gout
- Arthritis (osteoarthritis, RA, gonococcal, septic)
- Bursitis
- Tendinitis
- Ankylosing spondylitis
- Fracture (stress or traumatic)
- Peripheral entrapment syndromes (carpal tunnel, thoracic outlet)
- Neuropathies
- Degenerative joint disease
- Disc problems
- Systemic causes (systemic lupus erythematosus, sarcoidosis, Lyme disease, hemophilia, Raynaud's disease, Paget's disease, hemochromatosis)

If the patient presents with an atypical case of joint pain, systemic disease may be the underlying cause.

Occurrence: More than one third of individuals 45 years old have joint discomfort ranging from joint stiffness to severe pain. The inability to maintain normal physical activity or alteration in mobility because of pain in a joint often leads patients to seek medical care for this complaint.

Age: Joint pain is found more frequently in the elderly patient as a result of age-related muscle atrophy, demineralization of trabecular bone, atrophy of cortical bone, chronic disease, and loss of bone density. Arthritis (degenerative and inflammatory) is the most common cause of disability in individuals >75 years old, and it affects >80% of individuals in this age group, with joint pain being the dominant symptom.

Ethnicity: No documentation is found specifically for joint pain; however, the prevalence of certain types of inflammatory joint disease and systemic disorders is higher in various ethnic groups.

Gender: Joint pain occurs equally in males and females.

Contributing factors: Factors that may lead to joint pain include overuse or strain, previous injury or trauma to the joint, alterations in gait or balance, past surgery or joint replacement, known history of arthritis or joint disease, and postmenopausal women with no hormonal replacement therapy. Weight, physical stature, smoking, and family history should be assessed in reviewing the risk factors for osteoporosis. Other contributing factors include obesity, poor nutritional habits, low calcium intake, alcohol consumption, medications, and exercise habits.

Signs and symptoms: The history should include the onset of the pain (sudden, insidious); character of the pain (dull, sharp); and duration and location of the pain (including radiation). Inquire about any associated symptoms, any alleviating or aggravating factors, and timing (e.g., worse in morning, better late in the day). Symptoms associated with joint pain may include general weakness, stiffness, decreased range of motion, and inflammation.

Discuss normal activity levels and the possibility of overuse or strain. Has there been any old or recent trauma to the joint? If there was an injury, did the patient hear any popping or clicking? Discuss the limitation in joint mobility, and note the presence of edema, redness, or fever. Review if there is any associated muscle fatigue, joint deformity, or inability to perform certain movements.

The physical examination includes a complete assessment of the patient, paying specific attention to any joint pain complaints. Inspect, palpate, and percuss (if needed) each joint, and assess the appropriate range of motion, noting any pain or limitations in movement. Note the patient's gait, balance, and posture. Inspect each joint, noting the musculature, any atrophy, contractures, nodules (Heberden's or Bouchard's nodes), asymmetry, or gross deformity. Note any erythema, inflammation, or soft tissue swelling on or near the joint. Palpate for any tenderness or effusions on or around the joint. Assess for any lymphadenopathy. Check for crepitus, clicking, or popping in or around the joint.

Diagnostic tests: No tests are specifically indicated with a complaint of joint pain. Problem-specific complaints and physical examination findings dictate which tests are required. A CBC with differential is needed to rule out infection (elevated WBCs). Normocytic, normochromic anemia is seen with RA. ESR helps determine inflammatory disease (normal values depend on the method and laboratory parameters). An elevated ESR is seen in patients with collagen vascular disease, infection, inflammatory disease, and RA. Marked elevations in alkaline phosphatase level (20–90 IU/L) are seen in patients with bone disease (e.g., Paget's disease, metastatic bone disease). Hypercalcemia with marked alkaline phosphatase is seen in patients with hyperparathyroidism or bone carcinoma. Serum creatine kinase (CK) isoenzymes are elevated in persons with muscle trauma and progressive muscular disease.

If indicated, obtain a complete electrolyte panel and urinalysis, checking blood urea nitrogen and creatinine, to assess renal function. Many causes of joint pain are treated with NSAIDs, which potentially can alter renal function. Because kidney function decreases with aging, routine testing is necessary. Other, more problem-specific tests include:

- Hepatitis B profile with liver function tests (patients with recent infection can present with arthritic joint pain)
- Uric acid levels in patients with suspected gout
- Antinuclear antibody testing (results positive in patients with systemic lupus erythematosus and in 25% of patients with RA)
- RA latex fixation test (reveals high titers with severe joint disease)
- Rheumatoid factor, which may or may not be present with RA, but is elevated in chronic infection, TB, and sarcoidosis

X-rays of the joint can be useful to detect fracture, joint space destruction or narrowing, erosion, arthritic changes, and degeneration. Joint effusions may require aspiration and culture of the aspirate to assess for sepsis. Further evaluation with CT scans or MRI may be necessary, although experience with the diagnostic value of these modalities is limited.

Differential diagnosis: The disease processes associated with joint pain are considered in the differential diagnosis. Morning stiffness points toward an inflammatory arthritis, whereas postexercise stiffness indicates a degenerative process. Some other conditions to rule out include psoriatic arthritis, connective tissue disease, Reiter's disease, multiple myeloma, and scleroderma.

Treatment: Medical management of joint pain depends on the findings of the comprehensive assessment. The goal to decrease pain may include physical therapy, analgesic and anti-inflammatory medications, moist heat, intra-articular steroid injections, assistive devices, and surgery. Pharmacological agents include NSAIDs, which primarily have a role in treating inflammatory pain notwithstanding the GI and renal adverse effects. Cyclooxygenase type 2 inhibitors and opioids may be used when other agents fail. Acetaminophen continues to be the first-line drug in osteoarthritis in that it has a low cost, has low toxicity, and has high efficacy. Newer agents useful in inflammatory arthritis include disease-modifying antirheumatic drugs and biological response modifiers. Nonpharmacological therapies proven useful in randomized clinical trials include transcutaneous electric nerve stimulation and acupuncture. Emergency intervention is required if you suspect a fracture, avascular necrosis, or sepsis.

 Clinical Pearl: Capsaicin, an enzyme found in hot pepper, depletes substance P when applied to the painful area three times a day for several weeks.

Follow-up: Monitoring of patients depends on findings. Patients with acute or severe joint pain may need emergency care and intervention. Monitor patients with chronic pain frequently until the clinical workup is completed. Management of chronic joint pain or disease requires routine visits to monitor medications and laboratory and diagnostic test results.

Sequelae: The condition and prognosis relate to the etiology of the joint pain.

Prevention/prophylaxis: Prevention methods depend on the etiology of the joint pain. When applicable, use weight reduction to decrease stress on the joint; physical therapy and exercise for strengthening; and moist heat, topical medications, and steroid injections to reduce pain and spasms. Explore alternative methods of pain control (acupuncture, yoga, medication, or massage therapy). Address fall prevention for patients using assistive devices (canes, crutches, or walkers). Instruct the patient concerning joint protection and preservation. Discuss proper nutrition, calcium supplements, and smoking cessation.

Referral: Refer patients to a specialist pending the results of the workup. Refer patients to the appropriate emergency service if you suspect sepsis, fracture, or avascular necrosis.

Education: Teach patients about the appropriate dose of medications and the potential side effects that need to be reported. Instruct patients about appropriate follow-up and referrals. Tell the patient to report any persisting or worsening joint pain and any systemic involvement. Instruct patients on the appropriate methods for pain control. Review the use of any adaptive equipment and the role the patient plays in avoiding disability and slowing progression of the disease.

NAUSEA AND VOMITING

| Nausea | ICD-9-CM: 787.02 |
| Nausea with vomiting | ICD-9-CM: 787.01 |

Description: Nausea is entirely subjective and described as the unpleasant sensation that immediately precedes vomiting. It often is accompanied by increased parasympathetic activity, such as pallor, diaphoresis, salivation, and other vasovagal signs such as hypotension and bradycardia. Vomiting is a physical event that results in the rapid, forceful evacuation of gastric contents in retrograde fashion from the stomach up to and out of the mouth. Although usually preceded by nausea, vomiting may occur in the absence of nausea.

Etiology: The history helps to determine the etiology of the nausea and vomiting. Generally, toxins cause acute symptoms, whereas established illnesses cause chronic symptoms. Nausea is caused by alterations in the motility of the stomach and small intestine. The vomiting reflex involves visceral and somatic components and is integrated in the vomiting center and the chemoreceptor trigger zone of the medulla oblongata. The vomiting reflex begins in the stimulation of receptor sites in the mucosa of the upper GI tract, the labyrinth apparatus (inner ear), higher cortical centers (e.g., emotional stimuli), or the chemoreceptor trigger zone (dopamine receptors), which is stimulated by specific mediators in the blood. The afferent nerves carry the impulses to the vomiting center, then the efferent pathways (including the phrenic nerves to the diaphragm, spinal nerves to the abdominal musculature, and visceral nerves to the stomach and esophagus) carry the impulses to the effector muscles, resulting in relaxation of the gastric fundus and gastroesophageal sphincter, contraction of the gastric pylorus, and reverse peristalsis in the esophagus. The glottis closes, preventing aspiration and increasing intrathoracic pressure; the abdominal wall muscles and the diaphragm contract, causing an increase in intra-abdominal pressure, resulting in the forcing of the stomach contents through the mouth.

Adverse medication reactions are common causes of nausea and vomiting. Generally, nausea in response to a drug presents early in the course (within 24 hours) of its use. Medications cause acute rather than chronic nausea and vomiting. The most extensively studied form of medication-related nausea and vomiting is that caused by cancer chemotherapeutic agents. Risk factors for acute chemotherapy-induced nausea include lower socioeconomic status, prechemotherapy nausea, female gender, and absence of antiemetic therapy.

Radiation therapy for malignancy can produce emesis by its effect on the GI tract. Other substances that are ingested may produce nausea and vomiting. Alcohol, when consumed in excess, provokes vomiting by a local action on the GI tract and centrally in the brainstem. Excess intake of vitamin A also may cause nausea and vomiting.

GI and systemic infections may cause an acute onset of nausea and vomiting. Non-GI infections associated with nausea include otitis media, meningitis, and hepatitis.

Occurrence: Nausea and vomiting are common, particularly in terminally ill cancer patients, in whom the incidence is estimated to be 40% to 70%.

Age: Nausea and vomiting occurs at all ages. Certain causes (i.e., adverse drug reaction, terminal cancer) occur more often in advanced age.

Ethnicity: Not significant

Gender: Nausea and vomiting may occur more often in younger women than in younger men because of the incidence of nausea and vomiting during pregnancy. The evidence for this is expert opinion.

Contributing factors: The following contribute to the development of nausea and vomiting:

Medications and toxic etiologies
Cancer chemotherapy
    Severe: cisplatin, dacarbazine, nitrogen mustard
    Moderate: etoposide, methotrexate, cytarabine
    Mild: fluorouracil, vinblastine, tamoxifen
Analgesics
    Aspirin
    NSAIDs
    Opioids
    Antigout drugs
Cardiovascular medications
    Digoxin
    Antiarrhythmics
    Antihypertensives
    β-Blockers
    Calcium channel antagonists
Diuretics
Hormonal preparations/therapies
Oral antidiabetics

Antibiotics/antivirals
    Erythromycin
    Tetracycline
    Sulfonamides
    Antituberculous drugs
    Acyclovir
GI medications
    Sulfasalazine
    Azathioprine
Nicotine
Narcotics
Antiparkinsonian drugs
Anticonvulsants
Antiasthmatics
    Theophylline
Radiation therapy
Ethanol abuse
Hypervitaminosis
Infectious causes
    Gastroenteritis
    Viral
    Bacterial
    Non-GI infections
    Otitis media
Disorders of the gut and peritoneum
    Mechanical obstruction
    Gastric outlet obstruction
    Small bowel obstruction
Functional GI disorders
    Gastroparesis
    Chronic intestinal pseudo-obstruction
    Nonulcer dyspepsia
    Irritable bowel syndrome
Organic GI disorders
    Pancreatic adenocarcinoma
    Peptic ulcer disease
    Cholecystitis
    Pancreatitis
    Hepatitis
    Crohn's disease
    Mesenteric ischemia
    Mucosal metastases
Central nervous system causes
    Migraine
    Increased intracranial pressure

Malignancy
Hemorrhage
Infarction
Abscess
Meningitis
Seizure disorders
Demyelinating disorders
Emotional responses
Psychiatric disease
Psychogenic vomiting
Anxiety disorders
Depression
Pain
Anorexia nervosa
Bulimia nervosa
Labyrinthine disorders
Motion sickness
Labyrinthitis
Tumors
Ménière's disease
Iatrogenic
Endocrinological and metabolic causes
Uremia
Diabetic ketoacidosis
Hyperparathyroidism
Hypoparathyroidism

Signs and symptoms: Symptom duration, frequency, and severity are important. Acute onset of nausea and vomiting suggests gastroenteritis, pancreatitis, or cholecystitis. A more insidious onset of nausea without vomiting suggests gastroparesis, a medication-related side effect, metabolic disorders, or GERD.

The timing and description of the vomiting should be noted. Vomiting that occurs before breakfast is typical of uremia, alcohol ingestion, and increased intracranial pressure. Intracranial disorders may present with projectile vomiting versus ordinary emesis. The onset of vomiting caused by gastroparesis tends to be delayed by ≥1 hour after eating.

Details regarding the quality and quantity of vomitus are important. Vomiting of partly digested food suggests gastroparesis. Bilious vomiting is characteristic of small bowel obstruction. A feculent odor to the vomitus also is a sign of intestinal obstruction.

The physical examination is important in determining the underlying cause of the nausea and vomiting. Signs of weight loss and dehydration should be assessed. The abdominal examination is important, with emphasis placed on detection of abdominal distention, tenderness, visible peristalsis, and hernias.

Diagnostic tests: The patient's history and physical examination should direct the diagnostic testing. The goals are to assist in identifying the underlying cause of nausea and vomiting and to assess the consequences of vomiting. Basic laboratory testing might include a CBC with electrolyte and standard chemistry profiles to assess the need to correct any deficiencies, such as hypokalemia. Further laboratory studies include screening for abnormal thyroid function and drug levels for patients who are taking digoxin, theophylline, or salicylates to rule out toxicity. If vomiting is acute a flat and upright abdominal radiograph may reveal an obstruction as a cause.

Differential diagnosis: Self-limiting nausea and vomiting should be differentiated from acute and chronic nausea and vomiting.

Treatment: Treatment of the patient with nausea and vomiting must address:

- Correction of any fluid, electrolyte, or nutritional deficiencies
- Identification and elimination of the cause if possible
- Suppression or elimination of the symptoms if cause cannot be identified easily and eliminated

Two broad categories of pharmacological agents are used, antiemetics and prokinetics.

Antiemetics: Antiemetics act primarily within the central nervous system to suppress nausea and vomiting. The principal classes of drugs are phenothiazines, antihistamines, anticholinergics, dopamine antagonists, and serotonin antagonists. Dopamine antagonists, such as haloperidol and metoclopramide, act primarily on the chemoreceptor trigger zone. Serotonin antagonists, such as ondansetron, act together with dopamine antagonists in the chemoreceptor trigger zone and additionally act in the gut. Antihistamines may be useful adjuvant agents when combined with either serotoninergic or dopaminergic agents, although their side effects (sedation, urinary retention, delirium) may limit their usefulness in the elderly. Muscarinic blockers, such as scopolamine, are useful for patients with disturbed vestibular function.

Prokinetics: Prokinetic agents are used primarily in GERD, gastroparesis, and other dysmotility syndromes. Examples include metoclopramide, domperidone, erythromycin, and cisapride. Prokinetic agents such as metoclopramide can potentiate cholinergic activity in the GI tract, which is beneficial if the cause is gastroparesis. Corticosteroids enhance the effects of other antiemetics and may be useful in nausea and vomiting with increased intracranial pressure. For terminally ill elderly cancer patients, nausea can be controlled by many drugs. Administer trimethobenzamide (Tigan) suppositories, 200 mg every 6 hours, or prochlorperazine (Compazine) suppositories or tablets, 25 mg every 8 hours rectally or orally. Other useful drugs include promethazine, lorazepam, metoclopramide, and haloperidol.

 Clinical Pearl: Marijuana has been used as an appetite stimulant and antiemetic. THC (tetrahydrocannabinol) is the major active ingredient available in the prescription as dronabinol.

Nonpharmacological approaches to nausea and vomiting include dietary manipulation, such as eating cold foods, consuming clear liquids, and avoiding strong or spicy foods. Heated foods sometimes create strong odors and might be avoided. Frequent oral care is comforting. Distraction, relaxation, and other behavioral approaches might be helpful.

Follow-up: See the patient for follow-up as indicated for nausea and vomiting and management of the consequences of the nausea and vomiting, such as electrolyte disturbances.

Sequelae: Possible complications depend on the cause of the symptoms and may include dehydration, metabolic acidosis, electrolyte imbalances, and aspiration.

Prevention/prophylaxis: Prevention strategies depend on the cause of the symptoms. Dietary modification and medication modification may be necessary.

Referral: Refer the patient to a specialist appropriate for the cause and management of the symptom.

Education: Explain causes of symptoms, measures taken to determine cause, and symptomatic treatment. Advise patient when to seek medical care.

PERIPHERAL EDEMA

Peripheral edema	ICD-9-CM: 782.3
Due to venous obstruction	ICD-9-CM: 459.2
Localized lower extremity	ICD-9-CM: 459.2

Description: Peripheral edema is an increase in the interstitial fluid component as a result of an expansion of the extracellular fluid volume. When an accumulation of lymph in the extremities causes an increase in hydrostatic pressure, the term *lymphedema* is used.

Etiology: Normally the distribution of water between the blood and interstitial tissues is maintained by equilibrium. Starling's concept—the osmotic pressure of the plasma proteins balances the hydrostatic pressure in the capillaries—helps in the understanding of fluid dynamics. Fluid flows from the vessels to the interstitial area in response to intravas-

Table 2–5   Causes of Leg Edema

Bilateral	Unilateral
Cardiovascular disease (heart failure, pulmonary hypertension, valvular disease, chronic venous insufficiency)	Impaired lymphatic flow Venous obstruction Inflammation
Renal insufficiency	Infection
Hyperthyroidism, hypothyroidism	Tumor
Liver disease	Trauma
Obesity	Compartment syndrome
Drug induced	Ruptured cyst, tendon, or muscle
Chronic anemia	Reflex sympathetic dystrophy
Nephrotic syndrome	
Hypoproteinemia	
Allergic	
Idiopathic edema	

cular hydrostatic pressure and the colloid osmotic pressure of the interstitial fluid. In the opposite direction, fluid enters the blood because of the interstitial tissue tension and the oncotic pressure of the plasma proteins. Interstitial fluid also is returned to the blood as lymph. Under steady-state conditions, net fluid flux out of the capillary is balanced by lymph flow back into circulation. Alteration in any of these compartments (intravascular, extravascular, lymphatic) upsets the equilibrium, and leg edema occurs. Two basic steps occur in edema formation: sodium and water are retained, and capillary hemodynamics are altered.

Leg edema, common in elderly persons, often has diverse etiologies (Table 2–5), and more than one disorder can be causing edema in the same patient. In elderly patients with leg edema, the most common causes are venous insufficiency; congestive heart failure; drug-induced edema; and other conditions including lymphedema, ovarian and prostate cancers, postphlebitic syndrome, nephrotic syndrome, and chronic anemia.

Occurrence: The frequency of occurrence completely depends on the underlying etiology and combined etiologies.

Age: Peripheral edema occurs frequently in older adults.

Ethnicity: Not significant.

Gender: No documented significance is found, but gender statistics vary according to the specific etiology (e.g., idiopathic edema is more common in women; heart failure edema is more common in men).

Contributing factors: Physiological age-related changes increase the vulnerability to fluid retention. The older adult has a smaller amount of total body water overall (80% of body weight for a newborn, 60% for a young adult, 50% for an older adult), and of this, two thirds is intracellular and one third is extracellular fluid. As more intracellular fluid is lost over time, extracellular fluid volume starts to comprise more body water.

Risk factors for leg edema from age-related changes include a decrease in:

- Serum albumin
- Glomerular filtration rate
- Hepatic blood flow
- Sodium-concentrating ability of the kidney
- Myocardial contractility and cardiac output
- Baroreceptor sensitivity

Additional contributing factors include dependent positioning of the lower extremities; excessive intake of sodium; hot weather; and use of medicines that contribute to sodium retention, particularly hormones, NSAIDs, and antihypertensives.

Signs and symptoms: The patient may complain of fullness, discomfort, aching pain, shoes that are too tight, or weight gain. The history should elicit the seven dimensions of the signs and symptoms of edema, emphasizing location (unilateral or bilateral) and chronological evolution (acute or chronic progression). Associated symptoms need to be elicited, particularly shortness of breath. The presence or absence of pain is helpful in determining the differential diagnosis. Ask about aggravating and alleviating factors, including the effect of prolonged sitting or standing, and determine the effect of passive leg elevation. A history of cardiac, renal, liver, or peripheral vascular disease is important.

The physical examination begins with weight. Assess skin changes, including pigmentation and thickening, lesions, discoloration, texture, temperature, and induration. Evaluate the venous and arterial circulation, checking pulses throughout, capillary refill, and dependent rubor. Varicose veins are usually readily apparent with the inspection of the legs while the patient stands.

Assess the extremity for local or diffuse tenderness and for pitting or nonpitting edema. Measure and compare the circumference bilaterally from a fixed reference point above the ankle to the area of maximal edema (e.g., patella, calf, midcalf). Assess any localized enlargement.

 Clinical Pearl: In unilateral edema, a 1-cm difference in size above the ankle or 2-cm difference at the calf is significant and should lead to further investigation.

Examine body systems indicated by the history (e.g., cardiac, renal, endocrine, pulmonary).

Diagnostic tests: Diagnostic tests depend on the probable etiology of leg edema. Cardiac causes may warrant a chest x-ray, ECG, or echocardiogram. Thyroid panel evaluates TSH and free thyroxine. CBC with differential, serum protein albumin level, and electrolyte values should be obtained. Renal and liver panels usually are done as part of an automated chemistry test. Additional studies include ultrasound, venogram, venous

Doppler studies, lymphoscintigraphy, or the more invasive lymphangiography. CT scans for pelvic masses and lymphoma may be indicated.

Differential diagnosis: Leg edema is an important clinical sign, and its causes are diverse. The differential diagnosis is facilitated in part by noting if edema is unilateral or bilateral and recognizing distinctions between lymphedema, lipedema, and venous stasis.

 Clinical Pearl: Lipedema is a bilateral, symmetrical deposition of fat in the lower extremities that spares the feet (a distinguishing feature) and occurs exclusively in obese women.

Treatment: Always direct treatment at the cause of leg edema: diuretics for heart failure, a high-protein diet for hypoalbuminemia, ACE inhibitors for proteinuria, and thrombolytics for acute deep venous thrombosis. Any drugs known to cause edema should be discontinued or decreased in dosage.

Behavioral modifications include intermittent periods of recumbency, the avoidance of environmental heat, and sodium and water restriction as indicated. Exercise and compression garments may help to mobilize fluids.

Follow-up: Closely monitor patients for effectiveness of therapy and adverse events. Monitor the weight and limb circumference measurements using the same reference points.

Sequelae: When administering diuretics, the health-care professional must be alert to potential volume depletion (e.g., dizziness and metabolic abnormalities). Patients with edema as a result of deep venous insufficiency are prone to recurrent ulceration.

Prevention/prophylaxis: For patients with recurrent lymphangitis and cellulitis, prescribe intermittent long-term antibiotic prophylaxis. For patients with leg swelling secondary to deep venous thrombosis, thrombolytics may limit the tissue loss, pulmonary embolus, and more extensive thrombosis of the deep venous system.

Referral: Regardless of the cause of leg swelling, you can achieve the best fluid removal while the patient is hospitalized. This is particularly true when the process is an acute one, such as deep venous thrombophlebitis or cellulitis. When thrombolytic therapy is indicated, consult a vascular specialist.

Education: Patients need specific information related to the edema and the management of symptoms. Typically the patient with edema is instructed to avoid highly salted foods. If compression stockings are recommended, emphasize the importance of proper sizing and application technique to avoid excessive pressure. Instruct patients to elevate the legs to decrease peripheral vascular pressure. Periodic active muscle contraction exercises are important for individuals who must sit for long periods. Teach patients with peripheral vascular disorders to avoid excessive heat and to reduce weight if indicated. Special care of the skin, including proper shoes and prevention of trauma, is important.

SYNCOPE

Syncope	ICD-9-CM: 780.2
Anginosa	ICD-9-CM: 413.9
Bradycardia	ICD-9-CM: 427.89
Cardiac	ICD-9-CM: 780.2
Carotid sinus	ICD-9-CM: 337.0
Fatal	ICD-9-CM: 798.1
Heart	ICD-9-CM: 780.2
Heat	ICD-9-CM: 992.1
Laryngeal	ICD-9-CM: 786.2
Tussive	ICD-9-CM: 786.2
Vasoconstriction	ICD-9-CM: 780.2
Vasodepressor	ICD-9-CM: 780.2
Vasomotor	ICD-9-CM: 780.2
Vasovagal	ICD-9-CM: 780.2

Description: Syncope is defined as a sudden and transient loss of consciousness and postural tone resulting from a reduction in oxygen to the brain.

Etiology: In most instances, the loss of consciousness reflects a temporary decrease in cerebral blood flow that is usually secondary to a fall in the systemic arterial blood pressure. Interruption of cerebral blood flow for 8 to 10 seconds or <30 mL of blood flow/100 g of brain tissue per minute results in syncope. Most etiologies of syncope can be separated into cardiovascular and noncardiovascular causes (see Table 2–6 under Differential Diagnosis).

Occurrence: The Framingham Heart Study showed that 3% of men and 3.5% of women had experienced at least one syncopal episode. Syncope accounts for about 3% of all emergency department visits and 6% of all hospital admissions.

Age: The lifetime incidence of syncope may be 25% in the elderly. Some forms of syncope (i.e., vasovagal, carotid sinus hypersensitivity) are more common in younger persons than in older persons; other forms of syncope (i.e., cardiac, orthostatic, micturition-related) occur more often in older than in younger individuals.

 Clinical Pearl: Aortic stenosis is the most common structural lesion associated with syncope in the elderly.

Ethnicity: Not significant.

Gender: Among younger adults, women have nearly twice the rate of syncope as men; among elderly adults, men have the greater incidence. This likely reflects the most common etiologies in the different age groups.

Contributing factors: Cerebral blood flow has been reported to decline 25% with physiological aging, thought to be related to vascular stiffening.

Hormonal regulation of extracellular volume may become impaired with age. Cardiac reflexes and baroreceptor sensitivity also may become impaired. The kidneys' ability to conserve sodium and water declines. Chronic diseases, such as heart disease, diabetes, renal insufficiency, hypertension, and chronic pulmonary disease, are predisposing conditions. Medications used to treat these chronic diseases, such as diuretics, β-blockers, vasodilators, nitrates, antiarrhythmics, and antihypertensives, also may be offenders. Alcohol is a contributing factor in vasovagal syncope. An emotional response can cause neurally mediated syncope in susceptible individuals in stressful circumstances. Dehydration and orthostatic hypotension may be factors. Situational syncope can occur when the Valsalva maneuver is produced (micturition, defecation, cough, lifting heavy objects, or after meals related to postprandial hypotension).

 Clinical Pearl: Prolonged recumbency can contribute to micturition syncope. Men with prostate enlargement who awaken from a supine sleep and stand to urinate are at highest risk.

Signs and symptoms: Because the patient may not be able to recall the event precisely, gather corroborating history and the patient's witnessed appearance from others. Obtain the patient's description of symptoms preceding the event and of activities that may have precipitated the event. Cardiac-related syncope may be sudden and without warning. A brief prodrome of symptoms, such as nausea, pallor, or diaphoresis, may suggest a vasovagal episode. Determine if any focal neurological symptoms were present (i.e., diplopia, motor and sensory symptoms). Review significant past medical history, all medications being used, and alcohol intake. The history is important in distinguishing actual syncope from dizziness, vertigo, seizure, pseudovertigo, and disequilibrium.

First check the patient for evidence of trauma, then focus the physical examination on the cardiovascular and neurological components. Check blood pressure in both arms and positionally. Determine the compensatory pulse rate. Check the carotids for bruits. Examine the heart, assessing for signs of arrhythmia, vascular disease, and left ventricular dysfunction. Perform a thorough neurological examination, paying particular attention to focal abnormalities that may suggest neurological syncope. Generalized anxiety disorders can cause hyperventilation and trigger a vasodepressor reaction; this should be evaluated during the physical examination. Test the stool for blood.

Diagnostic tests:

Test	Result Indicating Disorder	CPT Code
ECG	Ischemia, rhythm disturbance, QRS pathology, structural heart disease. Common positive findings include bundle-branch block, previous myocardial infarction, left ventricular hypertrophy	93000

Additional cardiac diagnostic studies may include echocardiogram, ambulatory ECG monitoring, and electrophysiological studies. Carotid sinus compression sometimes is used to provoke symptoms, but this should be done cautiously and selectively and is contraindicated in patients with a bruit or a history of stroke. A chest x-ray, which may reveal cardiomyopathy, is indicated in patients with new abnormal findings, patients with dyspnea, and patients without a recorded baseline. Electroencephalogram and CT scan of the head is reserved for patients with focal neurological abnormalities. Tilt-table testing is useful in patients with syncope of unknown etiology or patients with recurrent syncope. Vasovagal syncope may be induced with this procedure; this may be done with or without isoproterenol. Laboratory evaluation is generally of low yield but may include a CBC with differential if infection or anemia is suspected. Renal function studies and electrolytes also may be considered.

Differential diagnosis: Distinguish syncope from seizures, dizziness, and drop attacks. Dizziness does not involve a loss of consciousness and is often characterized further as vertigo, lightheadedness, disequilibrium, or presyncope (sensation of impending loss of consciousness). Drop attacks are sudden drops without warning and may be due to transient basilar artery insufficiency at times precipitated by head movement or neck hyperextension. Metabolic disorders (hypoglycemia, hypoxemia) cause coma/somnolence rather than syncope. When a true syncopal event has been determined, the differential diagnosis is primarily cardiac and noncardiac etiologies (Table 2–6).

 Clinical Pearl: Syncope needs to be distinguished from seizures. During a syncopal event, the patient may have tonic-clonic movements or muscle twitching. The best discriminatory symptom of a seizure is disorientation after the event, with others being urinary incontinence and tongue biting.

Treatment: When you identify the specific cause of syncope, you can initiate the appropriate treatment. This may include β-adrenergic blockade,

Table 2–6   Differential Diagnosis: Syncope in Older Adults

Cardiovascular	Noncardiovascular
Arrhythmias	Hypoxemia
Carotid sinus hypersensitivity	Vasovagal attack
Valvular heart disease	Vagal glossopharyngeal neuralgia
Aortic arch syndrome	Situational syncope (micturition, cough, postprandial defecation)
Orthostatic hypotension	
Transient ischemic attacks	
Aortic dissection	Medications
Myocardial infarction	Psychiatric
Pulmonary embolism	Neurologic (i.e., migranes)

scopolamine, or theophylline for vasovagal syncope. Fludrocortisone, although not tested in randomized clinical trials, is used often in patients with autonomic failure. Antiarrhythmic therapy is initiated, if indicated, and drug-induced or idiopathic orthostatic hypotension is treated appropriately. Cardiac pacing may be appropriate. Cardiac surgery is the treatment of choice for obstructive heart disease. Always correct underlying anemia and metabolic imbalance, and optimize cardiac and pulmonary status in the elderly patient. Address any age-related, disease-related, or disuse-related changes that impair the patient's compensation for hypotensive stressors, such as dehydration, deconditioning, and orthostatic hypotension.

Follow-up: Unknown causes precipitate a high incidence of syncopal events, and in one third of patients syncope is a recurring event. Because recurrences may reflect lack of effective therapy or a failure to diagnose correctly, close monitoring is indicated.

Sequelae: Syncope from cardiovascular causes tends to be more dangerous, having a 1-year mortality of 20% to 30% compared with 5% for noncardiovascular or unknown causes. Sudden death with syncope has been attributed to arrhythmia. Patients with syncope are at risk for fall-related injury (fracture, subdural hematoma) and reduced functional capacity.

Prevention/prophylaxis: Patients with vasovagal syncope are taught to avoid triggers and, if premonitory symptoms occur, to lie down immediately and elevate the feet higher than the chest. Adequate fluid intake is a precaution, and for selected individuals with vasovagal syncope, a higher salt intake may be advised. Support hose may help prevent reduction in central plasma volume. Patients are encouraged to avoid a sudden change in position. For syncope caused by atrial fibrillation, low-dose warfarin or aspirin therapy may be prescribed. Micturition syncope can be avoided by advising men to sit down to urinate.

Referral: Hospitalization is necessary for patients in whom you suspect an arrhythmia or myocardial infarction as the cause of the syncope and for patients who sustain significant injury during the syncopal event. Consultation may be appropriate with a cardiologist for managing cardiac syncope and with a neurologist for managing neurally mediated syncope.

Education: In addition to teaching preventive strategies and the avoidance of triggering events, teach individuals with recurrent syncope safety precautions related to driving or the use of dangerous machinery.

TREMOR

Tremor	ICD-9-CM: 781.0
Essential	ICD-9-CM: 333.1
Familial	ICD-9-CM: 331.1
Flapping	ICD-9-CM: 572.8

Hereditary	ICD-9-CM: 333.1
Hysterical	ICD-9-CM: 300.11
Intention	ICD-9-CM: 333.1
Mercurial	ICD-9-CM: 985.0
Muscle	ICD-9-CM: 728.85
Parkinson's	ICD-9-CM: 332.0
Psychogenic	ICD-9-CM: 306.0
Senile	ICD-9-CM: 797
Specified type	ICD-9-CM: 333.1

Description: Tremor is the most common form of involuntary movement and is characterized by rhythmic oscillation of a body part that can be classified according to the circumstances under which it occurs. Only a small fraction of persons with tremor seek medical attention. Tremors may result from normal (physiological) or pathological processes.

Etiology: Because of the vast number of causes of tremor, etiologic classification is not helpful, whereas classification based on the following features is more useful to the clinician.

- Clinical phenomenology
- Anatomic or topographic distribution
- Activities that activate tremor
- Relative tremor frequency measured in cycles per second
- Medical and drug history and clinical evaluation (i.e., to detect concomitant neurological conditions, drug-induced or toxic tremors)

Terms used to describe the clinical phenomenology of tremor include rest tremors and action tremors. *Rest tremor* occurs when muscle is not activated voluntarily, and the relevant body part is fully supported against gravity, whereas *action tremor* is present with voluntary contraction of muscle. Action tremors can be subclassified further into postural, kinetic, intention, task-specific, and isometric tremor. *Postural tremor* is present while voluntarily maintaining a position against gravity. *Kinetic tremor* may occur during any form of voluntary movement of the affected body part. *Intention or terminal tremor* refers to exacerbation of kinetic tremor toward the end of a goal-directed movement. *Task-specific kinetic tremor* occurs exclusively during the performance of a specific task, such as writing or playing a musical instrument.

Occurrence: Everyone has a low-amplitude physiological tremor that can be observed when the arms are extended. Present in all muscle groups, it persists throughout the waking state. Estimates suggest that 3 to 4 million people in the United States have the most common form of tremor, essential tremor. In 50% of cases, the disease is familial (autosomal dominant, meaning 50% of an affected individual's children have it). The incidence of familial tremor is estimated at 415 in 100,000.

Age: The mean age of onset for familial tremor is 45. Essential tremor begins in young to middle-aged people and gradually intensifies with age. Most studies report a significant age-associated increase in the prevalence of essential tremor. Aging also is associated with a decrease in rate of the tremor and an increase in amplitude.

Ethnicity: Tremor is more prevalent in whites than in blacks and is of intermediate prevalence in Hispanics.

Gender: Tremor afflicts both genders equally, with perhaps slightly more frequency in men than in women.

Contributing factors: During times of stress, the amplitude of a physiological tremor increases. Fatigue, anxiety, hyperthyroidism, systemic illness, use of medications, drug withdrawal (especially from alcohol), use of methylxanthines, and excess caffeine intake can exaggerate tremor.

Signs and symptoms: Careful history taking is the first step in evaluation of tremor.

Clinical Pearl: To distinguish properly between resting and action tremors, patients should be evaluated while supine and when seated with the arms fully supported. (If patients are in a position that does not provide complete support, certain muscles may be active against gravity, producing a tremor that may be classified improperly as a resting tremor.)

Determine the duration and age of onset of symptoms, exacerbating or alleviating factors, and any family history of tremor or other neurological disorders. Include any associated symptoms, such as bradykinesia or rigidity (suggesting Parkinson's disease) or ataxia and nystagmus (suggesting cerebellar disease).

Clinical Pearl: Presence of abrupt tremor onset or concomitant neurological disease may suggest an alternative diagnosis.

The patient's medication history, any exposure to toxins, and the presence of other illnesses should be noted.

Clinical Pearl: Tremor may occur in various body parts, such as the hands, head, facial structures (chin, tongue, lips, and ears), vocal cords, trunk, and legs. Of all tremors, 94% occur in the hands, either unilaterally or bilaterally.

It is important to determine the anatomical distribution, type, and severity of tremor. The effect of ethanol on tremor symptoms may be a helpful assessment finding. Consuming even small quantities of alcohol leads to transient improvement of tremor in many essential tremor patients. Other tremor patients, such as those with Parkinson's disease, only rarely may experience such an alleviation of symptoms.

During a thorough tremor-focused neurological examination:

Muscle tone is checked throughout the body.

Cranial structures (including the mouth and jaw) are examined at rest and in action.

The tongue is observed during rest and protrusion.

The upper extremities are examined in an outstretched position with the hands supine (palms up), prone (palms down), and in the wing position (i.e., with apposition of the index fingers close to each other but not touching).

Goal-directed activities are performed, such as finger-to-nose, heel-to-shin, and toe-to-finger movements. In addition, tests such as measuring the amount of water spilled while pouring water from one cup to another or holding a cup for 1 minute are simple and objectively evaluate the performance of actions involved in ADLs.

The patient is asked to recite a standard paragraph and enunciate a sustained vowel.

Handwriting samples are obtained (e.g., script, numbers, Archimedes spirals).

Gait is evaluated, and Romberg (station) and balance testing are conducted.

Careful evaluation is performed for signs of other neurologic disease, including PD and dystonia.

 Clinical Pearl: Patients with essential tremor typically have handwriting that is shaky and large, whereas the handwriting of patients with Parkinson's disease initially may be of normal size and progressively become smaller (micrographia). Archimedes spirals drawn by essential tremor patients tend to illustrate natural fluctuations in tremor magnitude.

In assessment of the impact of tremor on patients' lives, functional disability in performing ADLs and the patient's subjective assessment of his or her quality of life are useful.

The Movement Disorder Society (MDS) consensus criteria describe several syndromes based on clinical observations of specific tremor elements. Important in the differential diagnosis of tremor, these syndromic classifications are as follows:

Physiological tremor: A normal phenomenon, physiological tremor occurs in all contracting muscle groups. Ranging in frequency from 8 to 12 Hz, it is subtly detectable on electromyography. Although seldom visible to the naked eye, physiological tremor often may be detected when the fingers are firmly outstretched with a piece of paper placed over the hands.

Enhanced physiological tremor or an intensification of physiological tremor to detectable levels: Physiological tremor may be enhanced under conditions of stress, anxiety, fatigue, exercise, cold, hunger, stimulant use, alcohol withdrawal, or metabolic disturbances, such as hypoglycemia or hyperthyroidism. Although the tremor is typically low in amplitude and high in frequency (8–12 Hz), it may be clinically indistinguishable from essential tremor.

Essential tremor (4–12 Hz): Essential tremor is a persistent postural and kinetic tremor that predominately affects the hands

and forearms. Classically, to show the tremor, the patient is asked
to extend the arms in front of the body. The legs are affected less
often. Although less frequently involved, the presence of tremor in
either or both the head and voice is a strong indication of essential
tremor and is especially useful in differentiating the syndrome from
Parkinson's disease. Head tremor, which is also postural,
disappears when the head is supported. Listening to the patient
speak or having the patient hold a musical note as long as possible
may reveal a quivering intonation. A resting component is present
only rarely and typically occurs in the most advanced cases.

Primary orthostatic tremor: Primary orthostatic tremor is a
postural tremor of lower limb, trunk, and, possibly, upper limb
muscles while standing, but tremor is absent when sitting or
reclining. In most patients, orthostatic tremor is suppressed on
walking. This tremor can be evoked by strong contraction of the
leg muscles against resistance. Also, have the patient stand with the
feet together and observe for rapid rhythmic contractions of leg
muscles that cause the kneecaps to bob up and down. On
electromyography, tremor frequency is 13 to 18 Hz.

Dystonic tremor: Although consensus has not been reached
concerning the definition of dystonic tremor syndrome, authors of
the MDS consensus criteria have proposed many definitions within
this general category. *Dystonic tremor* refers to primarily postural
and kinetic tremor occurring in a body part affected by dystonia.
Dystonia is a neurological movement disorder characterized by
sustained muscle contractions that frequently cause repetitive,
twisting, or writhing movements and distorted, sometimes painful,
postures or positions. Dystonic tremor may affect any voluntary
muscle in the body.

Task-specific and position-specific tremors: Tremors occur on
performance of specific, highly specialized motor activities. These
include primary writing tremor, defined as tremor occurring solely
or primarily while writing yet not with other hand activities;
occupational tremors, such as specific tremors affecting athletes or
musicians; or isolated voice tremors. Voice tremor may be
characterized by tremulousness of the voice in the absence of other
tremor manifestations—or by focal dystonia of the vocal cords.

Parkinsonian tremor syndromes (4–6 Hz): Parkinsonian tremor
syndromes involve resting tremor that is often asymmetrical.
Tremor may be observed when muscles are relaxed, such as when
the hands are resting on the lap, and may affect hands, feet,
mandible, and lips. Tremor disappears during sleep. Typical is an
alternating tremor of the thumb against the index finger—*pill-
rolling* tremor. Although rest tremor is a diagnostic criterion for
Parkinson's disease, other forms of tremor also may be present.

Cerebellar tremor syndromes: Cerebellar tremor syndromes are described as pure or primary intention tremors with a frequency predominantly <5 Hz, possibly in association with postural (but not resting) tremor. Other forms of tremor, such as postural tremor, are deemed of cerebellar origin only when coexistent with other cerebellar signs.

Holmes tremor: Traditionally known as *rubral or midbrain tremor,* Holmes tremor is defined as a symptomatic rest, intention, and possibly postural tremor resulting from lesions affecting the cerebellothalamic and dopaminergic systems—such as involving the brainstem, cerebellum, and thalamus and, possibly, their pathways.

Neuropathic tremor syndrome: Certain peripheral neuropathies, particularly dysgammaglobulinemic neuropathies, are commonly associated with tremor, primarily kinetic and postural tremor of the affected extremities.

Drug-induced and toxic tremor syndromes: Pharmacological agents used to treat other medical conditions may induce tremor. These medications include theophylline, valproate, lithium, tricyclic antidepressants, neuroleptics, sympathomimetics, amphetamines, steroids, certain agents used to treat endocrine and metabolic disorders, and other miscellaneous agents. Toxic tremor, such as seen in manganese, arsenic, or mercury intoxication or poisoning, occurs in association with other neurological symptoms, such as gait disturbances, rigidity, dystonia, ataxia, dysarthria, and confusion.

Psychogenic tremor: This form of tremor may be suggested by a history of somatization, the presence of unrelated neurological signs, and sudden tremor onset or remissions. Additional signs may include a decrease of amplitude or variation of frequency on distraction, unusual combinations of postural/intention and rest tremors, and coactivation resembling voluntary cocontraction during passive movements of a trembling limb about a joint.

Diagnostic tests: No specific tests are routinely ordered for tremors. Electromyography is used to subdivide tremors according to their rate and their relationship to posture of limbs and volitional movement. Tremor frequency usually is categorized as low frequency (<4 Hz), medium frequency (4–6 Hz), and high frequency (>6 Hz).

Laboratory testing may be necessary to exclude certain conditions that may be associated with tremor, such as metabolic disturbances, including hyperthyroidism (e.g., through thyroid function tests) and Wilson's disease. Brain imaging may be indicated for select patients, particularly patients with tremor that is unilateral, of sudden onset, or associated with atypical clinical features.

Differential diagnosis: The differential diagnosis, in general practice, is almost always between Parkinson's disease and essential tremor. Many hereditary and idiopathic disorders, metabolic conditions, cerebral diseases, and peripheral neuropathies comprise the differential diagnosis for tremor.

Treatment: First-line treatment for tremor is oral medication. β-Blockers, anticholinergic medication, and levodopa are useful modalities for resting tremor. Kinetic tremor may respond to β-blockers, primidone, anticholinergics, and alcohol. When there is a lack of response to medical treatment or when tremor results in severe disability, a patient may be considered for neurosurgery.

Physiological tremor: Usually no treatment is required for physiological tremor. When exaggerated, however, it may interfere with activities requiring extreme precision. Identifying and removing precipitating causes, such as thyrotoxicosis; hypoglycemia; emotional stress; pheochromocytoma; and use of tricyclic antidepressants, neuroleptics, and lithium, is the treatment. If the precipitating cause cannot be removed, propranolol *may be* effective.

Essential tremor: Varying degrees of control in essential tremor have been obtained with the β-blocker propranolol and the anticonvulsant agent primidone. Either agent may be considered an appropriate first-line therapy for the symptomatic management of essential tremor. When appropriate, these agents may be administered in combination with benzodiazepines, such as lorazepam or clonazepam. If the medication is of no benefit at a dose that causes adverse effects, dose levels should be tapered down gradually and eventually discontinued. If a medication is documented to be beneficial, it may be continued at the regulated doses, and the next medication may be added to the drug regimen. If the response to a drug is adequate and the dose is well tolerated, you may continue to monitor tolerance and possibly increase the dose. Physical and psychological measures may be helpful in managing mild tremor. Physical measures may include the application of weights to affected limbs to decrease tremor amplitude. Some patients have experienced benefits with biofeedback, relaxation methods, and other behavioral techniques through alleviation of anxiety or stress that may exacerbate tremor. As discussed previously, alcohol consumption may lead to transient improvement for many with essential tremor. The potential risk of alcohol dependence and abuse among essential tremor patients who drink alcohol to control symptoms is controversial.

Orthostatic tremor: This tremor rarely responds to β-blocker therapy, but clonazepam or primidone has been shown to be effective.

Dystonic tremor: Pharmacological treatment of dystonic tremor is usually disappointing; however, clonazepam or anticholinergics may be tried. Treatment of the underlying dystonia with botulinum toxin often results in significant improvement of tremor.

Task-specific and position-specific tremor: Propranolol, primidone, and botulinum toxin all have been advocated for treatment.

Parkinsonian tremor: The tremor of Parkinson's disease results from a loss of striatal dopamine, and this is the rationale for treatment with either the dopamine precursor levodopa or dopamine receptor agonists. Dopaminergic and anticholinergic agents are equally effective, but dopaminergic substances additionally improve other parkinsonian signs, and the potential side effects of anticholinergic medications make these drugs undesirable in the elderly. The combination of levodopa and carbidopa reduces levodopa-induced nausea; a typical starting dose is one tablet of Sinemet 25/100 three times daily.

Cerebellar tremor: There is no effective treatment of cerebellar tremor; however, some success has been reported with clonazepam.

Holmes or rubral (midbrain) tremor: This tremor is typically resistant to medical treatment, but occasionally is relieved by levodopa or anticholinergics. Benefit from clonazepam or a combination of propranolol and valproate has been reported.

Neuropathic tremor: Treatment of neuropathy may or may not improve neuropathic tremor. The tremor of hereditary motor-sensory neuropathy often responds to treatment with propranolol and alcohol.

Drug-induced and toxic tremors: Treatment of tremors induced by drugs or toxins should focus on identification and elimination of the offending agent.

Psychogenic tremor: Psychogenic tremor often carries a poor prognosis. Consultation with a mental health professional is indicated.

Follow-up: Patients should be evaluated for therapeutic effects and side effects within 1 week of starting treatment. Annual monitoring for weight loss, depression, and decline in functional status are necessary.

Sequelae: Functional disabilities may occur in ADLs, including compromised eating, drinking, and preparing food. Decreased caloric intake and weight loss may be observed. Ambulation, especially on stairs, may be hazardous. Withdrawal from social situations may occur, and depression is common.

Clinical Pearl: Of patients with essential tremor, 25% retire or change jobs as a result of tremor.

Prevention/prophylaxis: Reduce factors that can exacerbate the tremor. Continue medication regimen.

Referral: A neurologist should be consulted for cerebellar tremors, mixed tremors, or parkinsonian tremor or when a focal neurological deficit is identified. An ophthalmologist should be consulted when Wilson's disease is suspected. A mental health provider or psychiatrist should be consulted when a hysterical tremor is suspected. Physical therapy or occupational therapy may be helpful in advanced or disabling cases.

Education: Some patients, particularly patients with severe, disabling tremor, may limit their contact to only people with whom they are extremely close, such as immediate family members. Patients must be encouraged to learn as much as they can about their disease to help them cope better with the condition's progression. When a diagnosis has been established, the natural history of the condition should be explained to patients. Because many patients fear that their tremor may be associated with Parkinson's disease, clinicians may reassure their patients by explaining the distinction between the two. It also may be appropriate to recommend counseling. Use of appropriate coping strategies may reduce stress substantially, preventing possible augmentation of tremor owing to anxiety. Referral to appropriate patient-support organizations is helpful for most patients. These organizations provide detailed educational materials and access to local or regional support systems. The International Tremor Foundation and WE MOVE (Worldwide Education and Awareness for Movement Disorders) are international nonprofit organizations that may assist patients.

URINARY INCONTINENCE

Urinary incontinence	ICD-9-CM: 788.30
Hysterical	ICD-9-CM: 300.11
Mixed (urge and stress)	ICD-9-CM: 788.33
Overflow	ICD-9-CM: 788.39
Paradoxical	ICD-9-CM: 788.39
Stress, female	ICD-9-CM: 625.6
Stress, male	ICD-9-CM: 788.32
Urethral sphincter	ICD-9-CM: 599.84
Urge	ICD-9-CM: 788.31
Male (stress and urge)	ICD-9-CM: 788.33
Neurogenic	ICD-9-CM: 788.39
Nonorganic origin	ICD-9-CM: 307.6

Description: Urinary incontinence is the involuntary loss of urine sufficient to be a problem. Types of incontinence include transient and persistent. Acute urinary incontinence usually is of sudden onset and is related to an illness, treatment, or medication. When the illness resolves or the identified cause is addressed, this condition usually resolves.

Persistent urinary incontinence includes disorders of storage (stress and urge), disorder of emptying (overflow), and functional and mixed incontinence.

Urge incontinence: Now often called *overactive bladder,* urge incontinence is the involuntary loss of urine in association with a strong sensation of urinary urgency. The pressure in the bladder (detrusor) exceeds the pressure in the urethra. This results from detrusor instability, hyperreflexia, or uninhibited bladder contractions usually caused by lower urinary tract irritation or a neurological problem.

Stress incontinence: This is the involuntary loss of usually small amounts of urine that occurs when intra-abdominal pressure is increased by coughing or sneezing and the pelvic floor and urethral muscles are weak. Resulting from a decrease in the tone of internal and external sphincters, stress incontinence usually occurs in women, but men may experience it secondary to sphincter damage.

Mixed incontinence: Mixed incontinence, a combination of stress and urge incontinence, is especially common in elderly women.

Overflow incontinence: This is characterized by involuntary loss of frequent or constant dribbling and a failure to empty the bladder completely, resulting in overdistention.

Functional incontinence: This is characterized by an inability to get to the toilet on time as a result of chronic cognitive or physical impairments, environmental or physical barriers, or the lack of needed caregiving assistance.

Etiology: Urinary incontinence can be caused by several factors affecting the anatomy or physiology of the lower urinary tract or both or by other factors, including changes in cognition and mobility.

Occurrence: Approximately 25 million people in the United States have urinary incontinence.

Age: In the community-dwelling older population, the prevalence of urinary incontinence is about 30%, and at least 50% of nursing home residents leak urine.

Clinical Pearl: The economic costs of urinary incontinence are significant. A study done at two New Jersey nursing homes showed an additional cost of $17.21/day or >$6000/year. Extrapolated to the United States as a whole for community care and nursing home care, the cost would be >$16 billion in annual direct costs.

Ethnicity: Not significant.

Gender: Urinary incontinence is twice as prevalent in women as in men; however, overflow incontinence is more prevalent in men.

Contributing factors: The many contributing factors for urinary incontinence include pelvic muscle weakness, multiparity, estrogen depletion

Table 2–7 Drug Classifications That Contribute to Urinary Incontinence

Diuretics	Caffeine
Anticholinergic agents	Psychotropics
Tricyclic antidepressants	Phenothiazines
Antispasmodics	Antiparkinsonian agents
Narcotic analgesics	Sedative/hypnotics
CNS depressants, including alcohol	Angiotensin-converting enzyme inhibitors
β-Agonists	
α-Adrenergic agents, including antihistamines, sympathomimetics, sympatholytics	
Calcium channel blockers	

CNS, central nervous system.

(menopause), diabetes, stroke, multiple sclerosis, spinal cord injury, benign prostatic hypertrophy, urinary tract infection, fecal impaction, poor fluid intake, excessive fluid intake, smoking, cognitive impairment, immobility or impaired mobility, environmental barriers, and high-impact physical activities. The side effects of many medications also can contribute to urinary incontinence (Table 2–7).

Signs and symptoms: Because urinary incontinence is not life-threatening and may be a source of embarrassment, the patient may not seek evaluation and treatment unless the health-care provider broaches the question. Asking "Do you ever have difficulty getting to the bathroom in time?" or "Do you ever have a problem with leaking urine when you cough, sneeze, or laugh?" may yield more results than asking directly about incontinence. Other helpful questions include:

How frequently do you get up at night to use the bathroom?

Do you have any problems with constipation?

Do you visit the bathroom frequently during the day?

Do you feel like you are not emptying your bladder completely?

Do you wear a pad to prevent wetness?

Urge incontinence manifests as a sudden, strong urge to void, as a loss of urine on the way to the bathroom, or as a loss of urine without any symptoms. The history with stress incontinence includes leakage of small amounts of urine with a cough, sneeze, laugh, or other physical exertion; in some cases, urine is lost with postural changes. Mixed incontinence presents with a blend of urge and stress symptoms, with one troubling the patient more than the other. Patients with overflow incontinence may report several symptoms, including urgency, frequency, dribbling, or urge or stress incontinence symptoms; men often talk about hesitancy or slow stream.

Functional incontinence may present as urgency, or the functional limitations may be obvious, such as in patients with arthritis, Parkinson's disease, or post–cerebrovascular accident residual. Patients with cognitive impairment or depression may not have the ability to describe their symptoms; the history of the problem in these patients may come from a family member or caregiver.

Patients with unconscious or reflex incontinence may experience postvoiding or continual incontinence; some may have urgency and bladder irritability. A history of the problem should include onset, duration, aggravating and relieving factors, associated symptoms, and current self-management. Obtain a thorough drug history, including use of prescribed and OTC medications, herbal remedies, homeopathics, caffeine, and alcohol. A surgical history, including gynecological, colorectal, urological, and neurosurgical procedures, should be explored. Ask about a past history of urethral structure with dilation. A history of any concurrent chronic diseases, such as diabetes mellitus, multiple sclerosis, stroke, spinal stenosis, parkinsonism, congestive heart failure, hypertension, or cancer (particularly with past radiation therapy), is essential. Note if the patient has been hospitalized recently or had an indwelling catheter. Investigation of nutritional status and fluid intake, as well as recent changes in functional status, is also helpful.

The mnemonics *DRIP* and *DIAPERS* (see under Differential Diagnosis) may help you differentiate between transient and persistent incontinence. Having the patient keep a bladder diary, including voiding patterns, frequency, amount, episodes of incontinence, activity, and fluid intake, is also helpful in differentiating symptoms. A visit to the patient's residence helps to assess for environmental barriers to continence.

Physical examination should include functional assessment, with special attention to mobility, to the person's ability to remove necessary clothing in time to use the toilet, and to toileting hygiene. Vital signs should be completed looking for the presence of fever. Mental status, including cognition and evidence of depression, should be assessed. The abdomen should be examined for clues such as bladder distention, pelvic masses, or tenderness in the suprapubic region. Distention can be found in overflow incontinence secondary to some type of obstruction. A malignancy, benign myoma, or prolapse in the pelvic region creates pressure on the bladder seen in urge, stress, or mixed incontinence. A vaginal examination may reveal poor perineal hygiene, skin breakdown from urine soaking, or redness and thinning of tissue typical of atrophic changes. Prolapse of genitourinary structures or rectum may be seen. To assess for pelvic floor muscle strength and relaxation, instruct the patient to bear down as though having a bowel movement, then tighten or squeeze by pulling up on pelvic floor muscles; in patients with pelvic floor relaxation, you can see the inability to contract or weak contractions. Have the patient cough and determine if leakage occurs. Positive neurological findings in the perineal area include hypersensation, hyposensation, or absence of the bulbocavernosus (anal wink) reflex. A rectal examination may uncover fecal impaction, rectal prolapse, hemorrhoids, masses, or, in men, prostatic enlargement. Whenever possible, the examiner should observe the patient voiding, having the patient void into a measurable receptacle. This should be followed by evaluation of a postvoiding residual (PVR). Studies are inconclusive with respect to the amount of PVR that is significant, with values ranging from >50 mL to >200 mL. Use of a bladder scanner (ultrasound) allows the clinician to obtain estimates noninvasively.

Diagnostic tests:

Test	Results Indicating Disorder	CPT Code
Urinalysis	Leukocytes or nitrates suggest infection Blood suggests infection or obstruction Protein in the urine suggests a problem with renal filtration	81002

These findings necessitate other studies to determine the source of the problem. For suspected infections, a urine culture and sensitivity is indicated to identify the causative organism and the appropriate antibiotic treatment. If renal problems are likely, a creatinine clearance test yields further information. If diabetes is a consideration, order a fasting glucose test. Further diagnostic studies are considered individually in patients who are unsuitable for presumptive diagnosis and treatment, who do not respond to trial management after the basic evaluation, who have comorbid conditions, or who are candidates for surgical intervention. Specialized testing includes urodynamic testing, ultrasound, and cystoscopic procedures designed to identify the cause of urinary incontinence.

Differential diagnosis: Urinary incontinence is a symptom, not a diagnosis. The two mneumonics *DRIP* and *DIAPERS* often are used to differentiate transient (acute) from persistent urinary incontinence.

DRIP:

Delirium
Restricted mobility
Infection
Pharmaceuticals, polyuria

DIAPERS:

Delirium
Infection, impaction, inflammation
Atrophic vaginitis
Psychological, pharmaceuticals, psychotropics
Endocrine problem
Restricted mobility
Stool impaction

Treatment: The treatment depends on the cause of the incontinence. The first step in the treatment is to define the management goals. These goals may include managing comorbidities, decreasing or eliminating all episodes, improving ADLs and quality of life, and preventing complications. For transient urinary incontinence, treating, eliminating, or modifying the cause usually alleviates the symptom. Guidelines from the Agency for Health Care Policy and Research (AHCPR) address this area comprehensively. For persistent incontinence, treatment is categorized as behavioral, pharmacological, environmental, containment, or surgical. AHCPR guidelines advise going from the least invasive treatment to the most invasive treatment. Frequently used behavioral interventions include pelvic muscle exercises or Kegel exercises, performed alone or in combination with biofeedback, to help strengthen periurethral muscles, and toileting programs such as timed voiding, prompted voiding, and bladder training. The degree of independent participation by the patient in these programs depends on cognition and mobility. Electrical stimulation using intravaginal or intra-anal electrodes to inhibit bladder instability and improve sphincter and levator ani contractility is also useful as an adjunct therapy. If nocturia is a problem, limiting fluids before bedtime is helpful. Physical devices such as a pessary may be indicated for women with organ prolapse for whom surgery is not recommended or desired. Requirements for pessary use include intact cognition, manual dexterity, and the ability to follow instructions.

Always approach pharmacological therapy cautiously in older patients. Consider comorbidities and potential interactions with other prescribed medications before deciding on an agent. Treat stress or mixed incontinence associated with atrophic vaginitis with estrogen preparations, applied topically or taken orally. Various estrogen preparations are available, with new developments constantly in progress. Topical estrogen preparations are preferred because of the decreased incidence of side effects. A 2-g amount of vaginal estrogen cream contains 1.25 mg of conjugated estrogens per applicatorful. Dosage is one applicator daily, which may be reduced in frequency or given in a 3-weeks-on, 1-week-off regimen. Oral estrogen dosage is 0.3 to 0.625 mg daily. Progesterone must be given to women with an intact uterus, to prevent endometrial hyperplasia and malignancy; medroxyprogesterone, 2.5 mg daily continuously or intermittently, may be prescribed.

Estrogen is contraindicated in patients with suspected or confirmed uterine or breast cancer, undiagnosed vaginal bleeding, or a history of thrombophlebitis. Patients receiving estrogen therapy should have annual Pap tests and mammograms.

Phenylpropanolamine and pseudoephedrine are sympathomimetic drugs with α-adrenergic agonist properties; these drugs are thought to increase bladder outlet resistance, which is desirable in stress incontinence. The dosage of phenylpropanolamine is 25 to 100 mg orally twice daily in a sustained-release form. Pseudoephedrine dosage is 15 to 30 mg orally three times daily. This class of medications has many significant side effects, including tachycardia, elevated blood pressure, anxiety, insomnia, agitation, cardiac arrhythmia, sweating, and respiratory difficulty, and should not be used by patients with cardiac problems, hypertension, or any type of obstructive syndromes. Imipramine, discussed farther on, can be used as a second-line agent for stress incontinence when other drugs are ineffective.

Urge incontinence and detrusor hyperreflexia have been treated successfully with pharmacological therapy. Anticholinergic agents and tricyclic antidepressants (with anticholinergic properties) are the agents of choice. These drugs are contraindicated in patients with glaucoma or prostatic hypertrophy. Tricyclics, which cannot be taken concomitantly with monoamine oxidase inhibitors, should be used selectively in patients with heart disease. Common side effects include dry mouth, blurred vision, constipation, dry skin, confusion, and postural hypotension. Oxybutynin (Ditropan), 2.5 mg orally twice daily, which is recommended for older patients, has an antispasmodic effect on bladder smooth muscle, delaying the urge to void. Tolterodine (Detrol) is another potential drug to use. Propantheline (Pro-Banthine) is also used, in dosages of 7.5 to 30 mg orally three times daily, but it has an undesirable side-effect profile; monitor PVR to prevent urine retention. Flavoxate (Urispas), 100 to 200 mg three times daily, and dicyclomine (Bentyl), 10 to 20 mg three times daily, are other anticholinergic choices.

Imipramine (Tofranil), 10 to 25 mg orally taken one to three times daily, is the prototype tricyclic; it exerts a twofold action, decreasing bladder contractions and increasing outflow resistance. Doxepin, desipramine, or nortriptyline also can be used.

For overflow incontinence unrelated to obstructive uropathy (e.g., atonic bladder), bethanechol (Urecholine), 10 to 30 mg orally three times daily, can be prescribed. Its cholinergic effects include stimulation of the detrusor muscle. Because this drug has a high profile of undesirable side effects and is contraindicated in patients with asthma, Parkinson's disease, peptic ulcer, hypertension, cardiac disease, hyperthyroidism, or epilepsy, it is of limited usefulness in older patients.

For patients with overflow incontinence secondary to prostatic hypertrophy, surgery was previously the only available option. Now several drugs are being used, however, in selected patients. Urological consultation and workup is advised before prescribing these medications. Finasteride (Proscar), 5 mg orally daily, inhibits the enzyme that converts testosterone into its active form; this results in a regression of prostate tissue. Not all patients show an increase in urine outflow; some patients must take this drug for 6 to 12 months to determine its effectiveness. Use finasteride cautiously in patients with impaired liver function. Side effects include decreased libido and impotence. Measure prostate size and monitor for reduction through digital rectal examinations. Patients also should be monitored for changes in urine output and PVR volume, indicative of obstructive uropathy. The drug should not be prescribed to sexually active patients with partners of childbearing age because of potentially harmful effects on the male fetus; for this reason, also, it should not be crushed and handled by pregnant women or by women capable of becoming pregnant. Other drugs currently being used for treatment of prostatic hypertrophy include α_1-adrenergic blockers terazosin (Hytrin), prazosin (Minipress), and doxazosin (Cardura), antihypertensive agents that also relax the smooth muscle of the prostate and bladder neck, alleviating pressure on the urethra. Dosages for each of these are individualized, starting with 1 mg orally daily for terazosin and 1 mg orally twice daily for prazosin. Because older patients are sensitive to the hypotensive effects of these drugs, monitor carefully for safety and adverse events. Although not an approved usage, many older men use saw palmetto, an herbal product, for reduction of prostatic enlargement.

Other treatments for urinary incontinence include surgical interventions for stress incontinence in women or prostatic hypertrophy in men. Nonsurgical management of persistent urinary incontinence includes intermittent catheterization, use of pelvic organ support devices such as pessaries in women, physical and environmental modifications to improve access to the toilet, and use of absorptive products.

Follow-up: To evaluate the efficacy of the prescribed treatment, schedule follow-up visits biweekly initially and on an individualized basis thereafter. Patients following pelvic muscle exercise routines may need extra support to establish and maintain the program.

Patients taking replacement estrogen should have annual Pap smears. Medication therapy should be monitored for effectiveness, side effects, and drug interactions. Behavioral therapy requires patient or caregiver support and reinforcement to establish a desired habit or pattern.

Sequelae: Possible complications include urinary tract infection, hydronephrosis (with overflow or obstruction), renal failure secondary to hydronephrosis, adverse drug events, or failure of behavioral therapy. Skin breakdown is a significant complication with persistent urinary incontinence. Urosepsis can occur with unrecognized urinary tract infections. Falls can occur after episodes of urinary incontinence, particularly with individuals in a group residence or living alone.

Prevention/prophylaxis: Ways to help prevent incontinence include:

- Early identification and remediation of causes of acute or transient urinary incontinence
- Routine instruction of women in Kegel exercises after childbirth and in the early postmenopausal stage
- Teaching patient and family that urinary incontinence is not a normal aging change and is treatable
- Regular gynecological examinations for women to detect pelvic pathology

- Regular rectal examination in men to detect and treat early prostatic hypertrophy
- Careful attention to prescribing only essential drugs in the older population

Referral: Refer men with overflow incontinence for urological evaluation. If management is conservative (i.e., prescribing medications), it can be collaborative. If you have not studied the use of biofeedback or electrical stimulation, refer the patient to a knowledgeable nurse practitioner or to a health-care continence specialty group. In many long-term care facilities, consultations with and patient referrals to specialty groups for evaluation and management suggestions are routine. Refer for further evaluation patients with an uncertain diagnosis, patients for whom you are unable to develop a management plan from the basic diagnostic evaluation, and patients with a lack of correlation between symptoms and clinical findings. Refer patients for whom surgical intervention is considered, patients with hematuria without infection, patients who fail a therapeutic trial and desire further intervention, and patients with other comorbidities, including:

- History of prior surgery for incontinence or radical pelvic surgery
- Suspicion of prostate cancer
- Abnormal PVR urine
- Neurological condition, such as multiple sclerosis, spinal cord injury, or spinal cord lesions
- Persistent symptoms of difficulty emptying bladder
- Incontinence in conjunction with recurrent symptomatic urinary tract infections.

Education: Teach patients, family, caregivers, health-care providers, and the public that urinary incontinence is *not* a normal consequence of aging and *is* treatable. Teach the patient, family, and caregivers behavioral therapy techniques. Teach Kegel exercises, pessary use (when necessary), intermittent catheterization, medication actions, and medication side effects. Teach patients how to use a bladder record or incontinence monitoring record. Teach signs and symptoms of urinary tract infection, the role of diet in the prevention of constipation, avoidance of irritant and diuretic beverages, and good perineal hygiene to avoid infection. Patients should be instructed to avoid bladder irritation by keeping urine dilute; limiting caffeine and alcohol; and limiting citrus, spicy foods, and artificial sweeteners if these are contributors.

REFERENCES

Bowel Incontinence

Beers, MH, and Berkow, R (eds): The Merck Manual of Geriatrics, ed 3. Merck Research Laboratories, Whitehouse Station, NJ, 2000.

DeLillo, AR, and Rose, S: Functional bowel disorders in the geriatric patient:

Constipation, fecal impaction, and fecal incontinence. Am J Gastroenterol 95:901, 2000.

Ebersole, P, and Hess, P: Toward Healthy Aging, ed 5. Mosby, St. Louis, 1998.

Ham, RJ, et al: Primary Care Geriatrics, ed 4. Mosby, St. Louis, 2001.

Lueckenotte, AG: Gerontologic Nursing, ed 2. Mosby, St. Louis, 2000.

Matteson, MA, et al: Gerontologic Nursing, ed 2. WB Saunders, Philadelphia, 1997.

Romero, Y, et al: Constipation and fecal incontinence in the elderly population. Mayo Clin Proc 71:81, 1996.

Schiller, LR: Constipation and fecal incontinence in the elderly. Gastroenterol Clin N Am 30:497, 2001.

Schrock, TR: Fecal incontinence. In Lonergan, ET (ed): Geriatrics. Appleton & Lange, Stamford, 1996.

Chest Pain

Aisenberg, J, and Castell, D: Approach to the patient with unexplained chest pain. Mt Sinai J Med 61:481, 1994.

Bittner, V, and Clark, D: Chest pain of unknown origin: The differential diagnosis. Hosp Med 31:12, 1995.

Bittner, V, and Clark, D: Chest pain of unknown origin: Initial evaluation and management. Hosp Med 31:30, 1995.

Jones, ID, and Slovis, CM: Emergency department evaluation of the chest pain patient. Emerg Med Clin N Am 192:269, 2001.

Sams, R: Chest pain: Eight steps to definitive diagnosis. Adv Nurse Practitioners December:22, 2001.

Confusion

Chan, D, and Brennan, NJ: Delirium: Making the diagnosis, improving the prognosis. Geriatrics 54:28, 1999.

Foreman, MD, et al: Delirium in elderly patients: An overview of the state of the science. J Gerontol Nurs 27:12, 2001.

Inouye, SK: Prevention of delirium in hospitalized older patients: Risk factors and targeted intervention strategies. Ann Med 32:257, 2000.

Inouye, SK: Delirium in the hospitalized older patients. Clin Geriatr Med 14:475, 1998.

Inouye, SK, et al: Delirium: A symptom of how hospital care is failing older persons and a window to improve quality of hospital care. Am J Med 106:565, 1999.

Webster, JR, et al: Improving clinical and cost outcomes in delirium: Use of practice guidelines and a delirium care team. Ann Long-Term Care 7:128, 1999.

Winawe, N: Postoperative delirium. Med Clin North Am 85:1229, 2001.

Constipation

DeLillo, AR, and Rose, S: Functional bowel disorders in the geriatric patient: Constipation, fecal impaction, and fecal incontinence. J Am Coll Gastroenterol 95:901, 2000.

Romero, Y, et al: Constipation and fecal incontinence in the elderly population. Mayo Clin Proc 71:81, 1996.

Shiller, LR: Constipation and fecal incontinence in the elderly. Gastroenterol Clin N Am 30:497, 2001.

The Joanna Briggs Institute for Evidenced Based Nursing and Midwifery: Management of constipation in older adults. Best Practice 3:1, 1999. Contact:

http://www.joannabriggs.edu.au/bpconstip.pdf. Accessed December 18, 2002.

Cough

Ferri, FF, and Fretwell, MD: Practical Guide to the Care of the Geriatric Patient, ed 2. Mosby, St. Louis, 1997.

Healey, PJ, and Jacobson, EJ: Common Medical Diagnoses: An Algorithmic Approach, ed 3. WB Saunders, Philadelphia, 2000.

McCance, KL, and Huether, SE: Pathophysiology: The Biologic Basis for Disease in Adults and Children, ed 4. Mosby, St. Louis, 2000.

Seller, RH: Differential Diagnosis of Common Complaints, ed 4. WB Saunders, Philadelphia, 2000.

Dehydration

Bennett, J: Dehydration: Hazards and benefits. Geriatr Nurs 21:84, 2000.

The Joanna Briggs Institute for Evidenced Based Nursing and Midwifery: Maintaining oral hydration in older people. Best Practice 5:1, 2001. Contact: http://www.joannabriggs.edu.au/BPISHyd.pdf. Accessed December 18, 2002.

Yen, P: (2000) Focus on fluids. Geriatr Nurs 21:222, 2000.

Diarrhea

Chernecky, CC, and Bergey, BJ: Laboratory Tests and Diagnostic Procedures, ed 3. WB Saunders, Philadelphia, 2001.

Cole, MC: Chronic and acute diarrhea. In Rakel, RE (ed): Saunders Manual of Medical Practice, ed. 2. WB Saunders, Philadelphia, 2000.

Holt, PR: Diarrhea and malabsorption in the elderly. Gastroenterol Clin N Am 30:427, 2001.

LaForce, FM: Infections. In Jahnigen, DW, and Schrier, RW (eds): Geriatric Medicine, ed 2. Blackwell Scientific, Cambridge, MA, 1997.

Seller, RH: Differential Diagnosis of Common Complaints, ed 4. WB Saunders, Philadelphia, 2000.

Dizziness

Adelman, AM, and Daly, MP: 20 Common Problems in Geriatrics. McGraw-Hill, New York, 2001.

Beers, MH, and Berkow, R (eds): The Merck Manual of Geriatrics, ed 3. Merck Research Laboratories, Whitehouse Station, NJ, 2000.

Bickley, L: Bates' Guide to Physical Examination and History Taking, ed 8. Lippincott Williams & Wilkins, Philadelphia, 2002.

Ham, RJ, et al: Primary Care Geriatrics, ed 4. Mosby, St. Louis, 2001.

Hill-O'Neill, KA, and Shaughnessy, M: Dizziness and stroke. In Cotter VT, and Strumpf, NE (eds): Advanced Practice Nursing with Older Adults: Clinical Guidelines. McGraw-Hill, New York, 2002.

Jonsson, PV, and Lipsitz, LA: Dizziness and syncope. In Hazzard, WR, et al (eds): Principles of Geriatric Medicine and Gerontology, ed 4. McGraw-Hill, New York, 1998.

Kane, RL, et al: Essentials of Clinical Geriatrics, ed 4. McGraw-Hill, New York, 1999.

Seller, RH: Differential Diagnosis of Common Complaints, ed 4. WB Saunders, Philadelphia, 2000.

Dysphagia

Bickley, L: Bates' Guide to Physical Examination and History Taking, ed 8. Lippincott Williams & Wilkins, Philadelphia, 2002.

Domenech, E, and Kelly, J: Swallowing disorders. Med Clin North Am 83:97, 1999.

Firth, M, and Prather, CM: Gastrointestinal motility problems in the elderly patient. Gastroenterology 122:1688, 2002.

Gustafsson, B, and Tibbling, L: Dysphagia, an unrecognized handicap. Dysphagia 6:193, 1991.

Schindler, J, and Kelley, J: Swallowing disorders in the elderly. Laryngoscope 112:589, 2002.

Shaker, R, and Staff, D: Esophageal disorders in the elderly. Gastroenterol Clin N Am 30:355, 2001.

Fatigue

Beers, MH, and Berkow, R (eds): The Merck Manual of Geriatrics, ed 3. Merck Research Laboratories, Whitehouse Station, NJ, 2000.

Bickley, L: Bates' Guide to Physical Examination and History Taking, ed 8. Lippincott Williams & Wilkins, Philadelphia, 2002.

Rodriguez, T: The challenge of evaluating fatigue. J Am Acad Nurse Practitioners 12:329, 2000.

Valdres, RU, et al: Fatigue: A debilitating symptom. Nurs Clin North Am 36:685, 2001.

Headache

Dambro, M: Griffith's 5 Minute Clinical Consult 2002. Lippincott Williams & Wilkins, Philadelphia, 2002.

Evans, RW: Diagnostic testing for headache. Med Clin North Am 85:865, 2001.

Peroutka, SJ: Drugs effective in the therapy of migraine. In: Goodman and Gilman's the Pharmacological Basis of Therapeutics, ed 10. McGraw-Hill, New York, 2001.

Purdy, RA: Clinical evaluation of the patient presenting with headache. Med Clin North Am 85:847, 2001.

Rankin, LM, and Bruhl, M: Migraine in older patients: A case report and management strategies. Geriatrics 55:70, 2000.

Seller, RH: Differential Diagnosis of Common Complaints, ed 4. WB Saunders, Philadelphia, 2000.

Silberstein, SD, et al: Wolff's Headache and Other Head Pain, ed 7. Oxford University Press, New York, 2001.

Yoshikawa, TT, et al: Ambulatory Geriatric Care, ed 2. Mosby, St. Louis, 1998.

Hemoptysis

Ferri, FF, and Fretwell, MD: Practical Guide to the Care of the Geriatric Patient, ed 2. Mosby, St. Louis, 1997.

Healey, PJ, and Jacobson, EJ: Common Medical Diagnoses: An Algorithmic Approach, ed 2. WB Saunders, Philadelphia, 1994.

McCance, KL, and Huether, SE: Pathophysiology: The Biologic Basis for Disease in Adults and Children, ed 4. Mosby, St. Louis, 2000.

Seller, RH: Differential Diagnosis of Common Complaints, ed 3. WB Saunders, Philadelphia, 1996.

Involuntary Weight Loss

Kamel, HK, et al: Nutritional deficiencies in long term care: Part 2. Management of protein energy malnutrition and dehydration. Ann Long-Term Care 6:250, 1998.

Mansouri, A, et al: Pinpointing the causes of unexplained weight loss. Patient Care 28:46, 1994.

Marton, KI, et al: Involuntary weight loss: Diagnostic and prognostic significance. Ann Intern Med 95:568, 1981.

Morley, JE, et al: Nutritional deficiencies in long term care: Part 1. Detection and diagnosis. Ann Long-Term Care 6(suppl E):1, 1998.

Robbins, LJ: Evaluation of weight loss in the elderly. Geriatrics 44:31, 1984.

Uphold, CR, and Graham, MV: Weight Loss: Clinical Guidelines in Adult Health. Barmarrae Books, Gainesville, FL, 1993.

Joint Pain

Abrams, WB, et al (eds): Merck Manual of Diagnosis and Therapy, ed 17. Merck & Co, Rahway, NJ, 1997.

Barker, LR, et al: Principles of Ambulatory Medicine, ed 3. Williams & Wilkins, Baltimore, 1991.

Bates, B: A Guide to Physical Examination and History Taking, ed 5. JB Lippincott, Philadelphia, 1991.

Berg, D: Handbook of Primary Care Medicine. JB Lippincott, Philadelphia, 1993.

Doenges, ME, et al: Nursing Care Plans: Guidelines for Individualizing Patient Care, ed 4. FA Davis, Philadelphia, 1997.

Fischbach, F: A Manual of Laboratory Diagnostic Tests, ed 2. JB Lippincott, Philadelphia, 1984.

McCarberg, BH, and Herr, KA: Osteoarthritis: How to manage pain and improve patient function. Geriatrics 56:14, 2001.

Schwartz, M: Textbook of Physical Diagnosis, ed 2. WB Saunders, Philadelphia, 1994.

Nausea and Vomiting

Geriatric Review Syllabus: A Core Curriculum in Geriatric Medicine, ed 5. Blackwell Publishing, Boston, 2002.

Ham, RJ, and Sloane, PD: Primary Care Geriatrics: A Case-Based Approach, ed 3. Mosby, St. Louis, 1997.

Quigley, E, et al: AGA technical review on nausea and vomiting. Gastroenterology 120:263, 2001.

Peripheral Edema

Ciocon, J, et al: Leg edema: Clinical clues to the differential diagnosis. Geriatrics 48:34, 1993.

Ciocon, J, et al: Raised leg exercises for leg edema in the elderly. Angiology 46:19, 1995.

Galindo-Ciocon, D: Nursing care of elders with leg edema. J Gerontol Nurs 22:7, 1995.

Merli, G, and Spandorfer, J: The outpatient with unilateral leg swelling. Med Clin North Am 79:435, 1995.

Powell, AA, and Armstrong, MA: Peripheral edema. Am Fam Physician 55:1721, 1997.

Seller, RH: Differential Diagnosis of Common Complaints, ed 4. WB Saunders, Philadelphia, 2000.

Yale, SH, and Mazza, JJ: Approach to diagnosing lower extremity edema. Comp Ther 27:242, 2001.

Syncope

Hayes, O: The evaluation of syncope in the emergency department. Emerg Med Clin N Am 16:601, 1998.

Henderson, MC, and Prabhu, SD: Syncope: Current diagnosis and treatment. Curr Probl Cardiol 22(5):242, 1997.

Tremor

Barker, RB, et al: Principles of Ambulatory Medicine, ed. 6. Baltimore: Lippincott Williams & Wilkins, Baltimore, 2002.

Cooper, G, and Rodnitzky, R: The many forms of tremor: precise classification guides selection of therapy. Postgrad Med 108:57, 2000.

Evidente, VG: Understanding essential tremor: differential diagnosis and options for treatment. Postgrad Med 108:138, 2000.

Habib-ur-Rehman: Diagnosis and management of tremor. Arch Intern Med 160:2438, 2000.

International Essential Tremor Foundation. Contact: http://www.essential-tremor.org.

Movement Disorder Society. Contact: http://www.wemove.org.

Urinary Incontinence

ACOG Technical Bulletin #213: Urinary Incontinence. October 1995.

Agency for Health Care Policy and Research: Clinical Practice Guidelines: Overview: Urinary Incontinence in Adults, Clinical Practice Guideline Update. 1996. Contact: http://www.ahcpr.gov/news/press/overview.htm.

Chernecky, CC, and Bergey, BJ: Laboratory Tests and Diagnostic Procedures, ed 3. WB Saunders, Philadelphia, 2001.

Dambro, M: Griffith's 5 Minute Clinical Consult 2002. Lippincott Williams & Wilkins, Philadelphia, 2002.

U.S. Department of Health and Human Services, Public Health Service, Agency for Health Care Policy and Research: Clinical Practice Guideline Number 2: 1999 Update: Urinary Incontinence in Adults: Acute and Chronic Management. AHCPR Pub. No. 96-0682, Rockville, MD, 1999. Contact: http://www.nih.gov/ninr/research/vol3/Urinary.html.

Yoshikawa, TT, et al: Practical Ambulatory Geriatrics, ed 2. Mosby, St. Louis, 1998.

Chapter 3
SKIN

BURNS

SIGNAL SYMPTOMS ▶ erythema, swelling

| Burns | ICD-9-CM: 942–949 by region |

Description: Burns are injuries to tissues caused by thermal, chemical, or electrical contact. They may be classified by severity of injury to the total body surface area (TBSA), as follows:

- Small (<15% TBSA)
- Moderate (15–49% TBSA)
- Large (50–69% TBSA)
- Massive (≥70% TBSA)

The classification of burns is now designated as superficial, superficial partial thickness, deep partial thickness, and full thickness. A *superficial burn* can be caused by ultraviolet light or brief exposure to a flame. On examination, the area appears to be dry and red, yet blanches when pressure is applied. Although the area burned is painful, no scarring occurs. A *superficial partial-thickness burn* results from a scald or flame exposure. After the contact, the skin blisters, the color of the skin varies in tone, and the skin blanches with pressure to the area. The duration of pain from this type of burn may last a couple of weeks. The healed skin may have some pigmentary changes. A *deep partial-thickness burn* may result from exposure to flame, a scald, exposure to hot oil, or exposure to grease. The skin blisters but does not blanch with pressure. Patients report a sense of pressure in the area of the healing skin. It may take 3 weeks to 1 month for the skin to heal, especially in a thin-skinned older adult. Patients with deep partial-thickness burns are at risk for developing contractures at the site of injury. A *full-thickness burn,* the most serious type of burn, results from exposure to flame, steam, chemicals, high-voltage electricity, or scalding. The skin that is burnt appears whitish or leathery gray to charred black and does not blanch with pressure. Patients may experience a sense of deep pressure; it is unusual for them to feel pain.

Etiology: With a burn injury, wound edema and loss of intravascular volume, caused by increased vascular permeability, occur. Because of the normal aging changes of the skin, the older adult who suffers from a burn injury is at increased risk for morbidity and mortality. The decreased vascular response of skin in older adults contributes to poor wound healing and increased risk of infection.

Occurrence: An estimated 2.5 million injuries, 60,000 requiring hospitalization, and 6000 deaths occur annually in the United States from burns.

Age: Burns occur in all age groups, but the rate of fatal burns is much greater among persons ≥75 years old. Of fatal burns, 90% result from residential fires.

Ethnicity: Injuries from burns are more common in nonwhite populations.

Gender: Burns occur equally in men and women.

Contributing factors: Poverty is one of the strongest risk factors for fatality in a residential fire because of the overall poor living conditions. Cigarettes cause almost 50% of all residential fires. The use of space and kerosene heaters, fireplaces, faulty electrical wires, lack of smoke detectors and fire extinguishers, scalding liquids, heating pads, and prolonged exposure to the sun all contribute to burn injuries in older adults.

Signs and symptoms: A detailed history of the incident should be obtained from the patient or significant other, including any substances involved, duration of exposure, emergency treatment (if any), and overall condition of the patient before the incident (including medications, mental status, prior history of any burn injuries, and medical diagnosis). Ask the patient if he or she is coughing.

Physical examination should include assessment of vital signs and of the burn area and surrounding tissues. For patients with a suspected respiratory ventilation injury, conduct a nasal and oropharyngeal examination to discover any singed nasal hairs and a chest examination. In determining the extent of the burn injury, the rule of nines helps to assess the body surface area; however, only second-degree and third-degree burns are included when calculating the total burn surface. Of concern during an assessment of the patient with a burn is the likelihood of local edema. Remove objects clothing or jewelry as soon as possible to avoid constriction of the area surrounding the burned tissue and to promote circulation to the wound.

Diagnostic tests: Tests for extensive burn damage from inhalation/electrical burns include the following.

Test	Results Indicating Disorder	CPT Code
Electrolytes	Electrolyte imbalance, shock	80051
Urinalysis	Dehydration	81000
Blood urea nitrogen	Renal insufficiency	84550
CBC	Type and crossmatch for blood	85031
Chest x-ray	Smoke inhalation	71020 (frontal and lateral) 71030 (complete, minimum of 4 views)
Electrocardiogram	Evaluate for abnormal arrhythmias	93307
Type and crossmatch for blood products	Potential for blood, blood product transfusion	86900
Carboxyhemoglobin	An arterial level $>10\%$ indicates carbon monoxide exposure	82375
Xenon ventilation-perfusion scan	Diagnosis inhalation damage	78584
Urine myoglobin	Evaluate for rhabdomyolysis	81099
Creatine phosphokinase	Evaluate for rhabdomyolysis	82550
Fiberoptic bronchoscopy	Assess extent of smoke inhalation	31622

CBC, complete blood count.

General laboratory tests for a patient with an extensive burn injury include electrolytes, urinalysis, blood urea nitrogen, CBC, and type and crossmatching for blood products. Chest x-ray and electrocardiogram are also ordered. For patients with suspected respiratory inhalation injury, obtain arterial blood gas and carboxyhemoglobin levels to determine respiratory function. A fiberoptic bronchoscopy may be ordered to assess the extent of smoke inhalation damage A xenon ventilation-perfusion scan is beneficial in diagnosing inhalation damage. For patients with electrical burns, urine myoglobin and creatine phosphokinase levels are measured to determine if there has been muscle swelling and evidence of myoglobinuria.

Differential diagnosis:

- Toxic epidermal necrolysis
- Scalded skin syndrome

Treatment: Immediate treatment for a burn is to apply wet towels soaked in cold water to the burn or, if possible, to immerse the burned area in cold tap water. The burned area should be kept moist with cold water until the burn is pain-free in and out of the water. Ideally, cool saline-soaked gauze should be applied to the burns. Depending on the extent of the burn, it may take 30 minutes for this analgesic effect to occur. To guard against potential hypothermia in patients with large TBSA burns being treated with ice water or cold water, the unaffected part of the body should be covered with a blanket. Patients with superficial small TBSA burns and without inhalation injury may be treated on an outpatient basis; however, in older adults, the patient's overall health condition must be considered when determining the treatment plan. Generally, patients are hospitalized if the face, hands, perineum, or feet are injured. Refer any patient with a burn associated with electrical current. A burned area >10% to 15% of the TBSA or a full-thickness burn >3% of the TBSA needs to be referred for hospitalization.

Wounds need to be cleaned; however, the cleansing process may be painful. Assess the need for analgesics or local anesthesia. Mild soap and water can be used to clean the burned surface.

Superficial burns do not require infection prophylaxis; this type of burn can be treated with cold compress applications and analgesics, such as acetaminophen, as needed. A moisturizer that contains aloe vera cream can be applied to areas of intact burned skin to promote healing; no dressing is required. After the cold compresses have relieved the initial pain of a superficial partial-thickness burn, cleanse the wound with a gentle irrigation of sterile saline, apply a topical antibiotic such as silver sulfadiazine (except on the face or in patients with sulfonamide hypersensitivity), and wrap the wound in a sterile occlusive dressing. An oral analgesic may be administered to the patient before the irrigation of the wound. Bacitracin also can be used to prevent infections in burn patients. Biological dressings are also available; these dressings need to be applied within the first 6 hours after the injury. Older adults with deep partial-thickness and full-thickness burns should be referred after initial treatment; given the fragility of older skin and concomitant conditions such as diabetes, infection of the burn is of great concern. The older adult may require hospitalization for hydration as well as burn care.

Follow-up: Outpatients should be re-evaluated 24 hours after the burn injury. Examine the condition of the wound and surrounding tissues for signs of healing or impending infection. Re-examine respiratory status of patients with an inhalation injury to detect diffuse wheezing and rhonchi. Determine the adequacy of the current pain management regimen. Have the patient or significant other demonstrate proper dressing techniques. Depending on the severity of the burn, the patient may be asked to return once a week until progressive healing is noted; daily visits may be necessary. Have patients return periodically about every 4 to 6 weeks to determine healing, to assess progress/compliance with any physical therapy if required, and to assess coping mechanisms.

Sequelae: Immediate complications from a burn injury include burn wound sepsis, pneumonia, decreased mobility and function of an affected extremity, and gastrointestinal ulcer. Long-term complications from a burn include squamous cell carcinoma developing at the scar site of the original injury. Hypertrophic scarring and contractures are also common at the site of a complicated burn. Patients ≥ 70 years old have a poor prognosis for recovery from a burn injury. The survival rate from a burn injury is related to the severity of the burn, especially if respiratory ventilation injury accompanied the burn.

Prevention/prophylaxis: Antibiotic prophylaxis was discussed earlier. Tetanus prophylaxis is recommended for second-degree and third-degree burns because these wounds are tetanus-prone. A booster injection of tetanus toxoid should be administered intramuscularly topatients who have been immunized in the past but have not received a booster injection within the past 5 years. If the patient has not been actively immunized, give antitetanus globulin, 250 to 500 units intramuscularly in addition to the tetanus toxoid, depending on the severity of the burn.

Scalding injuries often can be prevented. Older adults should be instructed to set the hot water heater temperature at $43°C$ to $49°C$ $(110–120°F)$.

All homes should have an evacuation plan in case of an emergency. If the emergency phone number 911 is not available in the area, the numbers for all local emergency services should be either programmed on the telephone or listed within easy access. Encourage the use of functioning smoke detectors and home fire extinguishers. Although the use of a heating unit or fireplace in a home may be unavoidable, older adults should be rehearsed in safety precautions needed for these heating systems. Any home assessment should include an evaluation of fire prevention measures. Residents of long-term care facilities should be permitted to smoke only when supervised. A sunscreen with a sun protection factor (SPF) of ≥ 15 should be used and protective clothing worn during episodes of prolonged sun exposure. Anyone with a healed burn site should cover that area with a sunscreen throughout the year.

Referral: Outpatients being treated for a burn may require referral to a physical therapist for wound therapy. Older adults who have suffered a moderate or major burn injury require hospitalization and possibly admission to a specialized burn care unit. Anyone experiencing smoke inhalation should be referred to a respiratory physician specialist.

Education: After treatment for a burn, patients should:

Keep the wound clean and dry.

Keep the wound elevated, if applicable.

Change the dressing as directed.

Take antibiotics as directed.

Patients should be informed that using home remedies such as butter and mayonnaise are not effective for wound healing; these products may promote bacterial growth.

CELLULITIS

Cellulitis	ICD-9-CM: 682.9

Description: Cellulitis is a deep infection of the skin, most commonly caused by group A streptococci, *Staphylococcus aureus, Erysipelothrix rhusiopathiae, Vibrio vulnificus, Haemophilus influenzae,* or occasionally a gram-negative organism. Cellulitis also can be caused by specific pathogens from human or animal bites.

Etiology: Although cellulitis usually occurs when an organism enters the skin through an open area, it also can occur in intact but edematous skin. Cellulitis involves the dermis and subcutaneous tissue. A clear site of entry may not be evident in patients with obesity, edema, or alcoholism.

Occurrence: The occurrence of cellulitis is unknown.

Age: Cellulitis can occur at any age. Facial cellulitis is more common in people ≥50 years old.

Ethnicity: No known predominant ethnic group is associated with cellulitis incidence.

Gender: Cellulitis occurs equally among men and women.

Contributing factors: Cellulitis can occur in patients who have arterial insufficiency, diabetes mellitus, lacerations, lower extremity edema, human or animal bites, tinea infections, recurring cellulitis, burns, trauma, stasis ulceration, ischemia, and puncture wounds. It also is associated with certain surgical procedures and environmental and occupational hazards, such as occupations that involve regularly handling poultry, fish, or meat. Intravenous drug use is another factor contributing to the development of cellulitis. Acute and chronic sinusitis can lead to periorbital or orbital cellulitis. Patients with a history of coronary artery bypass graft surgery with removal of the saphenous vein are susceptible to cellulitis. Patients in septic shock are also susceptible to the development of cellulites.

Signs and symptoms: Patients may complain of fever, chills, malaise, anorexia, nausea, or headache, and, in severe cases, patients may have tachycardia, hypotension, and delirium. Cellulitis most often appears on the lower extremities after a skin aberration, such as dermatitis, ulceration, trauma, or tinea pedis. Scars from previous cardiovascular surgery are common sites for recurrent cellulitis. Examine for skin temperature, note any breaks in the skin and ulcerations, and determine presence of pulses and sensation. Local erythema with edema and tenderness elicited by palpation are presenting signs of cellulitis. The affected area may take on the appearance of an orange peel when the surface is infiltrated. Depending on the organism of origin, large hemorrhagic bullae may be present. Because lymphangitis and regional lymphadenopathy also may occur with cellulitis, the clinician should examine for red streaks extending proximally to the infected area. If gas gangrene (anaerobic cellulitis) is suspected, the skin should be inspected for crepitus and foul-smelling exudates, and the surrounding area should be palpated for muscle tenderness. A positive Homan's sign (pain in the calf on dorsiflexion of the ankle of affected limb) or palpable venous cord may suggest deep vein thrombosis. A cardiac examination is warranted to assess for a heart murmur.

Diagnostic tests:

Test	Results Indicating Disorder	CPT Code
Tissue culture	Determine organism in pus is present	87230 (toxin) 87073–87076 (anaerobic)
CBC with differential	Leukocytosis present in anaerobic cellulitis	85022–85025
Blood cultures	Determine severity of infection or suspected systemic toxicity	87040
Radiograph	Rule out presence of osteomyelitis	76006 (stress views any upper or lower extremity joint)

Unless pus has formed in the wound, a tissue culture is usually not necessary. In cases of extensive infection or suspected systemic toxicity, blood cultures and a CBC with differential should be obtained to determine the severity of illness. Leukocytosis is present in patients with anaerobic cellulitis, and the Gram's stain smear shows gram-positive encapsulated bacilli. Patients with diabetes mellitus should have a radiograph of the area to rule out the presence of osteomyelitis.

Differential diagnosis:

- Lipodermatosclerosis (tender red plaque on the medial lower legs in patients with venous stasis or varicosities)
- Acute severe contact dermatitis (edema is superficial, itching is more prevalent)
- Acute gout
- Necrotizing fasciitis (determined by magnetic resonance imaging or computed tomography; patient presents with diffuse swelling or an arm or leg with associated bullae with clear or seroosanguineous fluid)
- Thrombophlebitis (lower extremity Doppler ultrasound)
- Pseudogout
- Osteomyelitis (determined by radiographs)

Treatment: Patients with an open wound initially should be asked when their last tetanus toxoid booster was given; if the most recent booster was ≥10 years ago, 0.5 mL of tetanus toxoid should be administered immediately. If the wound is grossly contaminated and the patient's last tetanus booster was 5 to 10 years ago, the clinician should consider giving another booster at this time. An older adult who has not had primary immunization requires tetanus toxoid and tetanus immune globulin.

Patients with mild cellulitis may be given oral antibiotics. In a mild case of cellulitis found to be gram-negative bacilli in origin, antibiotics are not necessary unless the patient is at high risk (see under Referral). The drugs of choice include dicloxacillin, 125 to 500 mg four times daily; clindamycin, 300 mg four times daily; and a first-generation cephalosporin such as cephalexin, 250 to 500 mg four times daily. For streptococcal cellulitis, penicillin is the drug of choice. Oxacillin is also effective for streptococcus and staphylococcus. Oral therapy should be prescribed for 7 to 10 days. Patients with underlying tinea should be treated with topical antifungal medications as well as antibiotics.

Consider the patient's renal function before prescribing any medication. Tell the patient to elevate the affected area, keep the area as clean as possible, and avoid any trauma to the area. Moist warm soaks can be applied to the affected area. Patients may require analgesics in appropriate dosages for pain. Patients with edema should take measures to control the edema by elevating the extremity. Blood glucose levels need to be monitored carefully if the patient has diabetes. Patients with complications (see under Referral) should be hospitalized for monitoring and to receive intravenous antibiotics.

Follow-up: Outpatients should be requested to contact their health-care providers within 1 week if no improvement is noted or within 48 hours if fever or inflammation continues. On their return visit, patients should be examined for evidence of thrombophlebitis or recurrence of the cellulitis.

Sequelae: In patients with cellulitis of the lower extremities, thrombophlebitis is a potential complication. Additional problems arising from cellulitis include bacteremia and lymphangitis, especially in patients with recurrent cellulitis.

Prevention/prophylaxis: Preventive measures for cellulitis include reduction of chronic edema in patients with peripheral vascular disease, control of blood glucose in patients with diabetes, and meticulous hand washing. Wheelchair-bound patients should have protective measures to avoid trauma to their extremities.

Referral: Patients should be hospitalized if they have high fever, diabetes, alcoholism, human immunodeficiency virus (HIV), anaerobic cellulitis, necrotizing fasciitis, or cellulitis of the orbit or face or if they are experiencing extreme pain. Consultation with an infectious disease specialist may be necessary. Order a surgical consultation for patients who require incision and drainage of abscesses and débridement of necrotic tissue. Home intravenous treatment may be indicated to shorten hospital stay.

Education: Patients with cellulitis must be informed that completion of the antibiotic regimen is mandatory. Patients should not attempt to scratch the affected area but should keep the site meticulously clean to avoid superinfection. Advise patients with lower extremity involvement to maintain bed rest with bathroom privileges and to elevate the limb. Apprise them of the signs and symptoms of thrombophlebitis.

CORNS AND CALLUSES

SIGNAL SYMPTOMS hyperkeratotic overgrowths

Corns and calluses	ICD-9-CM: 700

Description: Corns and calluses are aggregations of hyperkeratotic skin on the foot. The hyperkeratotic nodules that occur on the sole of the foot are referred to as *plantar keratoses* or *clavi*.

Etiology: Increased rubbing of, pressure on, or friction to the foot causes corns and calluses. The most common cause is poorly fitting shoes. Individuals with foot deformities or gait disturbances, or both, are also at high risk for developing calluses, especially over bony prominences.

Age: Individuals >65 years old most commonly develop corns and calluses.

Gender: More common in women secondary to restrictive footwear.

Contributing factors: Gait disturbance or imbalance secondary to weakness, arthritis, normal aging changes of the foot, foot deformities such as hammertoe deformity, and use of improper footwear. High levels of ambulatory activity also can contribute to the formation of corns and calluses.

Signs and symptoms: Usually corns and calluses are asymptomatic. Thick calluses may cause a burning sensation in the foot. Depending on the location of the callus, tight-fitting shoes may cause severe pain.

Diagnostic tests:

Test	Results Indicating Disorder	CPT Code
Radiograph of the foot	Rule out abnormal bone structure	73620 (foot, 2 views)

Differential diagnosis:

- Plantar ulcers and plantar warts (verrucae)
- Tinea pedis (differentiate from soft corns)

Treatment: Mechanical paring of the corn, callus, or both is recommended. Improper footwear should be avoided. Use of accommodative padding, such as a metatarsal pad, helps to relieve pressure by changing the alignment of the toes. Silicone toe sleeves, polymer gel, cushions, and padding with foam or lamb's wool are available over-the-counter.

Follow-up: Periodic physical examination of the foot is needed, to assess the status.

Prevention/prophylaxis: Relief of the pressure on the affected area can prevent development of corns and calluses. Shoes should be wide enough at the toe to allow the toes to extend straight ahead. Encourage women to avoid wearing shoes with high heels.

Referral: Refer patients with complicated management to a podiatrist.

Education: Teach patients the importance of avoiding improper footwear. To prevent injury to the toes, 0.5 inch of extra space should be allowed in the toe box.

HERPES ZOSTER

SIGNAL SYMPTOMS▶ cutaneous eruption of a dermatome distribution, burning or tingling skin sensation

| Herpes zoster | ICD-9-CM: 053.9 |

Description: Herpes zoster is an acute vesicular eruption caused by a virus histologically identical to the varicella (chickenpox) virus. Herpes zoster is human (alpha) herpes virus 3 (varicella-zoster virus [VZV]), a member of the herpesvirus group.

Etiology: Recurrent VZV infection causes herpes zoster. The patient has initial contact with VZV in the form of chickenpox. The DNA virus resides within the neurons. During reactivation, the virus spreads across the ganglion to other neurons, which causes a cutaneous eruption of a dermatome distribution. Herpes zoster is self-limited. Although chickenpox is one of the most readily communicable diseases, herpes zoster has a much lower rate of transmission. Nonimmune persons are considered contagious 8 to 21 days after exposure to VZV. Mode of transmission is coming into contact with the vesicle fluid. Patients with herpes zoster may be sources of infection for 1 week after the appearance of vesicle lesions. Nonimmune individuals can transmit infection and should avoid contact with patients with herpes zoster.

Occurrence: Herpes zoster occurs worldwide, more commonly in older adults. An estimated half of the population is affected by age 85.

Age: This infection is most common in adults >55 years old.

Ethnicity: African-Americans are one fourth as likely as whites to develop herpes zoster.

Gender: Herpes zoster occurs equally in men and women.

Contributing factors: Individuals are more likely to develop herpes zoster if they are >55 years old, are immunosuppressed (e.g., HIV-infected patients), have certain malignancies, are receiving long-term corticosteroids, are receiving chemotherapy, or are taking radiation treatments. Physiological or psychological stressors can precipitate the development of herpes zoster.

Signs and symptoms: Patients usually experience burning or tingling pain at the site 4 to 5 days before the eruption appears. Pain in a dermatomal pattern may precede the appearance of the vesicles by weeks, however. The eruption is maculopapular for a few hours, then becomes characterized as grouped vesicles on an erythematosus base over one dermatome (usually). T5 and T6 are the most common vertebral dermatomes involved. Patients often experience a sense of anxiety and flu-like symptoms with the onset of herpes zoster. Patients may report sleep disturbances, decreased appetite, and depression. As vesicles age, they become pustular, then crust over after 3 to 4 days, finally healing in 2 to 4 weeks. Lesions may appear in irregular crops and are typically unilateral. Most common distributions are on the trunk or face in elderly persons. Regional lymph nodes may or may not be swollen and tender. The pain can last 6 to 12 months after disappearance of the rash (postherpetic neuralgia). Ocular complications occur in about half of patients with involvement of the ophthalmic division of the trigeminal nerve; these complications may include keratitis, anterior uveitis, and corneal ulceration. A precursor to corneal involvement in herpes zoster has been found to be vesicles on the tip of the nose (Hutchinson's sign).

Clinical Pearl: Patients with ≥20 lesions occurring outside of the primary contiguous dermatome have disseminated herpes zoster.
Patients with visceral herpes zoster also may have internal organ involvement, such as hepatitis, pancreatitis, or gastritis.

Diagnostic test: Diagnosis usually is based on clinical appearance and distribution of the eruption and careful history of when the rash appeared. The laboratory test listed is useful in complicated cases and epidemiological studies.

Test	Results Indicating Disorder	CPT Code
Immunofluorescence Antibody (IFA)	Positive for herpes zoster	87254

Immunofluorescence antibody test has been shown to be a rapid, sensitive test wich can confirm the diagnosis of herpes zoster.

Differential diagnosis: When the pain of pre-eruptive herpes occurs, the differential diagnosis depends on the dermatome involved:

- Migraine
- Myocardial infarction
- Acute abdomen

Once the rash or eruption appears:

- Contact allergic dermatitis (linear vesicles)
- Grouped vesicles (viral infection)

Treatment: Antiviral agents are recommended in the presence of significant pain, serious herpes zoster, or involvement near the eye. Postherpetic neuralgia is not reduced by antiviral therapy, but these agents may help with healing in the acute phase. Give acyclovir, 800 mg five times a day for 7 to 10 days; famciclovir, 500 mg orally every 8 hours for 7 days; or valacyclovir, 1000 mg orally every 8 hours for 7 days. These drugs must be given within 72 hours after onset of rash to be effective, and their use must be monitored in patients with reduced renal function. Topical agents are also effective in treating herpes zoster. The use of cool compresses with 1:20 Burow's solution, calamine lotion, and topical lidocaine (Xylocaine) is recommended for the soothing local effect.

Analgesics may be necessary for the initial pain associated with herpes zoster. Acetaminophen is recommended initially. Opiates, such as codeine and oxycodone-acetaminophen (Percocet), can be used for severe pain but are not generally recommended for elderly individuals.

For postherpetic neuralgia pain, capsaicin (Zostrix cream) can be applied topically. Also, nortriptyline 10mg orally or desipramine 10-25 mg orally both given at bedtime may be helpful and it may be necessary to gradually increase the dosage until reduction of pain; however because of the anticholinergic side effects, caution is warranted. Recently gabapentin received FDA approval for the treatment of postherpetic neuralgia. Initial dose is 300 mg on the first day and titrated up gradually until pain relief is safely reached; caution is advised when prescribing gabapentin to older adults given the side effects of dizziness and ataxia. The 5% lidocaine patch has been shown to be effective in treating the pain of postherpetic neuralgia. In cases of severe pain, a transcutaneous electrical nerve stimulator unit may be tried.

Follow-up: Patients should be re-examined in 2 to 4 weeks to monitor progression of rash and as needed for follow-up of postherpetic neuralgia.

Sequelae: Postherpetic neuralgia is the primary complication, occurring almost exclusively in people >60 years old. This pain persists at least 6 weeks after skin lesions. The pain, characterized as constant, severe, sharp, or burning, may develop into a long-standing, debilitating problem. Postherpetic neuralgia usually lasts ≤1 year. Another consequence of herpes zoster is secondary bacterial infection leading to cellulitis, caused by staphylococcus group A or group A β-hemolytic streptococcus. Cutaneous or visceral dissemination, the appearance of numerous varicella-like lesions in extradermatomal sites, may cause pneumonitis or encephalitis.

Prevention/prophylaxis: The only effective prevention for herpes zoster is prevention of primary varicella infection (chickenpox) because latent varicella virus cannot be cleared from the sensory ganglia. Studies are currently evaluating the efficacy of a varicella vaccine for the older adult. High-risk individuals, such as immunosuppressed patients and individuals who have not had chickenpox, should be kept from exposure. In varicella-nonimmune individuals who have been exposed, passive immune treatment with varicella-zoster immune globulin should be used to modify the infection.

Referral: Refer to an ophthalmologist patients with lesions on the nose or in the eye area because of probable ocular involvement. Patients with disseminated herpes zoster should be referred to a specialist. Refer patients with severe uncontrollable postherpetic neuralgia to a neurologist.

Education: Emphasize to the patient the need to stay home and get plenty of rest. Teach patients proper infection control measures and proper disposal of dressings or clothing that contain vesicle fluid. Patients should avoid contact with immunosuppressed individuals, pregnant women, or individuals who have not had chickenpox. Emphasize that herpes zoster is self-limited.

PRESSURE ULCERS

SIGNAL SYMPTOMS▶▶   nonblanching erythema, red painful lesions

Pressure ulcers	ICD-9-CM: 707.0 by region

Description: Pressure ulcers (decubitus ulcers) are localized areas of tissue necrosis that tend to develop when soft tissue is compressed between a bony prominence and an external surface for a prolonged period. Pressure ulcers are characterized by four stages of severity:

Stage 1: Erythema, epidermis intact.

Stage 2: Partial thickness, skin loss. Extends into but not through dermis.

Stage 3: Full thickness through the dermis and into subcutaneous tissue. Shallow crater that may include exudates or necrotic tissue.

Stage 4: Deep penetration into the fascia or bone.

Etiology: Pressure is the major causative factor in pressure ulcer formation. Several factors play a role, however, in determining whether pressure is sufficient to create an ulcer. The pathological effect of excessive pressure on soft tissue can be attributed to:

- Intensity of pressure
- Duration of pressure
- Tissue tolerance (the ability of skin and its supporting structures to endure pressure without adverse sequelae

Injury occurs to the skin and underlying tissues. Ischemia and hypoxia result as the pressure is applied to the area. Waste products accumulate as the ischemia continues, which produces toxins that cause further tissue breakdown.

Occurrence: It is a cause of lengthy hospital stays and affects 17% to 56% of critically ill patients.

Age: The prevalence of pressure ulcers in the elderly population is 11.6% to 27.5% with the increased risk assigned to advancing age. The incidence in skilled-care and nursing home facilities approaches 23%.

Patients admitted to a hospital geriatric unit have a similarly high prevalence rate. Of patients <70 years old, only 6% have pressure ulcers, whereas of patients ≥70 years old, the prevalence almost doubles to 11.6%.

Ethnicity: There is no known prevalence among ethnic groups.

Gender: Pressure ulcers occur equally in men and women.

Contributing factors: The major contributing factors to pressure ulcer development are friction, shear, pressure over bony prominences, and nutritional debilitation. Moisture, specifically incontinence, is frequently cited as a related condition because moisture alters the resiliency of the epidermis to external forces. Other predisposing factors include advancing age, low blood pressure, smoking, elevated body temperature, dehydration, decreased mobility, decreased sensation, and dementia.

Signs and symptoms: A detailed history of the incident should be obtained from the patient or significant other, including chronic illness, hygiene status, nutritional status, immobility, constant skin moisture, incontinence, ability to perform activities of daily living, psychological factors, and sources of support. Ask the patient if he or she has pain over bony prominences, which occurs in stages 1 and 2; however, the patient may not experience pain in these areas if progression to stage 3 or 4 has occurred. Clinical presentation can vary from nonblanching erythema to ecchymosis and to frank necrosis. Nonblanching erythema results from damage to blood vessels and extravasation of blood into the tissues. Its presence suggests that the tissue damage is imminent or has already occurred. The color of the skin can be an intense bright red to a dark red or purple; pressure-induced nonblanching erythema is often misdiagnosed as a hematoma or ecchymosis. When deep tissue is also present, the area is often either indurated or boggy when palpated. Note ulcer size, depth, and presence of exudates; epithelialization; granulation tissue; and findings such as necrotic tissue, sinus tracts, undermining, tunneling, and purulent drainage or other signs of infection.

Diagnostic tests:

Test	Results Indicating Disorder	CPT Code
Wound culture and sensitivity	To determine specific pathogen and appropriate antibiotic	87230 (toxin)
Albumin	Decreased	87073-87076 (anaerobic)
3.2–4.6 g/dL	Ages 61-90, <3.2 g/dL	82040
2.9–4.5 g/dL	Ages >90 years, <2.9 g/dL	85031
CBC	Hemoglobin decreased <12 g/dL	85651 (non-automated)
Hemoglobin Men ages 65–75, 12.6–17.4 g/dL Women, 11.7–16.1 g/dL Red cell distribution, 11.6–14.8 Lymphocyte, 1.0–4.8 (34%) Leukocyte, 4.5–11.0 Neutrophils, 1.8–7.7 (59%)	Red cell distribution increased Decrease lymphocyte count <1.5 × 10^9 (malnutrition) Elevated leukocyte count (osteomyelitis) Neutrophilic leukocytosis	85652 (automated)
Erythrocyte sedimentation rate Men >50, 0–20 Women >50, 0–30	Increased >20 in men and >30 in women	76006 (stress views any joint)
X-ray of appropriate area	Bony rarefaction, periosteal elevation, and new bone formation	

General laboratory tests for the patient with a pressure ulcer include a wound culture and sensitivity, especially for any of the following: signs of local infection (erythema, edema, induration, purulent or foul-smelling drainage, pain, crepitus); signs of systemic infection (fever, leukocytosis); bone involvement (because of risk for osteomyelitis); and nonhealing wounds. This helps in determining the causative organism. Staging of pressure ulcers is done to classify the degree of tissue damage observed. Numerical identification of stages does not imply a progression of ulcer severity. Laboratory testing includes albumin to rule out malnutrition, CBC to rule out malnutrition and osteomyelitis, and erythrocyte sedimentation rate as well as an x-ray to rule out osteomyelitis.

Differential diagnosis:

- Skin cancers (atypical skin growth or mole)
- Fungal and yeast infections
- Venous stasis leg ulcers (edema, hyperpigmentation usually found in lower extremities)
- Arterial leg ulcers (pale atrophic skin, hair loss)
- Diabetic ulcer (red, tender, ulcerated tissue usually on foot or toes)
- Neuropathic ulcers may mimic pressure ulcers

Treatment: An effective ulcer treatment plan should have three components:

Nutritional assessment and support

Management of tissue loads (pressure, friction, and shear as well as moisture)

Ulcer care and management of bacterial colonization and infection (débridement, application of dressings, and measures to control bacterial colonization and treat infection

These components are equally important, so they should be addressed simultaneously.

Pharmacological Management

Débriding methods

Wet-to-dry dressings

Enzymatic ointments

Irrigate with saline

Whirlpool soaks

Dressings

Semipermeable transparent film dressings are best for stages 1 to 3 without heavy exudates

Hydrocolloid dressings are best for low-to-moderate exudate wounds

Hydrogels are best for wounds with eschar or dry wounds

Alginates: are best for stages 2 to 3 and bleeding wounds

Nonpharmacological Management

Prevention: Identify high-risk clients

Mobility impairment, incontinence, nutritional status, and level of consciousness

Braden scale or Norton scale

Body weight <58 kg

Nutritional support

30 to 35 calories/kg per day

1.25 to 1.5 g of protein per kilogram per day

Daily high-potency vitamin and mineral supplement

Reduce pressure and friction

Make sure the patient moves and walks regularly

Reposition every 2 hours from supine to side-lying position at 30° to the support surface

Alternating air-pressure pads

Regular toileting and incontinence care

Follow-up: Caregivers should evaluate the patient's progress toward healing at least weekly. If signs of ulcer deterioration are observed sooner, steps to reverse them should be taken immediately. If the patient's general condition deteriorates, the ulcer should be reassessed promptly.

Caregivers should monitor the patient's general health, nutritional adequacy, psychosocial support, and pain level and should be alert to signs of complications. Frequency of monitoring should be determined by the clinician, based on the condition of the patient, the condition of the ulcer, the ulcer's healing rate, and the type of health-care setting.

Sequelae: Cellulitis, bacteremia, osteomyelitis, and meningitis may occur secondary to pressure ulcers.

Prevention/prophylaxis: Screening test and risk assessment tools (Braden and Norton) are crucial to any pressure ulcer prevention program. The specific deficits contributing to a score must be considered, to implement a treatment plan. The negative effects of risk factors may be minimized by correct positioning, providing pressure reduction sleep or sitting surfaces, improving the nutritional status of the individual, and managing incontinence.

Referral: Refer the patient to a specialist (endostomal therapist nurse, plastic surgeon, infectious disease specialist, dermatologist) if the wound does not respond to therapy or for product recommendation, débridement, biopsy, or surgical intervention (i.e., graft or myocutaneous flap).

Education: Patients and family caregivers should be given enough information to enable them to understand the contributing factors of pressure ulcer formation, treatment modalities, and expected outcomes. Prevention is key. Discuss good hand washing and hygiene and keeping the skin clean and dry. Tell patients to sing the alphabet song while washing their hands with warm water and antibacterial soap. Discuss proper positioning, nutrition, and signs of secondary infection.

SKIN CANCER

SIGNAL SYMPTOMS▶ telangiectasia, abnormal symmetry of lesion, crusting and bleeding

Skin cancer	ICD-9-CM: 179.9
Basal cell carcinoma, site unspecified	ICD-9-CM: 173.3
Basal cell carcinoma, face	
Basal cell carcinoma, neck, scalp	
Basal cell carcinoma, trunk	
Basal cell carcinoma of the limb	
Basal cell carcinoma, lower limb	
Skin neoplasm, site unspecified	
Melanoma of the skin, site unspecified	

Description: Neoplasms of the skin are the most common type of cancers in humans. Three main types of skin cancer are basal cell carcinoma (BCC), which arises from the basal cell layer of the epidermis; squamous cell carcinoma (SCC), which originates in the squamous cells of the epithelium; and malignant melanoma (MM), which is a tumor arising in a pigmented area.

Etiology: The major risk factor for the development of skin cancers is exposure to ultraviolet sunlight. Patients who have or had an occupation requiring them to spend extensive time outdoors are susceptible to the development of skin cancer. There is a high recurrence rate for BCC.

Occurrence: Each year, >1 million new cases of skin cancer are diagnosed in the United States. BCC, the most common type of skin cancer, accounts for 65% to 80% of these cases. SCC constitutes 10% to 25% of all skin cancers. BCC and SCC are referred to as *nonmelanoma skin cancer* (NMSC). MM accounts for the remainder of skin cancers.

Age: The incidence of all types of skin cancers increases with age, owing to sun exposure over an extended period.

Ethnicity: All skin cancers are more prevalent in fair-skinned persons, especially people with blonde, red, or light brown hair and people of Celtic ancestry. SCC is more common than BCC in African-Americans.

Gender: Currently, more men than women have BCC, but the number of women with BCC is increasing. SCC and MM are equally prevalent in men and women.

Contributing factors: Besides sun exposure as a contributing factor, skin cancer may occur as a late sequela to burns, scars, chronic ulcers, or radiodermatitis. Inorganic arsenic exposure also has been linked to the development of BCC. Patients who have had a renal transplant and immunosuppression are also at risk for developing skin cancer. Human papillomavirus and xeroderma pigmentosum may play a role in the development of SCC. A familial tendency to develop melanoma exists.

Signs and symptoms: Patients need to be questioned regarding their history of sun exposure, severe sunburn, burns, scars, ulcers, radiation dermatitis, previous skin cancer, prior occupation, and family history of skin cancer. The presentation of the skin cancer depends on the type of tumor. BCC generally presents first as a dome-shaped, white-to-pink papule or nodule having a raised pearly border with prominent telangiectasia. Patients may describe this lesion as a pimple that did not heal. As the nodule enlarges, scaling, crusting, or central ulceration may become noticeable. Of BCC, >90% occurs on the head and neck.

SCC often originates at the site of chronic inflammation or old scars. Actinic keratoses, which appear as round or irregular-shaped erythematosus or tan plaques with a scaly or rough surface, are a precursor to SCC. Signs of malignancy include elevation, ulceration, or inflammation of the lesion; the original lesion also may have enlarged in size. In later stages of SCC, the surface may appear crusted, and a horn of keratin forms. SCC appears on sun-exposed as well as on non–sun-exposed areas of the body. These tumors may be tender to touch owing to their rapid growth and inflammatory process. Examine the scalp, ears, lower lip, and dorsa of the hands for SCC.

The clinical features of a lesion suspected to be MM (the *ABCDEs* of melanoma) are:

- Asymmetry
- Border irregularity
- Color variation
- Diameter >6 mm
- Elevation of a previously flat lesion

Whited and Grichnik (1998) developed a seven-point checklist for suspected MM:

Major signs: Change in size, change in shape, change in color. One or more major signs, refer for expeditious biopsy.

Minor signs: Inflammation, crusting or bleeding, sensory change, diameter of ≥7mm. Three or four minor signs with a major sign, consider referral.

Patients may be concerned about a new, pigmented lesion or a change in an already existing one. Patients may report associated itching, burning, or pain in a mole. Superficial spreading melanoma is a flat to slightly raised pigmented lesion with irregular borders, commonly found on the backs of men and the lower legs of women. Lentigo maligna melanoma, an irregularly pigmented macula with notched borders, occurs on sun-exposed areas, especially on the face of older adults. Nodular melanoma, brown or black papules usually located on the trunk, head, and neck, is characterized by rapid growth. Acral lentiginous melanomas, the most common type of melanoma in African-Americans, occur on the palms, soles, fingers, and toes; a pigmented streak of the cuticle is diagnostic (Hutchinson's sign) of this type of melanoma. Clinical evaluation for skin cancer also includes a total body skin examination and palpation of regional lymph nodes, liver, and spleen.

Diagnostic tests:

Test	Results Indicating Disorder	CPT Code
Skin biopsy: shave	Histological confirmation	11100
Skin biopsy: punch	Histological confirmation	11100

Biopsy of the suspected lesion is necessary to confirm the diagnosis via histological examination of the tissue; an adequate tissue sample should be excised.

Differential diagnosis:

- Actinic keratoses
- Seborrheic keratoses
- Keratoacanthoma
- Atypical nevi
- Blue nevus
- Dermatofibroma
- Venous lakes
- Pyogenic granulomas
- Warts

Treatment: Several factors need to be considered before skin cancer therapy begins: the patient's age and general health, size and location of the tumor, the pathology of the tumor, and the cosmetic concerns of the patient. BCC may be treated by excisional surgery, electrodesiccation and curettage, cryotherapy, ionizing radiation, and Mohs' micrographic surgery. A chemotherapeutic agent such as 5-fluorouracil is used as a topical agent for superficial or small BCCs.

SCC may be treated the same as BCC; however, because of its more truculent growth pattern, wider excision and Mohs' micrographic surgery are the preferred methods of treatment.

Treatment of MM is surgical. An excisional margin surrounding the tumor is made, depending on the thickness of the tumor. Chemotherapy and radiation are used for palliative measures in the treatment of metastatic disease.

Follow-up: Follow-up for a patient with diagnosed skin carcinoma is essential because the recurrence rate of skin cancer is high; 50% of persons with BCC and SCC have a reappearance of a cancerous lesion within 5 years. A person who is susceptible to skin cancer may develop another cancerous lesion at any time. Precancerous lesions should be examined regularly every 3 to 12 months using a head-to-toe skin examination, including a careful inspection of the previous site of a lesion. In patients with SCC, palpation of regional lymph nodes is suggested. During subsequent visits of patients with malignant melanoma, a thorough review of systems is imperative to elicit clinical signs and symptoms of metastasis.

Sequelae: BCC rarely metastasizes; however, if it is not treated early, the carcinoma may invade the surrounding tissue and bone. Advanced SCC lesions of the lips, pinna, and genitalia often metastasize. Recurrent NMSC has a higher rate of recurrence and eventually may lead to the development of metastatic disease. The larger the NMSC in size, the higher the rate of recurrence.

 Clinical Pearl: The anatomical location of the NMSC also influences the recurrence rate; lesions on the face, ears, vertex, and scalp are known as high-risk cancer areas.

Five-year prognosis for MM is determined by the Breslow thickness of the tumor. Tumors <0.76 mm are associated with a 98% 5-year survival rate; tumors 0.76 to 1.49 mm, with an 87% to 94% 5-year survival rate; and tumors 1.50 to 3.99 mm, with a 66% to 83% 5-year survival rate. Patients with tumors >4.0 mm have a <50% 5-year survival.

Prevention/prophylaxis: All older adults, especially those who are fair-skinned, should wear sunscreen with an SPF of ≥15 throughout the year. The yearly physical examination should include assessment of the head, scalp, and skin and an accurate recording of descriptions of any suspicious lesions. A dermatologist should evaluate all precancerous lesions. Lesions that have variegated colors, irregular elevations, or irregular borders should be examined by biopsy. Immunosuppressed organ recipients are at high risk for developing skin cancer at rates faster than the general patient population; they should be scheduled for regular skin examinations.

Referral: When a suspicious lesion is found, referral to a dermatologist for evaluation and possibly biopsy is necessary. Whole-body photographs and epiluminescence microscopy may be used to follow patients with suspicious lesions. Oncology referral is needed for metastatic SCC and MM.

Education: Advise older patients that skin cancers are a common occurrence as one ages, especially for patients at risk. Older adults should perform a monthly self-evaluation of the skin; suggest the use of mirrors to examine lesions on the back. Any suspicious open lesion that does not heal in a reasonable time needs to be examined by a primary care provider. Patients also need to report any slow-growing, flesh-colored or pigmented lesion, noting if the lesion has irregular borders, changes in color, ulceration, bleeding, or horn formation. Sun exposure, especially during the hours of 10:00 AM to 4:00 PM, should be avoided. Year-round broad-spectrum sunscreen that blocks ultraviolet A and ultraviolet B light is recommended. Vulnerable areas, such as the head and neck, should be covered with protective clothing. Patients can obtain written information from the American Cancer Society, 1599 Clifton Road NE, Atlanta, GA 30329, 1-800-227-2345, www.cancer.org and the Skin Cancer Foundation, PO Box 561, Department SEC, New York, NY 10156, 1-800-SKIN-490, www.skincancer.org/.

REFERENCES

General

American Medical Association: Current Procedural Terminology: CPT 2002, ed 4. AMA, Chicago, 2002.

Callahan, LF, and Jonas, BL: Arthritis. In Ham RJ, et al: Primary Care Geriatrics: A Case-Based Approach, ed 4. Mosby, St. Louis, 2002.

DeGowin, RL, and Brown, D: DeGowin's Diagnostic Examination, ed 7. McGraw-Hill, New York, 2000.

Goroll, A, and Mulley, AG: Primary Care Medicine: Office Evaluation and Management of the Adult Patient, ed 4. Lippincott Williams & Wilkins, Philadelphia, 2000.

Burns

Morgan, ED, et al: Ambulatory management of burns. Am Fam Physician 62:2015, 2000.

Richard, R: Assessment and diagnosis of burn wounds. [Electronic version.] Adv Wound Care 12:468, 1999.

Wiebelhaus, P, and Hansen, SL: Burns and scalds. RN 62:52, 1999.

Cellulitis

Brill, LR, and Stone, JA: Foot ulcers. [Electronic version.] Patient Care 35:13, 2001.

Fink, A, and DeLuca, G: Necrotizing fasciitis: Pathophysiology and treatment. Medsurg Nursing 11:33, 2002.

O'Dell, ML: Skin and wound infections: An overview. Am Fam Physician 1998. Contact: http://www.aafp.org/afp/98051ap/odell.html.

O'Donnell, JA, and Hofmann, MT: Skin and soft tissues: Management of four common infections in the nursing home patient. Geriatrics 56:33, 2001.

Corns and Calluses

Bedinghaus, JM, and Niedfeldt, MW: Over-the-counter foot remedies. Am Fam Physician 2001. Contact: http://www.aafp.org/afp/20010901/791.html.

Bryant, JL, and Beinlich, NR: Foot care: Focus on the elderly. Orthop Nurs 18:53, 1999.

Freeman, DB: Corns and calluses resulting from mechanical hyperkeratosis. Am Fam Physician 2002. Contact: http://www.aafp.org/afp/20020601/22277.html.

Herpes Zoster

Bawja, Z, and Ho, CC: Herpetic neuralgia: Use of combination therapy for pain relief in acute and chronic herpes zoster. Geriatrics 56:18, 2001.

Bezold, GD, Lange, ME, Gall, H, and Peter, RU: Detection of cutaneous varicella zoster virus infections by immunofluorescence versus PCR. European Journal of Dermatology 11:2, 2001.

O'Donnell, JA, and Hofmann, MT: Skin and soft tissues: Management of four common infections in the nursing home patient. Geriatrics 56:33, 2001.

Stankus, SE, et al: Management of herpes zoster (shingles) and postherpetic neuralgia. Am Fam Physician 2000. Contact: http://www.aafp.org/afp/2000415/2437.html.

Pressure Ulcers

DeGowin, RL, and Brown, DD: DeGowin's Diagnostic Examination, ed 7. McGraw-Hill, New York, 2000.

Dunphy, LH: Management Guidelines for Adult Nurse Practitioners. FA Davis, Philadelphia, 1999.

Humes, HD: Kelley's Textbook of Internal Medicine, ed 4. Lippincott Williams & Wilkins, Philadelphia, 2000.

Skin Cancer

Gudas, S: Skin cancer. [Electronic version]. Rehabil Oncol 19:15, 2001.

Jerant, AF, et al: Early detection and treatment of skin cancer. Am Fam Physician 62:357, 2000.

Martinez, J, and Otley, CC: The management of melanoma and nonmelanoma skin cancer: A review for the primary care physician. [Electronic version.] Mayo Clin Proc 76:1253, 2001.

Whited, JD, and Grichnik, JM: Does this patient have a mole or a melanoma? JAMA 279:696, 1998.

Chapter 4
HEAD, NECK, AND FACE DISORDERS

ACUTE GLAUCOMA

SIGNAL SYMPTOMS ▶ unilateral eye pain, visual blurring with halos around lights, conjunctival injection and photophobia

| Acute glaucoma | ICD-9 CM: 365.22 |

Description: Acute glaucoma, also known as *angle-closure or narrow-angle glaucoma,* is an obstruction to the outflow of aqueous humor from the posterior to the anterior chamber through the trabecular meshwork, canal of Schlemm, and associated structures. It results in an elevation of intraocular pressure, damaging the optic nerve and causing loss of peripheral vision, eye pain, and redness. This type of glaucoma is uncommon but may occur as a primary disease or secondary to other conditions and constitutes an ophthalmic emergency. Associated presenting symptoms may complicate diagnosis or result in misdiagnosis.

Etiology: The precise pathophysiology of glaucoma is unknown. In the acute form, pupillary blockage limits the progress of the aqueous humor through the trabecular network. The peripheral iris, which blocks the trabecular meshwork, is displaced forward. In susceptible persons, this may be precipitated by emotional stress, sudden darkness (such as in a theater when the lights go out), or the instillation of mydriatics.

Occurrence: Uncommon; <100 to 500 cases in 100,000. More common in families with prior history.

Age: The predominant age range is 55 to 70 years old.

Ethnicity: Acute glaucoma is more common in African-Americans, individuals of Asian ancestry, and individuals of Eskimo ancestry.

Gender: Occurs more often in women.

Contributing factors: Contributing factors include an anatomically narrow anterior chamber angle, requiring the use of a special examination technique called *gonioscopy* to identify. This examination technique is beyond the scope of the primary care practitioner, but the condition can be evaluated during the comprehensive eye examination. Other risk factors include sudden eye trauma; hyperopia; small cornea; shallow anterior chamber; Eskimo ancestry; female gender; family history of glaucoma (first-degree relatives have a 2% to 5% risk over a lifetime); cataract; neovascularization; and use of certain cold remedies, antidepressants, and other drugs with anticholinergic properties (e.g., atropine, preoperative medications, imipramine, inhaled ipratropium bromide). Rarely, sneezing or laser treatment can precipitate the condition.

Signs and symptoms: The presentation is often dramatic, but the diagnosis can be missed because of the associated symptoms. The history reveals severe, unilateral eye pain, blurred vision, lacrimation, reports of seeing colored halos around lights, and a red eye. Headache, nausea, and vomiting frequently accompany eye pain, causing eye pain to be overlooked. Emotional stress also is common. Examination reveals circumcorneal conjunctival injection, tearing, and a fixed semidilated pupil that is nonreactive to light; the cornea is steamy or cloudy. Visual acuity, if evaluated, shows a loss in the affected eye.

Diagnostic tests: Immediately refer patients for a complete ophthalmic examination, including gonioscopy and tonometry.

Differential diagnosis:

- Conjunctivitis
- Uveitis
- Corneal trauma or infection

Treatment: The patient with acute glaucoma needs an immediate consultation with and referral to an ophthalmologist; permanent visual loss occurs within 2 to 5 days if this condition is untreated. Surgical treatment includes peripheral iridectomy or laser iridotomy. Intraocular pressure must be lowered preoperatively, which may require the use of an osmotic diuretic intravenously or orally and miotic eye drops. As the primary health-care provider, you must communicate to the specialist any medical conditions that need monitoring with the use of these agents. Bilateral treatment is indicated because patients are at risk for developing the same problem in the other eye.

Follow-up: The ophthalmologist treating the patient determines follow-up treatment. Periodic eye examinations are recommended by preventive guidelines.

Sequelae: If treated promptly, acute glaucoma is not associated with sequelae. If untreated, permanent visual loss occurs.

Prevention/prophylaxis: Knowing the risk factors for acute glaucoma, the health-care provider should educate patients with those risk factors (see under Education). Periodic eye examinations are recommended for prevention.

Referral: Refer the patient immediately on presentation and evaluation of symptoms.

Education: Teach patients with known risk factors (see under Contributing Factors) the importance of regular eye examinations and reporting symptoms.

AGE-RELATED MACULAR DEGENERATION

SIGNAL SYMPTOMS insidious loss of central vision, blurred or fuzzy vision (late), straight lines appear wavy

Age-related macular degeneration (AMD)	ICD-9 CM: 362.50
Macular degeneration, dry, nonexudative	ICD-9 CM: 362.51
Macular degeneration, wet, exudative	ICD-9 CM: 362.52

Description: AMD or age-related maculopathy is a disorder affecting the macula in the middle of the retina. The macula comprises millions of photoreceptor cells containing visual pigments for central vision; these are nourished by the retinal pigment epithelium, part of a complex basement membrane that becomes sclerotic with age. There are two types of AMD, wet and dry. Dry AMD is most common, accounting for 90% of cases. Onset of visual loss is gradual and may not be noticed if only one eye is affected. The cause is unknown, but there is disintegration of the retinal pigment epithelium and light-sensing cells. Wet AMD occurs in 10% of cases but accounts for 90% of all AMD blindness. Neovascularization of the choroid area with leakage of new blood vessels and fluid into the retinal pigment epithelium causes scarring and damage to the macula.

Etiology: Unknown; see under Contributing Factors.

Occurrence: Common. Macular degeneration is the leading cause of legal blindness in adults >55 years old. Risk rises with age; occurrence is 30% in adults >75 years old.

Ethnicity: Whites are more likely to experience visual loss from AMD than African-Americans.

Gender: Women are at greater risk of AMD than men.

Contributing factors: Risk factors for AMD include family history, smoking, exposure to sunlight, and possibly nutritional deficits. History of AMD in one eye is a risk factor for developing it in the other eye; 10% have binocular AMD within 1 year.

Signs and symptoms: In dry AMD, there are no symptoms initially, particularly if it is monocular. Later, patients may note a decrease in visual acuity or blurred vision that improves in bright light. In wet AMD, straight lines appear wavy, and there may be a hole in central vision. White-yellow drusen spots are seen on funduscopic examination; Amsler grid test reveals wavy lines or missing lines in central vision (Fig. 4–1).

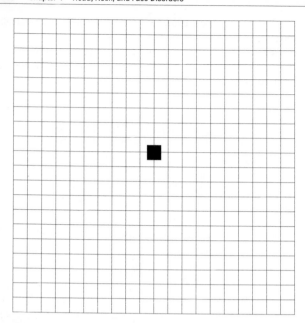

Figure 4–1 Example of Amsler grid.

Diagnostic tests:

Test	Results Indicating Disorder	CPT Code
Visual acuity with best correction (part of comprehensive eye examination)	Dramatic decrease in visual acuity may signal wet or exudative AMD	92004 (new patient) 92002 (established patient)
Funduscopic examination	Presence of drusen spots, neovascularization	92004 (new patient) 92002 (established patient)
Amsler grid	Wavy lines in wet AMD	Self-administered
Fluorescein angiography	Pattern of neovascularization and scarring	92235
Fundus photo (wet AMD)		92250

Differential diagnosis:
- Unexplained loss of visual acuity

Treatment: There is no treatment for dry AMD at present. The Age-related Eye Disease Study found that patients at high risk of advanced AMD lowered their risk by 25% when treated with high doses of vitamin C, vitamin E, beta carotene, zinc oxide, and cupric oxide; use of beta carotene is associated with an increased risk of lung cancer in smokers. There was no benefit to this therapy seen in patients without AMD or with early AMD. Low vision enhancement aids are available to help patients with dry AMD. Patients with wet AMD may benefit from laser photocoagulation treatment under certain circumstances, but inappropriate use of laser can cause further damage. A hot laser is used to seal the leaking vessels and prevent the growth of new vessels. A second treatment is photodynamic therapy with a cold laser for certain forms of wet AMD. It involves the intravenous injection of verteporfin (Visudyne), a light-sensitive drug. Verteporfin is taken up by the diseased blood vessels in the eye. A nonthermal or "cold" laser is applied in the eye via slit lamp, activating the verteporfin and destroying the neovascular cells. Current research is focused on retinal cell transplantation and submacular surgery.

Follow-up: All patients with AMD should be seen periodically by an ophthalmologist for re-evaluation of disease progression and, where applicable, further treatment. Patients may be given an Amsler grid to use weekly or monthly to check for visual changes.

Sequelae: Loss of central vision limits functional capacity and ability to read. Most AMD patients cannot drive. Environmental safety also is compromised; falls and hip fractures can occur in patients with AMD. Patients using high-dose vitamin and mineral therapy may have yellowing of skin; smokers are at increased risk of lung cancer from betacarotene.

Prevention/prophylaxis: There is no specific prevention. Annual eye examinations in persons >65 years old can facilitate early detection and, in the case of wet AMD, early intervention to limit visual loss. Smokers should be encouraged to quit.

Referral: All patients >65 years old should be referred to an ophthalmologist for annual eye examination. Patients <65 years old with visual symptoms also should be referred. Patients with AMD should be referred to the local chapter of the Blind Association for services, vision enhancement devices, and support groups.

Education: Teach patients the importance of seeking evaluation for visual symptoms as soon as they occur. Explain disease process and community support services. Educate family about need for environmental safety. Caution patients to avoid unproven remedies.

CATARACTS

SIGNAL SYMPTOMS diminished vision in one or both eyes, poor night vision, sensitivity to glare

Cataract, senile	ICD-9 CM: 366.10

Description: A cataract is an opacification of the lens that interferes with the passage of light through the lens, decreasing visual acuity. The location, size, and density of this opacity influence the degree of visual impairment. Nuclear sclerotic cataracts affect contrast sensitivity, progress slowly, and tend to preserve functional reading vision while frequently causing nearsightedness. In contrast, posterior subcapsular cataracts progress more rapidly and interfere with reading vision.

Etiology: Most cataracts are related to the aging process. The gradual thickening or hardening in the lens is believed to be due to oxidative damage to the lens protein.

Occurrence: The rate of visually significant cataracts in persons <50 years old is 2% to 5%. Of persons >75 years old, 92% have some cataract changes, with 46% experiencing a significant vision loss. Cataracts tend to be bilateral, although the rate of progression varies between the eyes.

Age: Although subtle changes in visual acuity related to cataract formation occur by age 50, people >75 years old experience most visually significant cataracts.

Ethnicity: No ethnic groups are significantly more prone to cataracts.

Gender: Cataracts occur equally in men and women.

Contributing factors: Diabetes mellitus, hypertension, poor nutrition, cigarette smoking, high alcohol intake, trauma to the eye, long-term exposure to ultraviolet (UV) B radiation (sunlight), and a strong family history of cataracts are risk factors. Use of certain substances, including haloperidol, iron, and glucocorticoids, also contributes to cataracts. An association between cataracts and glaucoma and intraocular inflammation exists.

Signs and symptoms: The patient with a cataract initially may present with an improvement in near vision requiring a new prescription for corrective lenses. Patients also may experience blurred vision or sensitivity to glare from bright light or from automobile headlights during night driving. Complaints of having difficulty reading and distinguishing contrast sensitivities and of seeing a yellow tint or washed-out colors are common. Some patients may not seek evaluation of their symptoms by a health-care provider owing to denial or fear of loss of independence (driver's license being revoked), whereas other patients seek prompt assessment in the hopes of early intervention. A recent history of falls, accidents, or injury is suspicious. On physical examination, visual acuity test results are abnormal for one or both eyes (evaluate near and distance vision). Examine the eye using an opaque light for opacification of the lens. The cataract may be visible to the naked eye. The red reflex may be absent, or the cataract may appear as a black area.

Diagnostic tests: No diagnostic testing is required other than that for visual acuity and examination of the eye, unless other visual problems are suspected. Refer the patient to an ophthalmologist for complete evaluation after initial screening.

Differential diagnosis:
- Corneal scarring
- Retinal detachment
- Macular degeneration
- Chronic glaucoma
- Diabetic retinopathy

Treatment: Treatment is determined after full evaluation by the ophthalmologist. Ultimately, surgical intervention is required with extraction of the cataract and immediate implantation of a plastic intraocular lens, unless contraindicated by other disease conditions. Patients with posterior capsular opacification may require neodymium yttrium-aluminumgarnet (Nd:YAG) laser capsulotomy; this should not be performed at the same time as other cataract surgery. Collaboration with the ophthalmologist is indicated for patients with severe cardiac, respiratory, or neuromuscular conditions that may prevent the patient from lying still or supine as required during the surgery. Patients receiving anticoagulant therapy also should be managed collaboratively. The degree of visual impairment and its influence on the patient's usual daily functioning determine the timing of the surgery. Initially a conservative treatment plan may include prescription of corrective lenses and periodic re-evaluation by the ophthalmologist, coupled with a plan for environmental safety and optimization of the patient's functional abilities within his or her visual limitations. Preoperative medical clearance is required before surgery. Surgery is performed in an outpatient or short procedure unit, with the patient returning home immediately after discharge.

Follow-up: Immediate postsurgical care includes eye protection and application of topical agents prescribed by the ophthalmologist. The patient should be cautioned to avoid straining, lifting, or bending. Postoperative follow-up is usually within 48 hours. The family or healthcare team should heighten precautions for environmental safety to avoid injury. Intensive supervision of mentally compromised patients is required to prevent damage to the operative site. Future follow-up includes a re-evaluation of visual acuity, prescription of corrective lenses as indicated, and monitoring of the unaffected eye for cataract development.

Sequelae: Possible sequelae to cataract surgery include faulty wound closure with aqueous humor leakage, blindness secondary to choroidal hemorrhage, infection, inflammation, retinal detachment, prolapse of the iris into the corneal wound, and secondary glaucoma.

Prevention/prophylaxis: The patient should be protected from exposure to UV B radiation by wearing sunglasses designed for this and by wearing a hat with a wide brim.

Referral: After the initial visual screening, refer the patient to an ophthalmologist for complete examination and treatment, including post-surgery follow-up.

Education: Provide the patient with information on age-related visual changes, the importance of protecting the eyes from sunlight with UV-blocking sunglass lenses, maintaining a nutritionally balanced diet, avoiding high alcohol intake, avoiding tobacco, and having periodic eye examinations every 2 years. Instruct the patient to seek prompt evaluation of any vision changes and reassure the patient that with proper treatment cataracts do not result in permanent loss of visual acuity.

CHALAZION

SIGNAL SYMPTOMS▶ increased lacrimation with lump on eyelid

Chalazion	ICD-9 CM: 373.2

Description: A chalazion is a mass on the eyelid caused by an inflammation of a meibomian (oil-secreting) gland of the upper or lower eyelid. Meibomian glands lubricate the lid margins.

Etiology: Blockage in a duct leading to the eyelid surface from the meibomian gland or obstruction of a gland results in inflammation, the formation of a hard mass, or infection (usually from *Staphylococcus*).

Occurrence: Common.

Age: Chalazion can occur at any age.

Ethnicity: No ethnic groups are significantly more prone to chalazion.

Gender: Chalazion occurs equally in men and women.

Contributing factors: Previously unresolved blepharitis, poor hygiene, immunosuppression, and skin conditions such as acne rosacea or seborrheic dermatitis all are contributing factors to development of chalazion.

Signs and symptoms: A slow-developing painless hard mass, with inflammation of the meibomian gland and possible involvement of the surrounding tissue, characterizes chalazion. Physical examination with inversion of the eyelid reveals a red elevated mass that may become large and press against the cornea.

Diagnostic tests: None unless recurrent, then biopsy of lesion to rule out malignancy.

Differential diagnosis:

- Foreign body
- Hordeolum
- Blepharitis
- Orbital cellulitis
- Sebaceous gland carcinoma

Treatment: Warm compresses are applied to the affected eyelid for 10 minutes, four times daily, to facilitate opening and drainage. Massage of the eyelid after warm compresses may help to soften secretions. In cases of secondary infection, antibiotic eye drops may be used. Incision and drainage by an ophthalmologist may be needed if there is no resolution after 2 months.

Follow-up: See patient in 2 to 4 weeks to evaluate treatment.

Sequelae: Complete resolution may take several weeks to months; frequent recurrence may indicate underlying malignancy.

Prevention/prophylaxis: Prevention strategies include advising the patient to perform proper lid hygiene (helps prevent recurrence) by gently scrubbing lids with diluted baby shampoo daily or directly applying baby shampoo with cotton-tipped applicator, then rinsing. Frequent hand washing is advised. Warm compresses should be initiated at the first sign of eyelid irritation or if chalazion starts to return; a clean cloth should be used for each warm compress to eye.

Referral: Refer to or consult with an ophthalmologist if the patient has a visual change, eye pain, or impairment to the eye or if the chalazion does not heal spontaneously in 6 weeks, as surgical removal may be necessary.

Education: Explain the problem and treatment. Discuss prevention strategies.

CHRONIC GLAUCOMA

SIGNAL SYMPTOMS ▶ none initially; tunnel vision, night blindness, halos around lights

Glaucoma, chronic open-angle   ICD-9 CM: 365.11

Description: Chronic open-angle or primary open-angle glaucoma is an insidious disease characterized by increased intraocular pressure severe enough to damage the optic nerve. Progressive over time with a gradual visual field loss, chronic glaucoma is called the *silent blinder* because it often goes unnoticed until the later stages. Variants occur in which intraocular pressure does not increase, but the optic nerve still becomes damaged. Secondary glaucomas are the result of prior or concurrent ocular disease or trauma; they may have open angles caused by steroid-induced pressure increases.

Etiology: The etiology of chronic glaucoma is unknown, but the disease is associated with increased intraocular pressure, optic nerve degeneration, and visual field loss. This condition is believed to result from impaired outflow of aqueous humor through the trabecular network or the canal of Schlemm.

Occurrence: Prevalence of chronic glaucoma increases in persons >40 years old, approaching 3% to 4% by age 75; 80% of cases are the open-angle type. Primary open-angle glaucoma causes 15% to 20% of all blindness in the United States and is the primary cause of blindness in African-Americans.

Age: The incidence increases in persons >40 years old, with another increase in incidence in persons between ages 60 and 75. Onset is earlier in African-Americans.

Ethnicity: African-Americans are at a higher risk than the general population for developing chronic glaucoma.

Gender: Chronic glaucoma occurs equally in men and women.

Contributing factors: Risk factors include age, a positive family history, African-American ancestry, diabetes mellitus, hypertension, and myopia. Risk factors for secondary open-angle glaucoma include long-term use of topical or oral corticosteroids.

Signs and symptoms: The disease is asymptomatic in the early stages; by the time symptoms develop, significant neural damage has occurred. Eye health specialists frequently discover chronic open-angle glaucoma during routine eye examinations. Patients may present with a complaint of blurred vision, needing a change in corrective lenses, or occasionally seeing a halo around lights.

On routine vision screening, visual acuity may be normal or unchanged from previous screening; visual fields may be decreased, however. The skilled examiner may detect changes in the cup-to-disk ratio on funduscopic examination. Because it is often difficult to perform a funduscopic examination on older patients without the benefit of a mydriatic agent, referral for specialized ophthalmologic examination is prudent. The ophthalmologic examination may reveal increased intraocular pressure or signs of optic nerve damage without increased pressure.

Diagnostic tests:

Test	Results Indicating Disorder	CPT Code
Visual fields with automated perimeters	Visual loss in nasal, inferior, or superior visual fields Tunnel vision	92081
Applanation tonometry with slit-lamp examination or hand-held Tonopen	Intraocular pressure >21 mm Hg	92100 (serial)
Gonioscopy	Abnormal angle structures in anterior chamber: extremely narrow, partially or totally closed, grade 1 or 0	92020
Comprehensive eye examination including funduscopic examination	Cup-to-disk ratio of >0.3 or asymmetry of cup-to-disk ratio of ≥0.2	92004 (new patient) 92002 (established patient)

Differential diagnosis:

- Cerebral neoplasia
- Vascular occlusive disease

Treatment: Chronic open-angle glaucoma cannot be cured; the goal of treatment is to halt progression of the disease and preserve existing vision by stabilizing the intraocular pressure. Topical eye drops that reduce aqueous production or encourage outflow are the mainstays of treatment.

β-Blockers: Reduce aqueous secretion

Betaxolol (Betoptic, Betoptic S) 0.25% to 0.5%, 1 to 2 drops twice daily; cardioselective for asthma patients

Carteolol (Ocupress) 1%, 1 drop twice daily

Levobunolol (AKBeta, Betagan) 0.25% to 0.5%, 1 drop twice daily

Metipranolol (OptiPranolol) 0.3%, 1 drop twice daily

Timolol (Timoptic, Betamol) 0.25% to 0.5%, 1 drop twice daily

Timolol gel (Timoptic-XE) 0.25% to 0.5%, 1 drop daily in morning

α-Adrenergic agonist: Reduce aqueous secretion

Apraclonidine (Iopidine) 0.5% to 1%, 1 to 2 drops three times daily

Brimonidine (Alphagan) 0.2%, 1 drop two to three times daily

Sympathomimetics: Improve aqueous outflow

Dipivefrin (Propine) 0.1%, 1 drop twice daily

Epinephrine (Epifrin,Glaucon) 1% to 2%, 1 drop one to two times daily

Direct-acting and indirect-acting parasympathomimetics/miotics: Improve aqueous outflow

Pilocarpine (Adsorbocarpine, Akarpine, Isopto Carpine, Pilagan, Pilocar, Piloptic, Pilostat) 0.25% to 10%, 1 drop four times daily

Pilocarpine gel (Pilopine HS), $^1/_2$ inch at bedtime

Prostaglandin agonist: Increases uveoscleral outflow

Latanoprost (Xalatan) 0.005%, 1 drop at bedtime

Topical carbonic anhydrase inhibitors: Reduce aqueous secretion

Brinzolamide (Azopt) 1%, 1 drop three times daily

Dorzolamide (Trusopt) 2%, 1 drop three times daily

Other topical agents:

Dorzolamide/timolol combination (Cosopt), 1 drop twice daily

Oral carbonic anhydrase inhibitors: Reduce aqueous secretion

Acetazolamide (Diamox), 125 to 500 mg orally two to four times daily

Acetazolamide sustained release (Diamox Sequels), 500 mg orally twice daily

Dichlorphenamide (Daranide), 25 to 50 mg orally one to three times daily

Methazolamide (Neptazane), 25 to 50 mg orally two to three times daily

If topical ophthalmic agents do not effectively lower intraocular pressure, systemic carbonic anhydrase inhibitors are added. These also may be used before surgery to lower the intraocular pressure. If medical therapy is unsuccessful, laser trabeculoplasty or filtration surgery, to improve aqueous outflow, is indicated. The laser treatment is considered for elderly patients who cannot tolerate surgery, although the outcome is not as desirable as with surgery. In either case, medication still may be required after surgery.

Follow-up: Monitor patients for compliance with the treatment regimen. If eye drops are used, ensure that the patient can instill these, or teach a family member or neighbor to do it. Monitor medications for adverse effects; the range and frequency of side effects to glaucoma medications are significant. Ensure that patients have regular ophthalmologic follow-up visits. If visual loss is severe, evaluate the environment for safety and risk of falls or injury. If the patient is still a licensed motor vehicle operator, driver's license retesting may be indicated in the interest of public safety.

Sequelae: If initial presentation is monocular, the other eye may become affected. Changes in the patient's overall health may have implications for the treatment plan.

Prevention/prophylaxis: Educate patients about risk factors, need for eye examinations, continued monitoring, and adherence to the prescribed regimen. Asymptomatic patients may question the need for regular treatment. Also, the frequency or complexity of the medication regimen may influence compliance. African-Americans should have periodic eye examinations every 3 to 5 years, beginning at age 40. Anyone with a family history of glaucoma should have an annual eye examination, beginning at age 40. Patients with hypertension or diabetes should have regular eye examinations, as recommended by their health-care provider. All patients >65 years old should have annual eye examinations.

Referral: Refer patients initially for ophthalmologic examination and diagnosis. Collaborate on the management plan if the patient has significant medical conditions that affect treatment options, particularly pharmacologic choices. Refer patients for periodic follow-up eye examinations or for treatment of complications if they arise.

Education: Educate the patient about the chronic and progressive nature of the disease, the need to follow the treatment regimen as prescribed, and the need for regular follow-up eye examinations and reporting of symptoms, if any. Reassure the patient that although the disease is not curable, it can be managed. Educate patients with known risk factors about the need for eye examinations despite the absence of symptoms.

HEARING LOSS

SIGNAL SYMPTOMS can hear but not understand, especially in a group; turning up radio or television louder to hear (noted by family or neighbors); inability to hear in one ear; tinnitus

Presbycusis	ICD-9 CM: 388.01
Conductive	ICD-9 CM: 389.00
Sensorineural with conductive (mixed type)	ICD-9 CM: 389.2

Description: Hearing loss is the decreased ability or complete inability to hear. The loss may involve the external, middle, or inner ear and can be unilateral or bilateral.

Etiology:

Sensorineural: A lesion in the organ of Corti or in the central pathways, including the eighth nerve and auditory cortex, causes sensorineural hearing loss. Presbycusis, noise-induced hearing loss, and ototoxic drug–related hearing loss all are sensorineural.

Conductive: Conductive hearing loss is caused by a lesion involving the outer and middle ear to the level of the oval window. Various structural abnormalities, cerumen impaction, perforation of the tympanic membrane, middle ear fluid, damage to the ossicles from trauma or infection, otosclerosis, tympanosclerosis, cholesteatoma, middle ear tumors, temporal bone fractures, injuries related to trauma, and congenital problems are some of the causes.

Mixed: Mixed hearing loss includes sensorineural and conductive components.

Retrocochlear: Retrocochlear hearing loss is caused by a lesion between the cochlea and the brain, such as an acoustic neuroma or meningioma.

Occurrence: One in three people >60 years old and half of people >85 years old have hearing loss. It is the most common sensory deficit in older adults.

Age: Sensorineural hearing loss increases with age.

Ethnicity: No ethnic groups are significantly more prone to hearing loss.

Gender: Presbycusis is more severe in men than in women; this is attributed to environmental causes.

Contributing factors: Exposure to loud noises; heredity; ototoxic drugs, such as aminoglycoside antibiotics, salicylates, loop diuretics, cisplatin, and quinine; eustachian tube obstruction; chronic middle ear infections; and chronic cerumen impaction are contributing factors. Most cases of sudden unilateral hearing loss in elderly persons are due to thrombotic or embolic obstruction of the internal auditory artery.

 Clinical Pearl: Inappropriate responses or lack of response in a previously responsive person may indicate cerumen impaction.

Always examine the ears for cerumen blockage as part of the diagnostic assessment.

Signs and symptoms: The patient may complain that people mumble. There may be difficulty hearing associated with pain, pressure, discomfort, vertigo, or loss of balance. Associated symptoms may include tinnitus, dizziness, blockage, popping, pressure, crackling, trouble hearing distant sounds, or stiffness. A history of noise exposure, prior ear problems, or familial hearing problems is significant.

Otoscopic examination and inspection of the external auditory canal and middle ear may reveal redness, foreign objects, discharge, scaling, lesions, or cerumen impaction. Expect to see minimal cerumen, a pink color, and hairs in the outer third of the ear. The tympanic membrane should have no perforations and be a translucent pearly gray; changes in the tympanic membrane may be consistent with conductive hearing loss.

Diagnostic tests:

Test	Results Indicating Disorder	CPT Code
Audiometry, pure tone	Presbycusis: bilateral mild-to-moderate, high-frequency loss	92551
Rinne	Bone > air suggests conductive or mixed hearing loss	92553
Weber	Sound heard better in one ear in conductive loss (lateralizes to ear with loss) No sound in one ear in neural loss	92553
Schwabach	Compares bone conduction in patient and examiner ears. If examiner hears longer, confirms sensorineural loss in patient	
Speech audiometry: word recognition and speech reception threshold	Misinterpretation of high-pitched consonant sounds and diphthongs: s, sh, p, f, t, th, k, g	92556
CT scan of head (if lesion is suspected)	Appearance of lesion between cochlea and brain or within brain	70460 (with contrast); 70450 (without contrast)

CT, computed tomography.

Differential diagnosis:

- Ménière's disease
- Acoustic neuroma (unilateral, with tinnitus)
- Cholesteatoma (unilateral)
- Embolic or thrombotic, associated with hypertension (sudden onset, unilateral)
- Meningioma (unilateral)
- Trauma (history of ear trauma, unilateral)
- Otitis media with effusion (retracted tympanic membrane, fluid behind tympanic membrane)

- Acute otitis media (unilateral, ear pain; bulging, immobile tympanic membrane)
- Central auditory processing disorder (seen in dementia)

Treatment: Treat the cause or refer the patient as appropriate. Encouragement, follow-up, and support are important for the patient with hearing loss.

Cerumen impaction: Use a 1:1 mixture of hydrogen peroxide and mineral oil or docusate liquid (Colace). Place 3 to 5 drops in the external ear and wait 1 hour, then lavage with warm water. Alternatively, patient may be instructed to use an over-the-counter softener such as carbamide (Debrox) or trolamine polypeptide oleate-condensate (Cerumenex).

Acute otitis media: Give amoxicillin/clavulanate (Augmentin), 875 mg orally twice daily for 10 days; an analgesic such as acetaminophen or acetaminophen with codeine may be indicated for pain initially.

In the presence of *tympanic perforation, ossicle damage, tumor, tympanosclerosis, otosclerosis,* or *temporal bone injury*, refer the patient to a specialist.

Presbycusis: Educate and support the patient so that no further damage occurs. Have the patient reduce noise exposure and avoid ototoxic medications. Refer to an audiologist for hearing aid evaluation. Teach the patient lip-reading when appropriate, and instruct the family to speak clearly. Consult a telephone equipment company about the availability of special audio equipment.

Follow-up: See patients as indicated by the cause of the symptom.

Sequelae: Possible complications depend on the cause of the symptom but may include permanent hearing loss. The patient may need a hearing aid. Middle ear problems may progress to chronic ear problems, such as perforations and cholesteatoma. Social isolation and depression may result from inability to communicate.

Prevention/prophylaxis: Advise the patient to use protective devices to guard against occupational or recreational hearing loss, to equalize ear pressure when diving, to chew gum or use decongestants in airplanes, to avoid flying or diving if upper respiratory infection is present, and to avoid ototoxic medications. Teach the patient proper techniques for cerumen removal. Hearing screening tests are recommended for persons >65 years old and persons who report hearing difficulty. A screening version of the hearing handicap inventory for the elderly is also helpful.

Referral: Refer to or consult with appropriate specialist, as indicated by cause of symptom. All patients with unexplained hearing loss should have an otoscopic and audiometric evaluation.

Education: Explain cause of symptoms, measures taken to determine the cause, and symptomatic treatment if any. Advise the patient when to seek medical care. Teach the importance of using hearing aids, if indicated, because this can make a significant difference in the patient's quality of life. Advise the patient to contact rehabilitation centers to learn lip-reading skills or sign language. Provide support, and help the patient resist the temptation to withdraw socially. See References for sources of educational resource materials.

ORAL CANCER

SIGNAL SYMPTOMS nonhealing sore in the mouth or on the lip, unexplained lymph node swelling

Neoplasm oral, primary	ICD-9 CM: 145.9
Secondary	ICD-9 CM: 189.89

Description: Oral cancer is a malignant tumor of the oral squamous epithelium. The most common sites are the floor of the mouth, tongue, oropharynx, and lips. The rare tumors of the upper gingiva and hard palate are usually salivary gland adenocarcinomas.

Etiology: Oral cancers are associated with chronic irritation of the squamous epithelial lining of the oral cavity. Tobacco (cigarette, pipe, cigar) smoking, use of smokeless tobacco, and heavy alcohol use are risk factors.

Occurrence: Oral cancer accounts for 3% to 5% of the malignancies diagnosed annually in the United States. Each year, 36,000 new cases are diagnosed. In recent years, the incidence of lip cancer has declined, whereas the number of tongue cancers has increased.

Age: Oral cancers usually are found in individuals >40 years old; approximately 50% of cases are in patients >65 years old.

Ethnicity: The incidence of oral cancer is declining among white men but is increasing among African-American men and all women.

Gender: Previously men were three to four times more likely to have oral cancer, but the gap is narrowing to 2:1.

Contributing factors: Tobacco use and heavy alcohol consumption, alone or synergistically, are strongly related to the development of oral cancer. Pipe smoking and sun exposure have been implicated in lip cancer. Leukoplakia or erythroplasia are often precursors to oral cancer. Relationships between oral cancer and Epstein-Barr virus, human papillomavirus, herpes simplex virus, and immunodeficiency states also have been found. No strong association exists between irritation from dentures or teeth and oral cancers.

Signs and symptoms: Nonhealing, ulcerative lesions on the lip, tongue, or oral mucosa usually are noted first. Leukoplakia, a white patch on the mucosa that cannot be rubbed off, is the most common precancerous lesion. Erythroplasia, a nonpainful, red, velvety lesion, typically on the floor of the mouth, can be carcinoma in situ. Patients may complain that dental appliances are not fitting properly and that they have difficulty chewing. Oral pain and bleeding lesions are usually late signs of malignancy. Occasionally patients may complain of numbness in the skin around the chin when the lesion involves a nerve. Enlarged submandibular or submental lymph nodes may be found in advanced disease. Unexplained weight loss may be a late symptom.

Diagnostic tests:

Test	Results Indicating Disorder	CPT Code
Biopsy of lesion after 2 weeks nonhealing	Squamous cell carcinoma	40808–41108
Complete blood count	Anemia in late stage or nutritional deficiency	85025
Chest x-ray to evaluate for lung involvement if smoker	Lesion suggestive of carcinoma	71010–71015
RPR or VDRL if syphilis is suggested	A positive result within 7 days of testing	86592

RPR, rapid plasma reagin; VDRL, Venereal Disease Research Laboratory.

The surgeon or oncologist also may order CT or magnetic resonance imaging.

Differential diagnosis:

- Oral candidiasis (white patches are scraped off and bleed underneath)
- Melanotic macule (rare)
- Oral lichen planus (lacy white lesions on buccal mucosa)
- Oral hairy leukoplakia
- Peutz-Jeghers syndrome (multiple lentigines of oral mucosa, associated intestinal polyposis)
- Secondary syphilitic lesion (split papules at the angle of the mouth, positive RPR or VDRL)

Treatment: Surgical excision and radiation therapy depend on the size and location of the tumor and on the presence or absence of metastases. Chemotherapy is currently not a first-line therapy in oral cancers. Most oral cancers have a cure rate nearly 90% if diagnosed when the size is ≤3 cm and before metastases occurs.

Follow-up: Lifetime surveillance is recommended; second primary cancers occur in 10% to 30% of cases. During the first year, the patient should be seen frequently for focused oral examinations and to assess for recurrence of symptoms, in addition to yearly complete physical examinations. Thereafter, follow-up visits should occur as scheduled by the surgeon or oncologist.

Sequelae: Complications of oral cancer include disfigurement and xerostomia from surgery and radiation treatments, malnutrition resulting from difficulty chewing, infection, second primary cancers, or metastases to lung, regional lymph nodes, or adjacent organs. Patients with dentures may need to abstain from wearing them for 1 year when radiation is performed.

Prevention/prophylaxis: Smoking cessation, treatment for alcoholism, adequate nutrition, and yearly oral examinations can help prevent oral cancer. Edentulous patients should remove dentures for oral examination. Wearing a hat with a brim or using lip gloss with sunscreen can prevent sun exposure of lips.

Referral: Refer the patient to an oral or maxillofacial surgeon and an oncologist. Also refer patient or family to National Cancer Institute Helpline (1-800-4-CANCER) for information resources and support and a local support group if available. If nutrition is a problem, refer to a nutritionist who works with cancer patients.

Education: Teach patients about the risk factors for developing oral cancer, including smoking and chewing tobacco, alcohol abuse, and poor nutrition. Discuss strategies to help the patient deal with these issues. Advise patients to report any nonhealing oral lesion within 2 weeks of initial occurrence.

RETINOPATHY

SIGNAL SYMPTOMS▶ blurred vision, painless visual loss, poor night vision, poor color vision, floaters

Retinopathy, diabetic	ICD-9 CM: 250.5
Hypertensive	ICD-9 CM: 362.11
Arteriosclerotic	ICD-9 CM: 440.8

Description: Retinopathy, a disease of the retina, includes hypertensive; diabetic; and, less commonly in older adults, sickle cell, polycythemia vera, and infectious causes such as toxoplasmosis or cytomegalovirus in human immunodeficiency virus (HIV).

Etiology: The pathology of the retinopathy relates to the underlying cause. Systemic causes common to older adults include hypertension (arteriosclerotic retinopathy), diabetes (diabetic retinopathy), and AMD (see earlier). Hypertensive or arteriosclerotic retinopathy is related to the severity of the hypertension. Diabetic retinopathy is a highly specific vascular complication of type 1 and 2 diabetes. It is related directly to the duration of diabetes, the patient's age at onset, and glycemic control. Diabetic retinopathy is either proliferative or nonproliferative. Nonproliferative retinopathy is most common in type 2 diabetics and is characterized by dilation of veins, microaneurysms, retinal edema and hemorrhages, and hard exudates. Proliferative retinopathy is common in type 1 diabetics and includes neovascularization, vitreous hemorrhage, and retinal detachment; secondary glaucoma also can occur because of blockage of outflow channels by new vessels. Diabetic retinopathy often coexists with hypertensive retinopathy.

Occurrence: Diabetic retinopathy is the leading cause of new blindness in people 20 to 74 years old. Type 1 diabetics usually have some retinopathy present within 5 years of diagnosis; it is found in 21% of type 2 diabetics at the time of diagnosis. Diabetic retinopathy develops earlier in older patients, but proliferative retinopathy is less common. Proliferative retinopathy is more common with insulin use. Hypertensive retinopathy is seen with poorly controlled hypertension.

Age: Elderly patients are more likely to have hypertensive or diabetic retinopathy because of the increase in chronic disease with age; approximately half of all diabetes cases occur in persons >55 years old.

Ethnicity: Diabetes is more common in Native Americans, Asian-Americans, African-Americans, Hispanic Americans, and Pacific Islanders than whites. Hypertension is also more prevalent among African-Americans.

Gender: Men develop diabetic retinopathy sooner than women.

Contributing factors: Contributing factors in diabetic retinopathy include age at onset, type of diabetes, duration of disease, poor glycemic control (persistent elevated glycosolated hemoglobin), and early detection of nonproliferative (background) retinopathy. Factors for other types of retinopathy include poorly controlled hypertension and AMD.

Signs and symptoms: The presenting symptom may be the insidious painless onset of decreased visual acuity. Patients may report blurred vision, poor night vision, poor color vision, or "floaters and flashers." All patients with known diabetes or hypertension should have regular comprehensive eye examinations, including a funduscopic examination. The funduscopic changes seen in patients with hypertension include arteriolar narrowing, arteriovenous nicking, changes in arteriolar light reflex, and tortuosity of vessels. Classic nonproliferative changes in patients with diabetes are microaneurysms and hard and soft exudate. Clinical findings in patients with proliferative retinopathy are cotton-wool spots, deep hemorrhages, and neovascularization.

Diagnostic tests:

Test	Results Indicating Disorder	CPT Code
Dilated funduscopic examination and comprehensive eye examination	Microaneurysms around macula, intraretinal hemorrhages, cotton-wool spots, hard exudates. With hypertensive retinopathy, vessel tortuosity, arteriovenous nicking, soft exudates, striae hemorrhages, and papilledema may be seen. With proliferative retinopathy, all of the above plus neovascularization	92004 (new patient) 92002 (established patient)

Although not specific for the diagnosis of retinopathy, regular monitoring of hypertension and blood glucose are essential in disease management and prevention of complications.

Differential diagnosis:

- Glaucoma
- Cataracts (lens opacity visible)
- Retinal detachment
- Cytomegalovirus retinitis (usually associated with HIV)
- Toxoplasmosis (associated with latent infection)
- Retinal vasculitis (related to sarcoidosis)

Treatment: Prevention and early detection is fundamental to preserving vision. Annual ophthalmologic examinations are required. For patients with diabetes, the goal is to optimize glucose control. Patients with hypertension or hypertension and diabetes should be treated to control blood pressure (goal is 130/85 mm Hg). The parameters and goal of treatment in patients with hypertension and diabetes should be clear and concise. For patients with neovascularization or vitreous hemorrhage, laser photocoagulation surgery is the treatment of choice.

Follow-up: Follow-up depends on the findings. A retinal specialist should follow-up patients with retinopathy. The primary care provider is responsible for regular disease management. The staging of retinopathy and the treatment plan require specialty follow-up.

Sequelae: Not all retinopathy is progressive. The condition and its outcome are related to the cause of the retinopathy and the degree of successful disease management.

Prevention/prophylaxis: Elderly patients should have an annual ophthalmologic examination. During routine office visits, perform a funduscopic examination on the eyes of diabetics and hypertensives. Promptly refer the patient to a retinal specialist at the earliest report of vision change or abnormal examination findings. Patients with diabetes and hypertension should be aware of the goals of treatment and the need to control blood pressure and blood glucose. Home monitoring of blood glucose and blood pressure may be advised.

Referral: A retinal specialist should see all patients with retinopathy. All patients with diabetes and hypertension need to see an ophthalmologist annually.

Education: Patients should report any alteration in vision. Patients should know how the goals of blood pressure and blood glucose control relate to prevention of complications. Finally, patients should understand the importance of follow-up care.

RHINITIS

SIGNAL SYMPTOMS▶ rhinorrhea, sneezing, postnasal drip, nasal congestion and itching

Chronic, purulent, ulcerative, hypertrophic	ICD-9 CM: 472.0
Allergic, nonseasonal, seasonal, vasomotor	ICD-9 CM: 477.9

Description: Rhinitis is an inflammation of the nasal mucosa.

Etiology: Rhinitis may be either allergic or nonallergic. Allergic rhinitis is due to the response of the nasal mucosa to airborne allergens in atopic individuals. This response is mediated by immunoglobulin E (IgE). IgE antibodies produced in response to the initial exposure to allergens bind to the nasal mucosa. Re-exposure to the allergens causes the release of histamine, leukotrienes, and prostaglandins, which results in local vasodilation and inflammation with increased mucus production. Allergic rhinitis may be seasonal, caused by pollens from trees, flowers, or grasses pollinating in the spring or fall. Perennial allergic rhinitis often is related to environmental exposure to pollutants, animal dander, dust, molds, or cigarette smoke.

Nonallergic rhinitis is defined as episodic or persistent perennial rhinitis symptoms that are not mediated by IgE immunopathology; there are several subtypes. Atrophic nonallergic rhinitis is probably due to degeneration and atrophy of nasal membranes and bony structures. Rhinitis medicamentosa is frequently due to the overuse of topical nasal decongestants. Other drug-induced rhinitis may occur with use of angiotensin-converting enzyme inhibitors, methyldopa, β-blockers, amitriptyline, chlorpromazine, aspirin, nonsteroidal anti-inflammatory drugs, and estrogens. Hormonal rhinitis can occur with hypothyroidism (pregnancy also). Gustatory rhinitis can occur after food or alcohol ingestion and may be mediated vagally. Infectious rhinitis is usually viral and can be acute or chronic, with secondary bacterial infection. Vasomotor rhinitis encompasses a heterogeneous collection of patients with symptoms that are nonallergic, noninfectious, and without nasal eosinophilia. Environmental conditions, including temperature changes, inhaled irritants, and odors, are implicated. In nonallergic rhinitis with eosinophilia (NARES), nasal eosinophils are present with perennial symptoms and anosmia but no evidence of allergic disease on testing.

Occurrence: Allergic rhinitis occurs in 9% to 21% of the population, or >20 million people in the United States. Nonallergic rhinitis occurs in 20% to 60% of the population.

Age: Allergic rhinitis is most common between ages 10 and 39, declining after age 40. Vasomotor rhinitis is a condition of adulthood and is more common in the elderly. Atrophic rhinitis is associated with aging.

Ethnicity: No prevalence for rhinitis exists among ethnic groups.

Gender: Men and women age 40 and older have roughly the same incidence of rhinitis.

Contributing factors: Risk factors for allergic rhinitis include family history of atopy, exposure to indoor allergens such as dust mites and animals, asthma, and higher socioeconomic class. Factors that may contribute to nonallergic rhinitis including infections, anatomic abnormalities, medications (especially in the elderly), immunodeficiency, tumors of the nasopharynx and paranasal sinuses, Wegener's granulomatosis, pregnancy, hypothyroid disease, and cerebrospinal fluid leak. Strong odors or fumes, temperature or barometric pressure changes, and psychological factors can trigger vasomotor rhinitis.

Signs and symptoms: Patients with allergic rhinitis report rhinorrhea, sneezing, obstructed nasal passages, and pruritic eyes, nose, and oropharynx. There is usually a family history of allergies, with symptoms during the spring or fall. Patients with perennial allergic rhinitis have the same symptoms associated with environmental irritants. Physical examination may reveal a pale, boggy nasal mucosa, injected conjunctiva, enlarged turbinates, dark discoloration or bags under the eyes, and mouth breathing; absence of pale, boggy nasal mucosa does not rule out allergic rhinitis.

Postnasal discharge and congestion are common complaints in vasomotor rhinitis; symptoms associated with allergic rhinitis may coexist. Individuals with atrophic rhinitis report a bad taste along with congestion and thick postnasal discharge. In nonallergic rhinitis, pink-to-red, dry nasal mucosa is found on examination. History is key in establishing diagnosis; physical examination includes EENT and respiratory examinations.

Diagnostic tests:

Test	Results Indicating Disorder	CPT Code
Skin tests for common allergens (more cost-effective than in vitro tests)	Presence of specific IgE antibodies to known allergens indicates allergic rhinitis. Negative response in the presence of ongoing rhinitis symptoms suggests a nonallergic cause if other conditions have been ruled out	95004
Nasal smear for eosinophils	Eosinophils are found in a high concentration in allergic rhinitis; skin test also is positive in most cases. Eosinophils are found in NARES, but skin test is negative. No eosinophils are found in other types of nonallergic rhinitis	89190

Differential diagnosis:

- Viral or bacterial upper respiratory infection (fever, purulent discharge, headache, sore throat, acute onset)
- Sinusitis (fever, purulent discharge, headache)
- Nasal polyps (visible with nasal specula examination)

- Deviated nasal septum (visible on examination)
- Hypothyroid disease (elevated thyroid-stimulating hormone)
- Tumor (visualized on x-ray or CT scan)
- Foreign body in the nose (visible with nasal specula examination)

Treatment:

Allergic Rhinitis

Environmental control measures are the key to management of allergic rhinitis. Patients with seasonal allergies should avoid outdoor activities during peak pollen periods, from 11 AM to 3 PM. Windows should be kept closed to decrease pollen levels indoors, and HEPA filters for the home may be helpful.

Dust mite control through protective covers on mattresses and pillows, frequent bedding changes, elimination of carpeting when possible.

Keep pets out of the bedroom and house when possible.

Individualized desensitization immunotherapy after allergy testing.

Pharmacologic therapy directed at control of the symptoms: Avoid first-generation antihistamines because of safety issues related to sedating effects. Anticholinergic effects may worsen benign prostatic hypertrophy, bladder neck obstruction, and narrow-angle glaucoma.

Second-generation antihistamines:

Loratadine (Claritin), 10 mg once daily (10 mg every other day in hepatic or renal insufficiency with glomerular filtration rate <30 mL/min).

Cetirizine (Zyrtec), 10 mg once daily (5 mg once daily with hepatic or renal insufficiency).

Fexofenadine (Allegra), 180 mg once daily, 60 mg twice daily (60 mg once daily with decreased renal function).

Azelastine (Astelin) nasal spray, 2 sprays each nostril twice daily.

Intranasal corticosteroids:

Budesonide (Rhinocort), 2 sprays each nostril twice daily.

Flunisolide (Nasarel, Nasalide), 2 sprays each nostril twice daily.

Fluticasone propionate (Flonase), 2 sprays each nostril once daily or 1 spray each nostril twice daily.

Mometasone furoate (Nasonex), 2 sprays each nostril once daily.

Triamcinolone acetonide (Nasacort), 2 sprays each nostril once daily.

Nonallergic Rhinitis

Avoid known irritants.

Nasal corticosteroids (see earlier) for NARES.

Nasal corticosteroids and elimination of topical decongestant sprays in rhinitis medicamentosa.

Ipratropium bromide(Atrovent) nasal spray 0.03%, 0.06%, 2 sprays each nostril two to four times daily, is an anticholinergic for local control of rhinorrhea.

Pseudoephedrine, 30 to 60 mg orally every 4 hours, a decongestant, decreases nasal mucosa swelling, but has little effect on other rhinitis symptoms; it is best used briefly and intermittently because of central nervous system side effects. It is contraindicated in elderly patients with poorly controlled hypertension, coronary artery disease, and a history of cerebrovascular accident.

Oral corticosteroids are recommended only for severe nasal obstruction, such as that caused by rebound rhinitis or nasal polyps; individualize dosing.

Follow-up: Have the patient return in 2 to 3 weeks to review response to medications and understanding of management and prevention.

Sequelae: Epistaxis and sinusitis are complications of rhinitis.

Prevention/prophylaxis: Teach patients to avoid irritants and to try to control environmental risk factors. Discuss the need to take antihistamines or use nasal sprays before exposure to irritants, to prevent symptoms.

Referral: When symptoms persist or worsen, refer the patient to an ENT specialist or allergist. Patients with comorbid conditions that affect treatment, patients who experience complications, and patients requiring oral corticosteroids or immunotherapy should be referred to an ENT specialist or allergist.

Education: Discuss environmental control and avoidance of known triggers. Avoid the use of over-the-counter nasal sprays for more than 3 consecutive days. Check with provider before taking any over-the-counter remedies, especially if on other medications.

REFERENCES

General

Beers, MH, and Berkow, R (eds): The Merck Manual of Geriatrics, ed 3. Merck Research Laboratories, Whitehouse Station, N.J., 2000.

Clinical Evidence: Issue 6. BMJ Publishing Group, London, 2001.

DeGowin, RL, and Brown, DD: DeGowin's Diagnostic Examination, ed 7. McGraw-Hill, New York, 2000.

Gallo, JJ, et al: Handbook of Geriatric Assessment, ed 3. Aspen Publishers, Gaithersburg, Md., 2000.

Gorroll, AH, and Mulley, AG: (eds.). Primary Care Medicine: Office Evaluation and Management of the Adult Patient, ed 4. Lippincott Williams & Wilkins, Philadelphia, 2000.

Molony, SL, et al: Gerontological Nursing: An Advanced Practice Approach. Appleton & Lange, Stamford, Conn., 1999.

Noble, J (ed): Textbook of Primary Care Medicine, ed 3. Mosby, St. Louis, 2000.

Pagana, KD, and Pagana, JT: Mosby's Diagnostic and Laboratory Test Reference, ed 5. Mosby, St. Louis, 2001.

Rakel, RE: Textbook of Family Practice, ed 6. WB Saunders, Philadelphia, 2001.

Reuben, DB, et al: Geriatrics at Your Fingertips: 2001 edition. Excerpta Medica, for the American Geriatrics Society, Belle Mead, N.J., 2001.

Seller, RH: Differential Diagnosis of Common Complaints, ed 4.WB Saunders, Philadelphia, 2000.

Stone, JT, et al: Clinical Gerontological Nursing: A Guide to Advanced Practice, ed 2. WB Saunders, Philadelphia, 1999.

Tallis, R, et al (eds): Brocklehurst's Textbook of Geriatric Medicine and Gerontology, ed 5. Churchill Livingstone, London, 1998.

Tierney, LM, et al (eds): Current Medical Diagnosis and Treatment 2001. Lange Medical Books/McGraw-Hill, New York, 2001.

Acute and Chronic Glaucoma

American Academy of Ophthalmology: Primary angle closure: complete summary. Contact: http://www.ngc.gov. Accessed February 2, 2002.

Beers, MH, and Berkow, R (eds): Glaucoma. In: The Merck Manual of Geriatrics, ed 3. Merck Research Laboratories, Whitehouse Station, N.J., 2000, p 1295.

Lesser, GR, et al: Glaucoma. In Noble, J (ed): Textbook of Primary Care Medicine, ed 3. Mosby, St. Louis, 2000, p 1663.

Lewis, PR, et al: Topical therapies for glaucoma: What family physicians need to know. Am Fam Physician 59:1871, 1999.

Reuben, DB, et al: Visual impairment. In: Geriatrics at Your Fingertips: 2001 edition. Excerpta Medica, for the American Geriatrics Society, Belle Mead, N.J., 2001, p 145.

Richter, CU: Management of glaucoma. In Gorroll, AH, and Mulley, AG (eds): Primary Care Medicine: Office Evaluation and Management of the Adult Patient, ed 4. Lippincott Williams & Wilkins, Philadelphia, 2000, p 1096.

Surgical Treatment of Coexisting Cataract and Glaucoma. Summary, Evidence Report/Technology Assessment: Number 38. AHRQ Publication No. 01-E049. Agency for Healthcare Research and Quality, Rockville, Md., 2001. Contact: http://www.ahrq.gov/clinic/epcsums/catarsum.htm.

Age-Related Macular Degeneration

American Academy of Ophthalmology: Age-Related Macular Degeneration. 2001. Contact: http://www.ngc.gov/FRAMESETS/guideline_fs.asp?view=full_summaryandguideline=002314andsynthesis_filename=andurl=andhidden=trueandsSearch_string=Age%2Drelated+macular+degeneration. Accessed March 6, 2002.

American Optometric Association: Care of the patient with age-related macular degeneration. 1997. Contact: http://www.ngc.gov/FRAMESETS/guideline_fs.asp?guideline=001215andsSearch_string=Age%2Drelated+macular+degeneration. Accessed February 2, 2002.

Beers, MH, and Berkow, R (eds): Age-related maculopathy. In: The Merck Manual of Geriatrics, ed 3. Merck Research Laboratories, Whitehouse Station, N.J., 2000, p 1304.

Fong, DS: Age-related macular degeneration: Update for primary care. Am Fam Physician 61:3035, 2000.

Gorroll, AH, and Mulley, AG (eds): Management of the patient with age-related macular degeneration. In: Primary Care Medicine: Office Evaluation and Management of the Adult Patient, ed 4. Lippincott Williams & Wilkins, Philadelphia, 2000, p 1094.

Tierney, LM, et al (eds): Age-related macular degeneration. In: Current Medical Diagnosis and Treatment 2001. Lange Medical Books/McGraw-Hill, New York, 2001, p 200.

Quillen, DA: Common causes of vision loss in elderly patients. Am Fam Physician 60:99, 1999.

Wormald, R, et al: Photodynamic therapy for neovascular age-related macular degeneration. Cochrane Review. In: The Cochrane Library, 1. Oxford: Update Software, Oxford, 2002. Contact: http://www.medscape.com/viewarticle/422494. Accessed February 10, 2002.

Contact: http://www.eri.harvard.edu/Documentation/md.html.

Contact: http://www.eyesight.org/.

Contact: http://www.macular.org/.

Contact: http://www.macular-degeneration.org/.

Contact: http://www.nei.nih.gov/publications/armd-p.htm.

Contact: http://www.ngc.gov.

Contact: http://www.southeasterneyecenter.com/visudyne_therapy_faq.html.

Contact: www.visudyne.com.

Cataracts

Agency for Healthcare Research and Quality, Rockville, Md., 2001. Contact: http://www.ahrq.gov/clinic/epcsums/catarsum.htm.

American Academy of Ophthalmology: Cataract in the adult eye. 2001. Contact: http://www.ngc.gov/FRAMESETS/guideline_fs.asp?view=full_summaryandguideline=002313andsynthesis_filename=andurl=andhidden=true andsSearch_string=Cataract. Accessed March 6, 2002.

Beers, MH, and Berkow, R (eds): Cataract. In: The Merck Manual of Geriatrics, ed 3. Merck Research Laboratories, Whitehouse Station, N.J., 2000, p 1293.

Quillen, DA: Common causes of vision loss in elderly patients. Am Fam Physician 60:99, 1999.

Schein, OD, et al: The value of routine preoperative medical testing before cataract surgery. N Engl J Med 342:168, 2000.

Surgical Treatment of Coexisting Cataract and Glaucoma. Summary, Evidence Report/Technology Assessment: Number 38. AHRQ Publication No. 01-E049, 2000.

Chalazion

Beers, MH, and Berkow, R (eds): Chalazion. In: The Merck Manual of Geriatrics, ed 3. Merck Research Laboratories, Whitehouse Station, N.J., 2000, p 1311.

Carter, SR: Eyelid disorders: Diagnosis and management. Am Fam Physician 57: 2695, 1998. Contact: http://www.aafp.org/afp/980600ap/carter.html. Accessed January 30, 2002.

Rakel, RE: Chalazion. In: Textbook of Family Practice, ed 6. WB Saunders, Philadelphia, 2001, p 1319.

Tierney, LM, et al (eds): Chalazion. In: Current Medical Diagnosis and Treatment 2001. Lange Medical Books/McGraw-Hill, New York, 2001, p 190.

Contact: http://www.southeasterneyecenter.com/visudyne_therapy_faq.html.

Contact: www.visudyne.com.

Contact: http://www.macular.org/.

Contact: http://www.eri.harvard.edu/Documentation/md.html.

Contact: http://www.eyesight.org/.

Contact: http://www.macular-degeneration.org/.

Contact: http://www.nei.nih.gov/publications/armd-p.htm.

Contact: http://www.glaucomaassociates.com/tests.html.

Hearing Loss

Guyla, AJ: Evaluation of hearing loss. In Gorroll, AH, and Mulley, AG (eds): Primary Care Medicine: Office Evaluation and Management of the Adult Patient, ed 4. Lippincott Williams & Wilkins, Philadelphia, 2000, p 1108.

Jackler, RK, and Kaplan, MJ: Ear, nose, and throat. Tierney, LM, et al (eds): Chalazion. In: Current Medical Diagnosis and Treatment 2001. Lange Medical Books/McGraw-Hill, New York, 2001, p 217.

O'Handley, JG, et al: Otolaryngology. In Rakel, RE (ed): Textbook of Family Practice, ed 6. WB Saunders, Philadelphia, 2001.

American Speech-Language-Hearing Association, 10801 Rockville Pike, Rockville MD 20852; 800-638-8255; website: http://www.asha.org/.

American Tinnitus Association (ATA), PO Box 5, Portland OR 97207; 503-248-9985; website: http://www.ata.org/.

Better Hearing Institute, PO Box 1840, Washington DC 20013; 800-327-9355; website: http://www.betterhearing.org/.

Hearing Aid Helpline, 20361 Middlebelt Road, Livonia MI 48152; 800-521-5247.

National Institute on Deafness and Other Communication Disorders, Clearinghouse Information Office, 9000 Rockville Pike, Bethesda MD 20892; 301-496-7243; website: http://www.nidcd.nih.gov; http://www.nidcd.nih.gov/health/pubs_hb/older.htm.

Oral Cancer

Kelly, JP: Screening for oral cancer. In Gorroll, AH, and Mulley, AG (eds): Primary Care Medicine: Office Evaluation and Management of the Adult Patient, ed 4. Lippincott Williams & Wilkins, Philadelphia, 2000, p 1106.

Kraus, DH, and Pfister, DG: Head and neck oncology. In Noble, J (ed): Textbook of Primary Care Medicine, ed 3. Mosby, St Louis, 2000, p 1173.

Contact: www.nci.nih.gov/cancer.

Retinopathy

Desai, UR, and Nussbaum, JJ: Retinal and choroidal diseases. In Noble, J (ed): Textbook of Primary Care Medicine, ed 3. Mosby, St Louis, 2000, p 1699.

Diabetic retinopathy: American Diabetes Association position statement. Diabetes Care 25(Suppl 1), 2002.

Doram, K, and Mishriki, Y: Primary care of the eye. In Noble, J (ed): Textbook of Primary Care Medicine, ed 3. Mosby, St Louis, 2000, p 1652.

Richter, CU: Management of diabetic retinopathy. In Gorroll, AH, and Mulley, AG (eds): Primary Care Medicine: Office Evaluation and Management of the Adult Patient, ed 4. Lippincott Williams & Wilkins, Philadelphia, 2000, p 1100.

Skyler, JS, and Hirch, IB: Diabetes mellitus. In Noble, J (ed): Textbook of Primary Care Medicine, ed 3. Mosby, St Louis, 2000, p 836.

Rhinitis

Dykewicz, MS, et al: Joint task force algorithm and annotations for diagnosis and management of rhinitis. 1998. Contact:http://www.jcaai.org/param/rhinitis/summary_statements.htm. Accessed February 10, 2002.

Dykewicz, MS, et al: Joint task force summary statements on diagnosis and management of rhinitis. Contact: http://www.jcaai.org/param/rhinitis/algorithm.htm. Accessed February 10, 2002.

Guzman, SE, in consultation with Fagnan, IJ, and Lanier, B: (2001). Diagnosis and management of allergic rhinitis. American Family Practice Monograph #3. American Academy of Family Physicians, Leawood, Kansas, 2001.

Chapter *5*
CHEST DISORDERS

CARDIAC DISORDERS

ARRHYTHMIAS

SIGNAL SYMPTOMS▶ may be absent; palpitations, symptoms of heart failure

Arrhythmias	ICD 9: 427.9
Bigeminal rhythm, bradycardia, coronary sinus, ectopic	ICD-9: 427.89
Block	ICD-9: 426.9
Contractions (premature)	ICD-9: 427.60
Extrasystolic	ICD-9: 427.60
Psychogenic	ICD-9: 306.2
Vagal	ICD-9: 780.2

Description: An arrhythmia is a disturbance of cardiac rhythm. Cardiac arrhythmias, which occur in the presence or absence of underlying heart disease, may be life-threatening or be an incidental finding. Arrhythmias may be differentiated by type or mechanism. Atrial fibrillation is the most common sustained rhythm disorder. Other prevalent forms of arrhythmias in a geriatric population are as follows:

Sick sinus syndrome: (1) Pathologic bradyarrhythmia with an alternating supraventricular tachyarrhythmia (bradycardia-tachycardia syndrome). (2) Supraventricular tachyarrhythmia—three primary categories.

Arrhythmias primarily of atrial origin: Atrial premature beats, ectopic atrial rhythms, multifocal atrial tachycardia, atrial flutter, and atrial fibrillation.

Arrhythmias arising primarily within the atrioventricular (AV) node: AV nodal reentrant tachycardia, junctional premature beats, and nonparoxysmal junctional tachycardia.

Arrhythmias partially supraventricular in origin: Pre-excitation syndomes.

Ventricular arrhythmias: Ventricular ectopic beats the most common variety.

Etiology: Most arrhythmias are thought to be caused by abnormalities in impulse formation (disordered automaticity or triggered mechanism) or in impulse conduction (allowing reentry) or by a combination. Increased automaticity is an accentuation of the inherent ability of many cardiac tissues to generate an independent rhythm. Reentry consists of a wave of excitation repeatedly circulating around a fixed anatomic obstacle. Triggered arrhythmias are caused by altered cellular depolarization.

Occurrence: Studies show that asymptomatic older patients with no known structural heart disease have an incidence of 40% of sinus arrhythmia, supraventricular or ventricular premature beats, or supraventricular tachycardia.

Age: The prevalence of ventricular arrhythmia increases with age, occurring in 80% of healthy older adults age 60 to 85. Atrial fibrillation is diagnosed in 4.8% of women and 6.2% of men >65 years old at baseline examination, and its prevalence increases to 10% in adults >80 years old. Although no specific data are available, the incidence of junctional arrhythmias and tachycardias related to the accessory pathway may be lower in elderly individuals because of an age-related reduction in accessory pathway conduction.

Ethnicity: Not available.

Gender: Arrhythmias occur more often in men than in women. (See under Age.)

Contributing factors: Preexisting heart disease and hypertension are contributing factors to arrhythmias, with structural disease becoming more prevalent with age. Fibrosis or calcification in the vicinity of the AV node causes conduction disturbances. Atrial arrhythmias may be caused by a mechanical obstruction to atrial emptying with subsequent left atrial dilation, myocardial ischemia, and increased sympathetic activity.

An age-related factor associated with tachyarrhythmias is increased left atrial size. This enlargement may contribute to the increase in supraventricular ectopy. Increases in ventricular ectopic beats may be related to left ventricular enlargement. The overload of ionized calcium in the older myocardium may contribute to ectopy. Age-related factors associated with bradyarrhythmias include an age-related decline in the number of pacemaker cells and presence of fat deposits around the sinoatrial node. His bundle cells are replaced with fibrous tissue, and adipose tissue and amyloid are deposited; this is also associated with conduction disturbance.

Systemic diseases (i.e., thyrotoxicosis, infection, hypoxemia, hypercapnia) can cause circulatory disturbances that may provoke an arrhythmia. Drugs that can cause an arrhythmia include digitalis and other antiarrhythmics, aminophylline, antihistamines, antipsychotics, macrolide antibiotics, and alcohol. Electrolyte disturbances, particularly hyperkalemia, hypokalemia, hypercalcemia, and hypocalcemia, can precipitate ectopic beats. Family history of sudden cardiac death may indicate a predisposing factor for rhythm disorder, such as hypertrophic obstructive cardiomyopathy, congenital prolonged QT syndrome, or presence of an aberrant conduction pathway.

Signs and symptoms: The history, physical examination, and electrocardiogram (ECG) represent the cornerstone to evaluation of arrhythmias. Arrhythmias may or may not cause symptoms. If they occur, symptoms are often due to a reduced blood flow or inadequate cardiac pump function. In the history, the patient may describe sensations that accompany abnormal cardiac rhythm, such as pounding, racing, or skipped beats. Other associated, although less common, symptoms may include shortness of breath, chest pain, or fatigue. Syncope or near-syncope may be experienced. Older adults are less likely to complain of palpitations and more likely to present with manifestations of heart failure or hypoperfusion (i.e., impaired mental function, dizziness, syncope). Along with the history of present illness, previous diagnosis and treatment for arrhythmia and cardiac disease should be elicited. Arrhythmias also may occur in response to reperfusion after thrombolytic therapy; electrolyte imbalance; hypoxic episodes; drug toxicity; and respiratory, endocrine, or metabolic disorders; a review of these systems and all prescribed and over-the-counter medications is in order.

In the physical examination, concentrate on the cardiac and peripheral vascular systems to determine the hemodynamic significance of an arrhythmia. Obtain the blood pressure reading, then check the pulses for 1 full minute to determine rate and regularity. Assess normal and extra heart sounds. S_1 intensity may provide information about the relation of atrial to ventricular contraction. The longer the PR interval, the softer the S_1. Note intermittent extra heart sounds (S_3 and S_4). The jugular vein must be assessed. In AV dissociation (when the atria and ventricles contract independently), giant A waves (cannon waves) may be observed—however, their absence does not rule out the presence of AV dissociation. Provoking maneuvers should not be attempted by the advanced practice nurse but may be attempted by a cardiologist. These maneuvers include carotid massage (for atrial arrhythmias only), mild exercise, psychological stress, pharmacological stress, and electrical programmed stimulation. Other indicators of hemodynamic response to an arrhythmia include level of consciousness and skin temperature and color. The history should guide the remainder of the episodic examination because it is also helpful in identifying the contributing factors that may precipitate or aggravate an arrrhythmia.

Diagnostic testing:

Test	Results Indicating Disorder	CPT Code
Rhythm strip 12-Lead ECG	Rhythm disturbance may be present, or if transient it may be absent Acute MI or ischemia, prolonged QT intervals, and pre-excitation may be identified as precipitators of an arrhythmia	93042 (evaluation) 93041 (tracing) 93040 (evaluation and tracing)
Ambulatory ECG monitoring	Quantifies arrhythmias with reference to symptoms Identifies patients at risk for sudden death by documenting ventricular arrhythmias and heart rate variability	93224–93237
Implantable loop recorder	In infrequent syncope this long-term device (14 months) may identify the precipitant	93727
Echocardiogram	Identifies structural, functional, and hemodynamic abnormalities in the cardiovascular system	93320–93350
Cardiac electrophysiological study	Evaluates specific arrhythmias to distinguish these, determine location and characteristics, and guide therapy	93600–93660
ICD	ICD firings may be due to recurrent arrhythmia	33240, 33245–33249
Electrolyte panel	Identify electrolyte disturbance (i.e., hypokalemia, hyperkalemia, hypomagnesemia, hypocalcemia) that may be causative or contributory	80051

MI, myocardial infarction; ICD, implantable cardioverter defibrillator.

Differential diagnosis: Clarify the diagnosis with precision. Note reversible and precipitating causes of an arrhythmia and coexisting diseases.

Treatment: The incidence of asymptomatic arrhythmias of questionable clinical significance is high. Arrhythmias are never treated in isolation; some are benign, and some are lethal. Patients with hemodynamic compromise resulting from arrhythmia need to be hospitalized as soon as possible. Prehospital care for threatening hemodynamic instability secondary to tachyarrhythmia may include direct current cardioversion, and the nurse practitioner should be skilled in this intervention. After thorough investigation, the goals of arrhythmia treatment include the alleviation of bothersome symptoms, the prevention of complications from sustained arrhythmias, and the avoidance of sudden death associated with certain arrhythmias.

The risk of treatment is considerable. Aggressive therapeutic treatment is indicated when patients are symptomatic, and the urgency of therapy depends on the associated hemodynamic disturbance.

Three major factors determine how well a patient tolerates an arrhythmia: heart rate, duration of the arrhythmia, and presence and severity of associated underlying heart disease. Arrhythmias often cannot be controlled unless underlying cardiac problems are discovered and treated. Antiarrhythmic drugs can reduce as well as increase cardiac arrhythmia. In addition, bothersome and potentially dangerous side effects necessitate precise indications and use of the utmost caution. Pharmaceutical agent selection is based on the electrophysiology of the rhythm disturbance, the mechanism of action, and the side effects of the drug. Drugs can only suppress arrhythmias; they do not cure or eliminate them. Conditions common in the elderly that can affect the choice, dosing, efficacy, and safety of antiarrhythmic therapy include decreased hepatic or renal function, decreased serum albumin levels, and electrolyte abnormalities.

The broad categories of arrhythmia treatment include medications, pacemakers, antitachycardia devices, ICDs, catheter ablative procedures, and certain surgical procedures. These interventions are often used in combination. At times, specific maneuvers may be attempted. Vagal maneuvers (carotid massage or the Valsalva maneuver) may terminate or slow AV nodal reentry or AV reentry types. These maneuvers are associated with high risk of emboli dislodgment. The carotid arteries should be assessed for bruit before administering massage. Because of the high mortality associated with antiarrhythmic surgery, this is not recommended in elderly individuals. The specifics of treatment are not detailed in this text because all assessment and management must be done in close collaboration with a physician; much of the treatment is initiated by the specialist in the hospital setting.

Follow-up: Because of their low therapeutic ratio, drug dosing and plasma concentrations of the antiarrhythmics are based on therapeutic monitoring. Side effects are significant, including the negative inotropic effect, which can precipitate heart failure or proarrhythmia in the presence of structural heart disease. Extracardiac side effects also can be significant, including anticholinergic effects, gastrointestinal effects, and neurologic toxicity with some antiarrhythmic agents. Monitor patients after pacemaker insertion with regular follow-up appointments and ECG testing, specifically looking for pacemaker failure, infection, thromboembolism, perforation or dislodgment, and complicating arrhythmias.

Sequelae: Regardless of age, the nature and severity of underlying heart disease are of much greater prognostic significance than the arrhythmia alone. The following rhythm disturbances have been reported to carry a poor prognosis in patients with coronary artery disease: frequent ventricular premature contractions (>10/min), multiform ventricular premature contractions, ventricular couplets, R-on-T phenomenon, and ventricular tachycardia.

Syncope can occur secondary to asystole. Bradycardia can contribute to complete heart block and to the development of heart failure in patients with associated ventricular dysfunction. Tachycardia can precipitate angina and circulatory arrest in patients with coronary artery disease. Bradyarrhythmias or tachyarrhythmias can cause systemic embolism and stroke. Atrial fibrillation can result in heart failure and a low cardiac output state. The risk of stroke related to atrial fibrillation increases with age.

The Cardiac Arrhythmia Suppression Trial (CAST) showed that patients treated for prognostically significant arrhythmias may have a higher mortality from sudden cardiac death if class IC (flecainide and encainide) agents are used (Greenberg et al, 1995). The risk of sudden death is significantly greater in patients with left ventricular hypertrophy.

Prevention/prophylaxis: All patients with atrial fibrillation should be considered for long-term low-intensity warfarin therapy. Aspirin, although less effective in preventing stroke, is an alternative for some patients in whom warfarin is contraindicated. Electrolyte imbalances should be monitored, and metabolic disturbances should be treated. Patients receiving digitalis should be monitored for toxicity.

Referral: All patients with treatable arrhythmias require collaborative management. Clinically significant ventricular arrhythmias or any symptomatic arrhythmia is managed by the specialist. A primary care physician may handle many atrial arrhythmias and low-grade ventricular arrhythmias; however, a specialist should be consulted for all clinically significant ventricular arrhythmias, arrhythmias resistant to routine therapy, or arrhythmias whose clinical significance is in doubt.

Education: Carefully instruct all patients receiving antiarrhythmics about the therapeutic effects, side effects, and potentially adverse effects of these medications. Because patients with pacemakers are vulnerable to external electrical fields, they should be instructed to recognize this potential and avoid exposure. Patients with pacemakers also must be aware of signs and symptoms of pacemaker failure.

HEART FAILURE

SIGNAL SYMPTOMS▶ dyspnea, nocturia, weakness

Heart failure	ICD 9: 428
Congestive heart failure	ICD-9: 428.0
Left heart failure	ICD-9: 428.1
Heart failure, unspecified	ICD-9: 428.9

Description: Heart failure is a syndrome in which the heart cannot pump an adequate supply of blood, in relation to venous return, to meet the metabolic needs of the tissues.

Etiology: Causes of acute and chronic heart failure in elderly individuals are essentially the same as those in the general adult population. Most patients with heart failure have coronary artery disease, chronic hypertension, or both. Common causes of heart failure in elderly adults include coronary artery disease, ischemic heart disease (IHD), aortic stenosis, mitral regurgitation, diastolic dysfunction, metabolic disorders such as diabetes or hyperthyroidism, arrhythmias, and fluid overload.

Distinction is made between systolic and diastolic dysfunction. Systolic dysfunction relates to the inability of the heart to contract normally and expel sufficient blood, whereas diastolic dysfunction is related to the heart's inability to relax and fill normally.

Occurrence: Of Americans, >4.7 million have heart failure, with an additional 500,000 new cases diagnosed each year. Systolic heart failure is the most common form with about two thirds of patients experiencing this form. Heart failure affects 10% of the population >70 years old and is the most common diagnosis in that group. Of patients with heart failure, 50% die within 5 years of the onset of symptoms.

Age: The average annual incidence for development of the first clinical evidence of heart failure in men and women increases more than four-fold from age 45 to 54 to age 65 to 74. Age is a significant independent risk factor for heart failure. Older adults increasingly are presenting with diastolic failure with preserved systolic function.

Gender: Postmenopausal women have an increased risk of cardiovascular disease, which can lead to heart failure. At present, women account for 50% of patients with heart failure.

Ethnicity: African-Americans have higher rates of heart failure discharges, perhaps from the higher prevalence of hypertension and dilated cardiomyopathy found in this group. No reports have been published on the prevalence of heart failure that are generalizable to a racially mixed population of older people.

Contributing factors: Aging is associated with changes in the heart and vasculature that may cause or exacerbate heart failure. As the heart begins to fail, the body compensates for impaired circulation in three ways: sympathetic nervous system stimulation resulting in a decrease in circulating neurohormones, activation of the renin-angiotensin-aldosterone system, and ventricular remodeling. These same mechanisms that help to preserve cardiac output initially eventually contribute to deterioration of myocardial function. Other contributing factors for heart failure include risk factors for heart disease in general, including hypertension, diabetes, smoking, obesity, hyperlipidemia, and elevated homocysteine levels.

Signs and symptoms: Initial symptoms of left-sided heart failure (left ventricular failure) are related to increased pulmonary pressures and pulmonary congestion. These include paroxysmal nocturnal dyspnea, orthopnea, dyspnea on exertion, decreased exercise tolerance, fatigue and weakness, and dry, hacking cough (especially when lying down). Signs may include extra heart sounds (S_3, S_4) and crackles in the lung bases. Because the two pumps of the heart form a circuit, eventually left-sided failure results in increased hydrostatic pressure on the right side. These signs include lower extremity swelling with weight gain, abdominal discomfort associated with ascites or hepatic engorgement, and neck vein distention. In elderly persons, the presenting symptoms of heart failure may be distorted by comorbid conditions, and dyspnea may not be experienced when the patient's physical activity is limited.

 Clinical Pearl: Because of a sedentary lifestyle, many elderly patients with heart failure may not experience progressive exertional dyspnea.

Instead of the classic dyspnea seen in younger patients, lethargy, fatigue, or restlessness may prevail. The decrease in peripheral perfusion may present as acute confusion or a cerebrovascular accident. The degree of functional impairment experienced by the patient with heart failure is an important parameter to be assessed initially and periodically. The New York Heart Association (NYHA) functional classification system is used most commonly.

Diagnostic tests:

Test	Results Indicating Disorder	CPT Code
CBC	Anemia/secondary polycythemia suggests alternative or additional diagnosis	85031
Electrolytes	Determine comorbidity (i.e., diabetes) and monitor treatment of heart failure	80051
BUN, creatinine	Nephritic syndrome may worsen volume overload	84520, 82565
Albumin	Hypoalbuminemia may worsen volume overload	82040
Liver function	Hepatic disease as component of heart failure or comorbid condition	80076
Thyroid levels (thyroxine, thyroid-stimulating hormone)	Thyroid disease may aggravate heart failure symptoms	84436, 84443
ECG	Presence of acute ischemic events, arrhythmias, medication effects, changes from old ECG results, and ventricular hypertrophy	93000
Chest x-ray	Pulmonary congestion and cardiac enlargement	71030
Echocardiogram	Differentiate between systolic and diastolic dysfunction, evaluation of heart wall motion, observation of pericardial effusions, measurement of the ejection fraction, determine valvular lesions	93303
Stress testing	May help show ischemia and underlying coronary artery disease	93015–93024
Cardiac catheterization	At times necessary to determine the severity of myocardial dysfunction and valvular lesions, assessment of heart pressures, and the presence of coronary artery disease	93526–93529

CBC, complete blood count; BUN, blood urea nitrogen.

Differential diagnosis: Heart failure is diagnosed based on a variable constellation of signs and symptoms. Misdiagnosis is common, particularly when the presentation is atypical. Dyspnea, the primary symptom of heart failure, can be caused by other conditions, including obstructive airway disease, parenchymal lung disease, pulmonary emboli, chest wall or respiratory muscle disease, heart disease, deconditioning, renal failure, anemia, abdominal masses, and anxiety neurosis. The primary care provider needs to differentiate if the dysfunction is systolic or diastolic or both by measuring the left ventricular ejection fraction by echocardiogram.

Treatment: Correction of the reversible causative factors and concomitant conditions is the primary therapy in heart failure. When heart failure develops, current pharmacological interventions are directed at the hemodynamic and the neurohormonal abnormalities. Diuretics are used to reduce volume overload and high ventricular filling pressures in systolic and diastolic failure. Use caution with diuresis in diastolic dysfunction because overdiuresis may increase symptoms of heart failure. Hydrochlorothiazide (usually 25 mg daily) is useful for patients with mild-to-moderate heart failure without severe renal impairment. Metolazone (2.5–5 mg daily), a thiazide-like agent, is a long-acting diuretic. Loop diuretics, such as furosemide (Lasix), are more potent than thiazide diuretics. Elderly patients should be started on 10 mg of furosemide daily initially. The usual maintenance dose is 40 mg daily but can be increased to 160 mg daily if necessary to achieve diuresis. Hospitalized patients with severe volume overload may require doses of intravenous furosemide, 240 mg twice daily, to obtain brisk diuresis. Bumetanide is 40 times more potent than furosemide and is less ototoxic, but some patients develop myalgias with it. Torsemide may be advantageous because absorption is unimpaired and the response is less variable than the other loop diuretics. For refractory volume overload, combination diuretic use may be effective. Spironolactone, in addition to a loop diuretic, has been associated with an improvement in diuretic response.

All patients with heart failure should be given angiotensin-converting enzyme (ACE) inhibitors unless the following contraindications are present: renal insufficiency (serum creatinine ≥ 3 mg/dL) or hyperkalemia (>5.5 mEq/L). For patients who develop hypotension (systolic pressure <90 mm Hg), decrease the diuretic first, then add the ACE inhibitor if blood pressure stabilizes. ACE inhibitor dosing in elderly patients is controversial. Several ACE inhibitors are approved for use in the United States. All should be started at low doses (captopril, 6.25–12.5 mg three times daily; enalapril, 2.5–5 mg twice daily; lisinopril, 2.5 mg once daily) and increased gradually to achieve target doses (captopril, 50 mg three times daily; enalapril, 20 mg daily; lisinopril, 10 mg daily) as tolerated, while monitoring closely blood pressure, renal function, potassium levels, and intractable cough. Ramipril, another ACE inhibitor, in the

HOPE study showed a reduced risk of death, stroke, and cardiac arrest. Patients who do not tolerate ACE inhibitors can be treated with an angiotensin II receptor blocker, such as losartan (although it is a less effective treatment) or vasodilators, such as hydralazine and isosorbide dinitrate.

β-Blocker therapy (carvedilol, metoprolol) has shown reduced morbidity and mortality and hospitalizations in patients with mild-to-moderate heart failure, but the elderly in particular need to be carefully evaluated clinically for worsening of volume status and side effects. Use of digoxin for patients in heart failure is controversial, although it is indicated sometimes for patients who persist with symptoms despite diuretics, ACE inhibitors, and β-blockers. It remains a risky drug to use, however. The pharmacokinetics of digoxin are altered in elderly adults because of reduced lean body mass and altered creatinine clearance. Patients with reduced renal function should be started on 0.125 mg daily or lower and titrated to an adequate serum digoxin level. Digitalis toxicity may occur at therapeutic serum levels in older adults so that serum concentration in the lower therapeutic range (0.7–1.2 ng/mL) may be advisable.

Patients with severe or intractable heart failure may be treated with β-adrenergic agonists (dopamine, dobutamine, amrinone, or milrinone).

Vasodilators are used in heart failure to relieve compensatory vasoconstriction. Intravenous nitroglycerin is the drug of choice for heart failure in the setting of IHD. Intravenous nitroglycerin is started at 5 μg/kg/min with an infusion pump and titrated to effect.

There is no consensus regarding standard therapy for the treatment of diastolic heart failure, although the mainstays of therapy include diuretics and nitrates. Calcium channel blockers, ACE inhibitors, and angiotensin II receptor antagonists may be helpful, although objective data are limited.

Patients with heart failure and coronary artery disease may be evaluated for revascularization. The goal of coronary artery bypass graft (CABG) surgery is to prevent further injury to the myocardium or to restore nonfunctional but still viable myocardium. Most studies evaluating the effect of CABG surgery on survival in heart failure patients have shown positive results, although a randomized controlled trial has not yet been done. Percutaneous transluminal coronary angioplasty (PTCA) has not been shown to improve survival.

Indications for valvular surgery in elderly patients include severe valvular lesion and symptoms. Mortality is increased when the patient has severely depressed left ventricular function, inoperable coronary disease, pulmonary hypertension, multiple medical problems, poor functional status, or a poor nutritional state. Balloon valvuloplasty has been used successfully in patients considered at too high a risk for surgery.

Heart transplantation is not indicated for heart failure patients of advanced age but is considered on a case-by-case basis in younger patients.

Follow-up: Ask the patient about the presence of symptoms of heart failure as noted previously. Determine and document the most strenuous activity that the patient can perform without significant symptoms. Ask general questions related to the patient's quality of life, such as sleep patterns, sexual difficulties, and coping behaviors. Complete review of all medications, including nonprescription medications, is necessary. Laboratory work should be done as needed, including electrolyte, creatinine clearance, and digoxin levels when indicated.

Sequelae: The most severe complication of heart failure is end-organ disease. Hepatic and renal failure can result from heart failure in final stages.

Prevention/prophylaxis: Reducing cardiac risk factors in elderly persons affects coronary disease as strongly as it does in younger age groups. Encourage risk factor reduction using age-specific guidelines to facilitate changes in lifestyle. Patients with heart failure are at risk for a vascular event, although the evidence that antithrombotic treatment (aspirin or warfarin) is indicated is controversial.

Referral: Warning signs for the need for hospitalization include prolonged weight gain, palpitations, persistent or recurrent dizziness, agitation or cognitive changes, inability to sleep because of paroxysmal nocturnal dyspnea, abdominal pain, and inability to walk.

Most patients with heart failure can be managed by the primary care provider. Referral to a cardiologist may be indicated when the diagnosis is unclear, if the patient remains symptomatic despite therapy, and in patients with significant cardiac disease.

Education: Education and the use of support groups are important in patients with heart failure because noncompliance is a major cause of morbidity and unnecessary hospital admissions. Instruct patients and their families about the nature of heart failure, necessary medications, dietary restrictions, worsening heart failure, and prognosis. Explain typical symptoms of worsening heart failure (orthopnea, paroxysmal dyspnea, leg edema, or exercise intolerance), and instruct patients to contact their health-care provider if these should occur. Mild aerobic exercise increases functional capacity and improves the quality of life for heart failure patients. Dietary sodium should be restricted to 2 or 3 g/day. Discourage alcohol use and smoking. Fluid restriction is not necessary unless there is hyponatremia, but patients with heart failure should avoid excessive fluid intake.

Have the patient contact the health-care provider if daily weight changes by more than 2 to 4 lb. Nurse practitioners should recommend that patients with heart failure receive vaccination against influenza and pneumococcal disease and avoid the use of nonsteroidal anti-inflammatory drugs, which can cause fluid retention. Encourage patients to complete advance directives regarding their health-care preferences.

HYPERTENSION

SIGNAL SYMPTOMS usually none

Hypertension	ICD 9: 401.0
Malignant	ICD-9: 401.1
Benign	ICD-9: 401.9 unspecified
With: 402–404.90; Due to 405.09–405.99	

Description: Hypertension may occur in two forms in elderly persons. Isolated systolic hypertension (ISH) is a systolic blood pressure >140 mm Hg and a diastolic pressure <90 mm Hg. Systolic-diastolic hypertension (SDH) is a systolic pressure >140 mm Hg and a diastolic pressure >90 mm Hg. Blood pressure is measured twice, separated by 2 minutes, then averaged. If the first two readings differ by >5 mm Hg, additional readings should be obtained and averaged.

Etiology: The pathophysiology of ISH and SDH in the elderly involves loss of vascular tissue elasticity, causing an increase in peripheral vascular resistance. Patients with ISH have increased aortic stiffness and high peripheral vascular resistance. Patients with SDH have a decrease in cardiac output and intravascular volume and an increase in peripheral vascular resistance and left ventricular mass. Secondary forms of hypertension may be due to renal parenchymal damage, primary aldosteronism, and pheochromocytoma.

Occurrence: Of adults in the United States, 15% to 20% are hypertensive. Of people >65 years old, >15 million (>60% of the U.S. elderly population) have elevated systolic pressure, with or without elevations in diastolic pressure. Nearly three fourths of adult Americans with hypertension do not control their blood pressure to less than the recommended 140/90 mm Hg.

Age: SDH hypertension usually begins in middle age and levels off at about age 55. The prevalence of ISH continues to rise even after age 80.

Ethnicity: The prevalence of systolic and diastolic hypertension is greater in African-Americans (>70% of elderly African-Americans) than it is in elderly whites or Mexican-Americans.

Gender: In adults >65 years old, African-American women have the highest rate, followed by African-American men, Mexican-American men, white men, Mexican-American women, and white women.

Contributing factors: A variety of factors contribute to elevations in blood pressure in the elderly. Physiologic age–related changes include reduced myocardial compliance, diminished β-adrenergic sensitivity, blunted baroreceptor reflexes, extracellular fluid volume contraction, decreases in renal functional capacity, and altered activity in the renin-angiotensin system.

Other factors include obesity (particularly intra-abdominal fat); physical inactivity (may raise blood pressure, owing to more constricted peripheral vessels); alcohol (daily consumption of more than two alcoholic drinks has a vasopressor effect); sodium consumption (salt-sensitive response greater in all persons >60 years old, in African-Americans, and in obese individuals). Additional influences include smoking (causes slow repeated rises in blood pressure) and insomnia (causes more sustained elevations in blood pressure, which normally is lowest late in the day and during sleep and highest in early morning hours).

Signs and symptoms: Usually no symptoms are associated with elevations in blood pressure, unless the hypertension is a malignant or accelerated type or is due to a secondary cause. The history should elicit the duration of the hypertension; previous treatment for hypertension; family history of hypertension; and presence of diabetes, renal disease, coronary artery disease, or peripheral vascular disease. Risk factors, including smoking, sedentary lifestyle, and high intake of sodium and fat, should be determined. Ask the patient about signs and symptoms of conditions such as stroke, transient ischemic attack, MI, angina, and renal disease, which could indicate target-organ damage. All medications (prescribed and over-the-counter [OTC]) should be reviewed thoroughly. Psychosocial history should be examined for potential stressors.

The physical assessment technique for measuring blood pressure includes having the patient be in a basal (resting) state for 5 minutes before measurement and using a relaxed bare arm supported at the heart level and the proper size cuff. Patients should have refrained from smoking or caffeine intake for 30 minutes before measurement. Measure the blood pressure with the patient lying or sitting; have the patient stand, wait 2 minutes, and recheck the blood pressure. The pulse should be checked as well, and if a drop in blood pressure is not followed by a compensatory rise in pulse (increase >10 beats/min), the patient may have baroreceptor reflex impairment. The initial physical examination should include two or more blood pressure measurements, each separated by 2 minutes. Measurement of the blood pressure is all that is required; if elevated, three blood pressure readings taken on different occasions should be averaged. Labile or white coat hypertension is blood pressure that is elevated when measured in the physician's office in association with a normal 24-hour blood pressure reading.

Diagnostic errors can be avoided in the elderly by checking for pseudohypertension. Blood vessels that have become rigid from arteriosclerosis are difficult to occlude with the sphygmomanometer; this can yield falsely high blood pressure readings. Perform Osler's maneuver by pumping the cuff to higher than the patient's recorded systolic blood pressure; if the radial or brachial artery is still palpable, pseudohypertension may be present. The utility of this maneuver has been questioned. If pseudohypertension is suspected, an electronic oscillometric device can be used to provide readings that more closely correspond to intra-arterial levels; otherwise, the more invasive intra-arterial measurement may be done.

A postprandial decrease in blood pressure is common in elderly persons, with the maximal decrease noted 60 minutes after eating (particularly a high-carbohydrate meal). Postprandial hypotension is thought to be due to increased splanchnic blood flow, which decreases systemic vascular resistance; it also may be due to a rise in plasma insulin levels.

The clinician must avoid an auscultatory gap error. In some elderly individuals, a wide gap between the first Korotkoff's sound and subsequent beats is noted. If the cuff is not inflated high enough, the systolic pressure can be underestimated. This can be avoided by palpating the radial pulse and inflating the cuff beyond the disappearance of the palpable pulse. Height, weight, and waist circumference should be measured.

The physical examination in the hypertensive patient also should include an assessment for target-organ disease, such as retinopathy, cardiac enlargement, arrhythmias, murmurs, extra heart sounds, abdominal masses, neck and abdominal bruits, weak or absent peripheral pulses, and edema.

Clinical Pearl: An elevated pulse pressure (systolic–diastolic), indicating reduced vascular compliance in the large arteries, is a better marker of increased cardiovascular risk than either the systolic or the diastolic blood pressure alone.

Diagnostic tests:

Test	Results Indicating Disorder	CPT Code
Blood pressure readings (taken twice at least 2 minutes apart, then averaged)	ISH: systolic >140 mm Hg with diastolic <90 mm Hg SDH: systolic >140 mm Hg with diastolic >90 mm Hg	Part of 99211
Urinalysis	Target-organ damage: proteinuria or hematuria	81000–81007, 81015
12-Lead ECG	Target-organ damage, past MI, ischemia, left ventricular hypertrophy	93040–93042
CBC	Anemia, polycythemia	85031
BUN/creatinine	Renal insufficiency	84520, 84540, 84525, 82565
Electrolytes (glucose, sodium, calcium)	Target-organ abnormalities	80048
Lipid profile (total, high-density, and triglycerides)	Elevations indicating cardiovascular risk	83718, 83721, 84478
Ambulatory blood pressure monitoring: ≥24 hours	Elevations as noted in above-noted criteria	93784–93790

Differential diagnosis: The differential diagnosis for hypertension includes the determination of the type (ISH, SDH, or secondary cause). A secondary cause for hypertension is suspected if the onset of SDH occurs after age 55, the hypertension is difficult to treat, or the clinical or laboratory findings suggest a cause. Pseudohypertension is suspected when target-organ damage is not found in patients with blood pressure readings that are consistently elevated or when patients complain of symptoms of low blood pressure, although the blood pressure readings are high.

 Clinical Pearl: Hypertension is not an inevitable consequence of aging; prevention and aggressive management of hypertension are warranted to reduce morbidity and mortality in the elderly.

Treatment: The aim of therapy is to reduce the systolic blood pressure to <140 mm Hg and the diastolic blood pressure to ≤90 mm Hg if tolerated. A specific challenge in the elderly is to reduce the systolic blood pressure to the appropriate range while cautiously reducing the diastolic blood pressure to avoid compromised coronary perfusion. Treatment strategies must take into account the patient's cardiovascular risk profile and the blood pressure level. Drug therapy may be initiated at high-normal blood pressure levels (130/85 mm Hg) in patients who have diabetes or evidence of target-organ damage. Lifestyle modifications are generally the initial mode of therapy unless the systolic blood pressure is >190 mm Hg or the diastolic blood pressure is >100 mm Hg, in which case pharmacological therapy is indicated immediately.

As a lifestyle modification, weight reduction is noteworthy because even small amounts of weight (10 lb) loss in obese persons can lead to significant reductions in blood pressure. This may be due to increased insulin sensitivity when weight is lost. Sodium restriction should be moderate (2.5–5 g sodium/day equivalent to ½–1 tsp table salt) because salt sensitivity in common in the elderly. Increased physical activity is encouraged because repetitive aerobic exercise lowers the blood pressure by dampening the sympathetic nervous system. The blood pressure remains lower for 12 hours as a result of persistent postexercise vasodilation. Moderate alcohol consumption is advised (≤1 oz/day). Discontinuation of smoking is advised strongly for improvement in cardiovascular health. Other lifestyle changes include increasing potassium intake from fresh fruits and vegetables, relaxing to decrease stress, reducing fat and caffeine intake, and maintaining adequate calcium and magnesium intake. Emotional stress can raise the blood pressure, so relaxation therapies and biofeedback may be helpful.

If after 3 to 6 months nonpharmacological therapy has not been effective and the blood pressure remains elevated, pharmacological therapy is added. Drug therapy may be initiated sooner if the patient has target-organ disease or multiple cardiac risk factors. Blood pressure reduction with pharmacological therapy should be done in slow increments of drug modifications every 3 to 4 months unless hypertension is severe.

Diuretics are the initial drug of choice for older adults because they are the only classification shown to reduce cerebrovascular and cardiovascular morbidity and mortality. A low-dose diuretic (hydrochlorothiazide, 12.5–25 mg/day) is recommended. The relatively few adverse reactions to this low-cost drug may include electrolyte depletion, glucose intolerance, hyperuricemia, and serum lipid elevations. Loop diuretics (furosemide, 20 mg, or bumetanide, 0.5 mg initially) may be necessary in elderly patients refractory to thiazides or patients with renal insufficiency.

β-Blockers are thought to decrease the blood pressure by decreasing cardiac output, interfering with rennin, and having a central effect. Findings from studies on the role β-blockers play in decreasing cardiovascular events are less impressive. β-Blockers remain the drug of choice, however, for patients with a history of MI or angina. Side effects include fatigue, exercise intolerance, worsened insulin sensitivity, glucose intolerance, and increased triglyceride levels. These agents are contraindicated in patients with chronic obstructive pulmonary disease, although they may be well tolerated in mild forms of lung disease. β-Blockers in combination with thiazide diuretics may work well for older patients.

Calcium channel blockers, which provide vasodilation and promote diuresis, are used widely as first-line drugs in ISH in the elderly, and studies have shown these to be equal to β-blockers and diuretics in efficacy. The few adverse effects found among older adults include conduction defects, peripheral edema, headache, and constipation.

Other drug classifications are preferred for certain patients. These include ACE inhibitors for patients with heart failure, patients post-MI, and diabetic patients with nephropathy. Diabetic patients are resistant to treatment and often require combination therapy to reach target blood pressure levels. α_1 and centrally acting antihypertensive agents are used cautiously in the elderly. Selected patients benefit from the addition of antiplatelet and statin therapies.

In the event of an inadequate response or compliance and quality-of-life issues related to the drug therapy, the drug dose may need to be increased, another drug substituted, or a second agent or third from another classification added. When the hypertension has been controlled for 6 months, the dose may need to be stepped down slowly and progressively. In some older, frailer individuals with poor prognosis and comorbidities, the benefits of drug therapy are too small to outweigh the risks involving the quality and quantity of life.

Follow-up: See the patient every 2 to 4 weeks until antihypertensive therapy stabilizes the blood pressure. After control has been established, a visit may be required every 3 to 4 months. Electrolyte, serum glucose, and lipid levels and measures of renal function need to be monitored in selected patients; orthostatic blood pressure must be measured at each visit. Assessment of target-organ damage and patient adherence is done. The clinician needs to monitor the J-curve phenomenon; this refers to the point at which mortality increases owing to compromised coronary filling, which appears to occur when the diastolic pressure is reduced to 70 to 85 mm Hg.

Sequelae: National clinical trials show that reductions in blood pressure decrease the rate of cardiovascular and cerebrovascular events, even in individuals >80 years old (Joint National Committee, 1997). The elevation in systolic blood pressure, which is the greatest risk factor for coronary artery disease in elderly persons, interacts with other risk factors to compound it. A well-documented relationship exists between blood pressure elevation and stroke, transient ischemic attacks, sudden death, congestive heart failure, aneurysms, and renal failure.

Prevention/prophylaxis: Compliance with antihypertensive therapy is the best way to reduce blood pressure. Prevention of obesity and avoidance of smoking are important primary prevention strategies.

Referral: In accelerated or malignant hypertension, end-organ damage from hypertension occurs over a brief period. Patients with a diastolic pressure >120 mm Hg or symptoms indicating a hypertensive emergency (e.g., hypertensive encephalopathy, intracranial hemorrhage, unstable angina, or acute MI) need an intensive care setting to monitor urine output and arterial and central venous and pulmonary capillary wedge pressure. Patients with associated conditions, including heart failure, high-grade retinopathy, acute cerebrovascular ischemia, and progressive renal insufficiency, also require close collaboration with the physician. Patients with resistive hypertension, on three drugs or more at maximal levels, should be referred to a specialist.

Education: Patients need specific information on the disease and management. If home blood pressure monitoring is advantageous, the patient or caregiver should be taught proper technique using an accurate device and encouraged to maintain a log that includes the reading, time of day, and source of the reading. On each visit, the patient should discuss the medication management and demonstrate the ability to comply with pharmacological management and lifestyle modifications. Consult a dietitian to provide the appropriate nutritional instructions; a psychotherapist for stress reduction may be appropriate.

ISCHEMIC HEART DISEASE

SIGNAL SYMPTOMS▶ chest pain, tightness, or discomfort

| Ischemic heart disease | ICD-9: 414.9 |

Description: IHD is the imbalance between the supply and demand for blood flow to the myocardium.

Etiology: The pathophysiology of myocardial ischemia in younger or older adults is related to an imbalance between myocardial demand and coronary perfusion. This imbalance precipitates ischemia, which frequently is manifested as angina but instead may present silently as an acute event (i.e., sudden death or MI). The main cause is coronary atherosclerosis with plaque formation. Specific pathologic mechanisms also may include spasms of the coronary arteries, changes in the normal arterial tone, thrombus formation, or arteritis.

The amount of oxygen required by the myocardium (demand) is determined by the blood pressure, heart rate, left ventricular size and thickness, and the contractility state.

Occurrence: Although IHD is decreasing in incidence, it remains the leading cause of death for elderly men and women. Among adults >70 years old, the prevalence of ischemia presenting as angina is estimated at 22%; however, estimated prevalence based on thallium test results is almost 60%. Some studies have estimated the ratio of silent-to-symptomatic ischemic episodes to be 7:1.

Age: The prevalence increases dramatically with age, peaking after age 70.

Ethnicity: The prevalence of coronary artery disease in men age 64 to 74 is higher in whites than in African-Americans. In women, coronary artery disease is almost twice as prevalent in African-American women, however, compared with white women. Among Native American men and women, the prevalence of coronary artery disease is twice that of white men and women.

Gender: The incidence of IHD is greater in men, peaking in the 50s and 60s. In women, IHD increases steadily with age, peaking in the 70s.

Contributing factors: Age-related changes in myocardial and circulatory pathophysiology include reduced left ventricular compliance, amyloid deposits, diastolic dysfunction, increased aortic impedance, and peripheral vascular resistance. Other factors predictive of risk for IHD include elevations in the systolic blood pressure, plasma glucose, body mass index, homocysteines, and total serum cholesterol and the presence of diabetes, obesity, and smoking.

Signs and symptoms: The key symptom of IHD is chest pain, but anginal equivalents in elderly individuals may include fatigue or breathlessness. Some patients may have no symptoms or atypical ones so that coronary artery disease may not be diagnosed until they experience an MI. The classic features of ischemic pain include characterizations of dull, crushing substernal pain associated with dyspnea, diaphoresis, nausea, and sometimes palpitations. Some individuals may describe the feeling as a heaviness or pressure sensation rather than pain.

Chest pain in elderly persons is more likely to be of mild intensity, to be located elsewhere than in the substernal region, and to last a shorter time than in younger individuals. The discomfort often is triggered by physical exertion, lasts a few minutes, and subsides with rest or sublingual nitroglycerin. The discomfort may radiate to the neck, left shoulder, arm, or lower jaw. Precipitants to ischemic episodes include emotional stress, consumption of a heavy meal, and exposure to cold air. The altered pain perception in older adults changes the classic presentation of ischemia, which may lead to misdiagnosis and undertreatment. IHD among elderly individuals is more likely to coexist with other conditions, particularly gastroesophageal reflux disease; it may be impossible to differentiate the two conditions.

Stable angina is described as discomfort associated with increased myocardial demand at a stable, constant, and predictable level. Often patients show signs of autonomic dysfunction, including elevated heart rate, elevated blood pressure, and diaphoresis. Unstable angina is characterized by angina occurring at rest, variant angina (Prinzmetal's angina), and discomfort patterns that change suddenly with less prediction.

Physical examination findings during an ischemic episode may be nonexistent or may include extra heart sounds, mild hypertension, tachycardia, or tachypnea. A paradoxical split of S_2 may indicate an alteration in left ventricular function associated with ischemic discomfort.

Diagnostic tests:

Test	Results Indicating Disorder	CPT Code
ECG	ST-segment depression or elevation or T-wave inversion in the absence of left ventricular hypertrophy supports the diagnosis of ischemia Q waves may be evidence of an old MI	93040–93042
Exercise stress testing	Reproduce ischemic symptoms Defects in myocardial perfusion with exercise Cardiac risk identified in patients with a decrease in the blood pressure, S_3, rales, or prolonged downsloping ST-segment depression after exercise	93015–93018
Myocardial perfusion imaging	Perfusion defects Left ventricular dysfunction	78460–78465, 78478–78480
Echocardiogram Stress echocardiogram	Assesses the severity of left ventricular dysfunction Multiple reversible wall motion abnormalities	93320–93350
Cardiac catheterization	For patients who fail pharmacological therapy, have had an MI, or have unstable angina, to determine the severity of disease	93526–93529

Differential diagnosis: IHD must be differentiated from other, super-imposed diseases that may increase myocardial oxygen demand and decrease its supply (i.e., anemia, infection, hyperthyroidism, and arrhythmias).

Chest pain from IHD must be differentiated from pleuritic, costochondral, or pericardial pain. This type of pain also can mimic gastroesophageal reflux disease, herpes zoster, and panic disorder.

Treatment: The immediate goal of treatment is to decrease oxygen consumption and increase the blood supply to the myocardium by reducing vascular tone, improving collateral flow, and preventing platelet plugs and thrombosis. The treatment regimens are similar for symptomatic and asymptomatic elderly persons. The primary drugs used include nitrates, β-blockers, calcium antagonists, thrombolytics, and aspirin.

Nitrates decrease the preload through venous dilation and decrease the afterload through arterial dilation. Nitroglycerin given sublingually, 0.3 to 0.6 mg, or used as a lingual spray, 0.4 mg, often provides relief during the ischemic episode. The anti-ischemic effect is diminished if nitroglycerin is given continuously because tolerance develops rapidly; intermittent dosing is preferred with a scheduled nitrate-free period. Longer acting nitrate preparations, such as isosorbide dinitrate (10–40 mg four times daily), exert an antianginal effect for 2 to 4 hours, and cutaneous application can be effective for 3 to 5 hours. Because elderly persons are particularly sensitive to vasodilators, they may show an exaggerated drug response; smaller doses and careful titration are recommended. Side effects include headache and dizziness, although after vascular adaptation these symptoms often subside in 1 or 2 weeks.

β-Blockers decrease myocardial oxygen demand by decreasing the heart rate, blood pressure, and myocardial contractility. Propranolol, 10 to 40 mg four times daily, is used to treat elderly persons; longer acting drugs (e.g., atenolol) can be given once a day. Contraindications to these agents include conduction disturbances and significant reactive airway disease and heart failure. These drugs may cause fatigue and lethargy, increase triglyceride levels, decrease high-density lipoprotein and cholesterol levels, and induce coronary spasm and must be tapered (abrupt withdrawal has been associated with exacerbation of angina, precipitation of MI, and sudden death). Switching from the highly lipophilic drugs propanolol and metoprolol to the more hydrophilic atenolol and nadolol may alleviate central nervous system symptoms. Calcium channel blockers are a chemically diverse group of compounds that work by decreasing coronary and peripheral vascular resistance and reducing coronary artery spasm; significant side effects include peripheral edema and constipation. The second-generation dihydropyridine group (amlodipine, felodipine) seems to be tolerated better in the elderly. Using various combinations of the three drugs (nitrates, β-blockers, and calcium channel blockers) may yield an additive effect; however, the patient needs to be monitored carefully for adverse effects.

Acetylsalicylic acid (ASA), 75 to 325 mg, affords a protective benefit to individuals with angina. ASA is given after an acute MI to reduce platelet aggregation. Daily doses of 20 mg of ASA are continued for at least 2 years after the MI and indefinitely for many patients. The risk of gastric irritation and gastrointestinal bleeding exists even with low doses of ASA. For ASA-sensitive patients, ticlopidine or clopidogrel might be options by blocking platelet aggregation and reducing reoccurrence and progression. Lipid-lowering drugs may be added. New data on the antioxidant effects of vitamin E are encouraging.

Invasive intervention therapy for elderly patients also includes intravenous thrombolytic therapy in patients with known or suspected acute MI (see under Myocardial Infarction). Mechanical intervention with PTCA is used to revascularize elderly patients with acute or chronic manifestations of coronary artery disease. Elderly patients with all forms of angina tolerate well and benefit from PTCA, particularly patients with comorbid factors that limit the appropriateness of a surgical procedure (i.e., CABG surgery). A high rate of restenosis occurs after PTCA. Other percutaneous interventions available include lasers, atherectomy devices, stents, and intra-aortic balloon counterpulsation.

The longer term goals for patients who have end-organ damage from IHD are to relieve symptoms and allow patients to resume their preferred lifestyle. CABG surgery is a revascularization procedure that is effective in alleviating ischemic symptoms. CABG surgery has an advantage over PTCA in that its results are more durable, and revascularization is more complete. The patient most likely to benefit maximally is one with the potential to return to an active lifestyle who can tolerate the 3 to 4 months of cardiac rehabilitation. Comorbid factors known to affect the outcome negatively include diabetes, cerebral and peripheral vascular disease, a history of recent MI, systemic hypertension, renal insufficiency, pulmonary disease, and obesity. Elderly women have a considerably higher risk of death and complications from IHD than their male counterparts.

Follow-up: Patients with IHD must be monitored for the effectiveness of prescribed drugs and any potential adverse effect. Changes in features of symptoms and disease progression should be determined.

Sequelae: Silent ischemia has the same prognosis as symptomatic ischemia. Angina is associated with a twofold to threefold increase in the risk of death when ECG abnormalities are also present. ECG abnormalities compatible with ischemia are associated with mortality even in the absence of chest pain.

Complications from coronary artery disease include congestive heart failure, acute MI and associated problems, arrhythmias, and sudden death.

Prevention/prophylaxis: Risk factor modification includes control of systolic hypertension, cholesterol levels, and elimination of smoking. A sedentary lifestyle predisposes an individual to coronary artery disease, particularly in the presence of other risk factors. Physical conditioning tends to lower the blood pressure; individuals who are physically active have slightly higher plasma high-density lipoprotein levels than sedentary individuals. Other strategies to manage risk include weight control, stress reduction, hypolipidemic therapy if indicated, and perhaps estrogen therapy in postmenopausal women. Low-dose aspirin therapy (325 mg every other day) may reduce the risk of MI; however, its use is associated with adverse effects. Its risk and benefits must be examined individually in patients. Studies show potential benefit of ACE inhibitors after MI in reducing risk of future coronary events.

Referral: Unstable patients with IHD require hospitalization because approximately 20% of these patients have MI. Collaborate closely with the physician regarding patients who are refractory to treatment.

Education: Advise patients to report changes in the pattern or intensity of angina. All patients should be instructed to call emergency services when experiencing chest pain because the differential diagnosis is difficult to determine without technological equipment.

MYOCARDIAL INFARCTION

SIGNAL SYMPTOMS *typical:* prolonged chest pain (>20 minutes' duration)
atypical: shortness of breath, neurological symptoms (confusion, weakness), worsening of heart failure

Myocardial infarction	ICD 9: 410–410.9

Description: MI is necrosis of heart tissue caused by lack of blood supply. MIs can be transmural or subendocardial (non–Q wave MI).

Etiology: MI generally occurs after the abrupt decrease in coronary blood flow to the myocardium following a thrombotic occlusion of a coronary artery already narrowed by atherosclerosis. In most cases, this atherosclerotic plaque ruptures or ulcerates, and a mural thrombus forms in the coronary artery.

Occurrence: A total of 1.5 million cases of acute MI occur in the United States every year and account for 400,000 to 500,000 deaths annually. Coronary disease is the most frequent cause of death in people ≥65 years old. Mortality rates from coronary artery disease are decreasing in the general population but remain high in the elderly population. More than one third of acute MIs occur in adults >75 years old, and 60% of MI deaths are in this age group. MIs in older adults are usually smaller in size, and non–Q wave infarcts occur more commonly than ST-segment elevation infarcts.

 Clinical Pearl: Silent MIs occur about 40% of the time in older adults and carry serious prognostic implications.

Age: Postmortem studies show that coronary atherosclerosis, which often begins to develop before age 20, is widespread even among asymptomatic adults. At autopsy, >50% of individuals >50 years old have significant stenosis in at least one coronary artery. Aging itself may be a risk factor for MI in men and women.

Ethnicity: Not available.

Gender: MI is much more prevalent in men than in women ≤74 years old; after age 74, the occurrence increases steeply with age in both genders. On average, women develop heart disease 10 years later than men and have MIs and sudden death 20 years later than men.

Contributing factors: Risk factors for heart disease and MI in elderly individuals are essentially the same as in younger individuals. Risk factors include hypertension, hyperlipidemia, diabetes, physical inactivity, obesity, and stress. Cigarette smoking is associated with new coronary events for elderly men and women. Whether postmenopausal women are at increased risk for MI because of the loss of estrogen and its cardioprotective effect is controversial.

Aging alters the cardiovascular system in ways that reduce cardiac reserve and efficiency, compromising the ability to respond to stress or illness. The cardiovascular system becomes less compliant as diastolic filling of the ventricles declines and afterload increases secondary to increased stiffness in the ascending aorta. This results in moderate hypertrophy of the left ventricle, causing a more precarious balance between myocardial oxygen supply and demand. Other changes in the elderly cardiovascular system include decreased responsiveness to β-adrenergic stimulation, decreased baroreceptor sensitivity, and an increased dependence on a higher end-diastolic volume to maintain cardiac output.

Signs and symptoms: With advancing age, the presentation of acute MI is less likely to include the classic symptoms of crushing substernal chest pain, nausea, vomiting, and diaphoresis. A vague ache or discomfort may be present. Elderly persons may not recognize that throat, shoulder, or abdominal pain may be referred cardiac pain. Dyspnea is the second most common symptom of MI in younger and older populations. For patients ≥85 years old, syncope, acute confusion, or stroke may be the only presenting symptom. Some elderly patients may present only with faintness, weakness, giddiness, or restlessness.

On physical examination, the patient may be anxious and weak and may appear gray or cyanotic. Mild tachycardia may be present, and arrhythmias may be noted on the ECG. The skin may be diaphoretic, cold, and clammy. Thrills, heaves, and an abnormal point of maximum impulse may be palpated. Peripheral pulses may be irregular, slow, fast, or thready, and capillary refill time may be prolonged. Auscultation may reveal an S_3 or S_4, pericardial friction rub, murmurs, or crackles. The physical examination must focus on ruling out diagnoses other than MI and in recognizing complications from MI.

Diagnostic tests:

Test	Results Indicating Disorder	CPT Code
12-Lead ECG	ST-segment changes Q waves New left bundle-branch block A normal or nondiagnostic ECG does not rule out MI	93040–93042
CK-MB enzyme profile	Elevations occur when myocardial cells are damaged typically 3–8 hours after the onset of chest pain Elderly may not have a significant rise owing to decreased muscle mass, particularly those with renal failure, hypothyroidism, or skeletal muscle injury	82550–82554
Troponin I and T enzyme profile	Test with greater sensitivity to degrees of myocardial necrosis, and levels remain elevated for 10–14 days post-MI Elevations indicative of abnormality	84512, 84484
Chest x-ray	Heart failure evidence	71010–71030
CBC	Leukocytosis	85025, 85027
Clotting profile	Increased clotting	85345–85348
Electrolytes	Marked hyperglycemia, ketoacidosis, potassium abnormalities	80048, 80053, 80051

Differential diagnosis: The pain from MI can be similar to that of acute pericarditis, pulmonary embolism, acute aortic dissection, or costochondritis. Many conditions can present as cardiac disease in the elderly, including cor pulmonale, pneumonia, esophageal spasm, gastroesophageal reflux disease, hiatal hernia, gallbladder disease, osteoarthritis of the spine, muscle injury, and panic disorder.

Treatment: Nitrates, once considered the cornerstone for therapy of ischemic pain, continue to provide symptomatic relief for individuals experiencing anginal pain, although randomized clinical trials have failed to show a consistent benefit from routine administration of them. Chest pain should be treated with sublingual nitroglycerin if the systolic blood pressure is >90 mm Hg. The drug can be repeated three times, 5 minutes apart, unless the patient becomes hypotensive. Intravenous nitrates are indicated for ongoing ischemia, heart failure, or hypertension. Nitrates should be used with caution in patients with right ventricular infarction or in patients taking sildenafil (Viagra). Morphine sulfate, 2 to

4 mg every 10 minutes, up to 20 mg, is also effective for pain relief. Supplemental oxygen should be given if oxygen saturation is <94%. Aspirin, 160 to 325 mg chewed or swallowed, should be given as soon as possible if there is no obvious contraindication (clopidogrel is an alternative if the patient is allergic to aspirin). Aspirin, 75 to 325 mg/day, should be continued for life after an MI. Glycoprotein IIb/III receptor blockers (abciximab, eptifibatide, tirofiban) have potent antiplatelet actions and may decrease complication rates in patients with unstable angina.

Thrombolytic agents, such as tissue-type plasminogen activator (tPA) and streptokinase, have become the standard treatments for MI, although newer agents, including anisoylated plasminogen-streptokinase activator complex (APSAC), recombinant tissue plasminogen activator (reteplase), and tenecteplase, also are being used. Indications for thrombolysis are based on the existence of chest pain and specific ECG changes, including ST-segment elevation or new left bundle-branch block. Studies show this therapy frequently is omitted for elderly patients; reasons include frequent delay in seeking medical care, atypical presentation of MI, and a higher prevalence of non–Q wave MIs. Fear of hemorrhage after use of thrombolytics must be weighed against the proven gains in survival for all age groups, especially for patients presenting early with MI. A variety of studies suggest that streptokinase may be as beneficial as tPA in treating the elderly MI patient. It is considerably less expensive.

Current practice includes heparin after tPA. For patients not receiving thrombolytics, unless contraindicated, low-dose subcutaneous heparin or low-molecular-weight heparin is used for prophylaxis of thrombosis. Elderly patients with large anterior MIs and heart failure and patients with documented left ventricular thrombus should receive full heparin anticoagulation for 3 to 5 days, followed by 3 months of warfarin.

β-Blockers, which have been shown to limit infarct size, decrease chest pain, and improve prognosis, are generally well tolerated in patients age 65 to 75. Some conditions that contraindicate the use of β-blockers in the elderly include acute bronchospastic lung disease, marked bradycardia, hypotension, acute decompensated heart failure, depression, and diabetes. Studies show that β-blockers are underused in the elderly; age alone should not determine their use. In acute MI, metoprolol is given slowly, 2.5 to 5 mg intravenously every 5 minutes, for a total of 15 mg (atenolol, esmolol, or propranolol also may be used).

At about 3 days after an MI, ACE inhibitors are recommended for elderly patients with ejection fraction <40% and no obvious contraindication to their use (if given earlier than the third day, they may cause hypotension and result in extension of the MI). Captopril is given first as a test dose of 6.25 mg. If tolerated, captopril, 50 to 100 mg, is given daily (enalapril or ramipril also may be used).

Clinical Pearl: Patients in whom cough develops as a result of an ACE inhibitor may be prescribed an angiotensin receptor blocker, although it has not shown a significant vascular protector effect.

Calcium channel blockers have limited use in the MI patient. Prophylactic use of lidocaine or other antiarrhythmics may cause more harm than benefit.

In terms of interventional management of elderly MI patients, direct PTCA with or without stenting may be a valuable alternative in patients for whom thrombolytics are contraindicated when done by qualified clinicians within 90 to 120 minutes. CABG surgery is preferred for patients with left main stenosis and patients with moderately severe left ventricular depression. Emergency PTCA or CABG surgery in elderly patients presenting with cardiogenic shock or heart failure is associated with high morbidity and mortality.

Follow-up: Risk stratification for future cardiac events after stabilization from MI is recommended by the American College of Cardiology. Tests to evaluate for ischemia or myocardium at risk include ECG stress testing at times with the addition of nuclear perfusion or echocardiographic imaging. Cardiac catheterization and coronary revascularization after MI is not routine but may be indicated in patients with spontaneous or easily provoked ischemia. Patients at high risk for sudden death from arrhythmias should undergo electrophysiological evaluation. An ICD is indicated for patients with ventricular arrhythmias post-MI.

Sequelae: Increasing age is associated with more complications after MI, including heart failure, arrhythmias, pulmonary edema, cardiogenic shock, cardiac rupture, and death. Many post–acute MI patients experience recurrent chest pain and depression.

Prevention/prophylaxis: Secondary prevention in the elderly MI patient includes use of aspirin (or clopidogrel), β-blockers, and ACE inhibitors, unless there are absolute contraindications to these agents. Lipid-lowering therapy is beneficial in slowing atherosclerotic progression. Reduction of risk factors is necessary. Nitrates may be useful for symptom control. Cardiac rehabilitation can be as beneficial in older MI patients as in younger ones and includes lifestyle, psychological, and social interventions.

Referral: Suspicion of acute MI should prompt transfer of the patient to an environment equipped with cardiac monitoring and the ability to administer advanced cardiac life support. As hospitalization continues, consultation with a variety of disciplines, such as surgery, social work, and physical therapy, may be necessary.

Education: Individualized teaching after MI for each patient and family should be provided, using age-specific teaching methods. Teach the basic definitions of coronary artery disease, angina, and MI. Patients need information on the healing process after MI, when to return to work or resume normal daily activities, and when to resume sexual relations.

Support exists for lifestyle modifications, including exercise, dietary modifications and weight loss, and smoking cessation, and these should be reinforced at each follow-up visit. Involve patients and families in a discussion of the psychological adjustment after MI. Health-care practitioners should work with patients to set goals and design plans. Give the patient information on community resources, such as the American Heart Association or support groups in their area.

Medication teaching and review is important. Health-care providers should be aware of all medications prescribed for the patient. Teach patients about the desired effects and common side effects of their medications. Review what to do if medication cannot be taken or obtained. Discuss interactions with OTC medications.

Teach elderly patients about altered pain perception that can occur with age and with diseases such as diabetes. Teach patients and their families about warning signs, such as chest pain or pressure, shortness of breath, indigestion, choking, sweating, dizziness, palpitations, severe weakness, and loss of consciousness. Establish a clear plan for obtaining prompt medical attention.

VALVULAR HEART DISEASE

SIGNAL SYMPTOMS▶   may be asymptomatic; cardiac symptoms may be present

Mitral	ICD-9: 424.0
Aortic	ICD-9: 424.1
Tricuspid	ICD-9: 424.2
Pulmonary	ICD-9: 424.3

Description: Valvular heart disease (VHD) is damage to a valve or valves of the heart, causing cardiac dysfunction. The most prevalent types of VHD in elderly persons are calcific and degenerative aortic valve disease.

Aortic stenosis: An abnormal narrowing of the aortic valve orifice.

Aortic regurgitation: Retrograde blood flow through an incompetent aortic valve into the left ventricle during ventricular diastole.

Mitral stenosis: An abnormal narrowing of the mitral valve orifice.

Mitral regurgitation: Retrograde blood flow during systole from the left ventricle into the left atrium through an incompetent mitral valve.

Mitral valve prolapse: Mitral regurgitation associated with a bulging of one or both mitral valve leaflets into the left atrium during ventricular systole.

Etiology: In the elderly, the predominant causes of VHD include age-related degenerative calcification, myxomatous degeneration, papillary muscle dysfunction, and infective endocarditis. There has been a decline in older adults with VHD secondary to rheumatic fever. Valvular stenosis usually results in elevated pressures in the chamber upstream from the stenosis. In valvular regurgitation, a portion of the ejected volume of blood leaks back into the upstream cardiac chamber.

Occurrence: Approximately 5 million Americans have VHD. Occurrence of VHD varies according to the type of disease; only limited information is available.

Age: Aortic stenosis, the most clinically significant valvular lesion in elderly persons, increases in frequency with age and is found in 5.5% of adults >75 years old. Isolated aortic regurgitation is seen rarely and usually is accompanied by some degree of mitral valve involvement. Bicuspid aortic valves are prone to regurgitation. Mitral regurgitation is more common than mitral stenosis in elderly individuals. About 6% of adults >60 years old have mitral annular calcification that causes mitral regurgitation. Mitral stenosis has a progressive slow course with latent symptoms over 20 to 40 years followed by rapid acceleration in later life.

Ethnicity: Not significant.

Gender: Mitral annular calcification (a frequent cause of mitral regurgitation) affects women two to three times more frequently than it affects men. Mitral valve prolapse is more common in elderly men than in elderly women.

Contributing factors: Age-related fibrotic thickening of valvular tissue or dilation and calcification of the valve annulus may contribute to and cause hemodynamic abnormalities. Valvular stenosis of rheumatic origin can progress gradually throughout adult life. Other factors that may contribute to or cause valvular disease include metastatic carcinoid tumors; drugs, including methysergide and ergotamine (used to treat migraines) and appetite-suppressing drugs fenfluramine and phentermine; rheumatoid arthritis (can produce nodules in the leaflets); systemic lupus (can cause small vegetations, thickening, and regurgitation in the leaflets); antipholipid syndrome; and radiation therapy.

Signs and symptoms:

Aortic Stenosis

Most patients are asymptomatic. For patients with symptoms, the prognosis is poor, with mortality rates of 50% at 3 years and 90% at 10 years. Chest pain is an early symptom. Presyncope followed by effort syncope occurs in about one third of patients with symptoms. Exertional dyspnea may herald the development of congestive heart failure.

Physical findings include a characteristic loud, rough systolic ejection murmur in the second right intercostal space at the midclavicular line that is well transmitted into the neck. This murmur, which peaks in intensity in mid to late systole, may be associated with a thrill. S_1 is often soft, and the aortic component of S_2 is soft or absent. An S_4 is common. The pulse pressure is narrow; there is a slow rise in the carotid pulse and a sustained brachial or apical beat.

Aortic Regurgitation

In chronic aortic regurgitation, patients are asymptomatic for many years. When the left ventricle no longer can manage the increased stroke volume, patients may experience effort intolerance and dyspnea/orthopnea.

The presentation of acute severe regurgitation is different in that left ventricular compensation and stroke volume changes have not yet occurred. The presenting symptoms may include tachycardia and dyspnea owing to pulmonary venous congestion, and at this point patients decompensate quickly.

Physical findings with chronic aortic regurgitation include a wide pulse pressure and possibly bounding pulses. Systolic and diastolic thrills may be present on the precordium. S_1 is normal or soft. S_2 may be physiologically split, but A_2 may be soft or not heard owing to a high-frequency, early diastolic blowing murmur heard best at the left sternal border. An atrial gallop and S_3 are often present. An apical diastolic rumble, the Austin Flint murmur, may be heard.

The clinical features of acute aortic regurgitation are dominated by sudden severe heart failure. The pulse pressure may be narrowed because of elevated left ventricular diastolic pressure. The cardiac impulse is displaced, vigorous, and diffuse. S_1 is soft, a prominent summated gallop is common, and the diastolic murmur is harsh and shortened by the elevated ventricular filling pressure.

Mitral Stenosis

The symptoms of mitral stenosis, dyspnea on exertion and lethargy resulting from elevated left atrial and pulmonary venous pressures, and a decreased cardiac output generally are associated with valve areas of <1.5 cm (normal 4 cm). Later symptoms include those of right ventricular overload, such as neck vein distention, ascites, and edema.

The clinical findings include a loud S_1 and an apical diastolic rumble with presystolic accentuation. An opening snap also may be present, but it may be soft or not heard at all because of valve stiffness and calcification.

 Clinical Pearl: The murmur of mitral stenosis can be accentuated by a brief walk or positioning the patient in the left lateral decubitus position and auscultation with the bell of the stethoscope.

Mitral Regurgitation

For patients with mitral regurgitation, the main complaints are fatigue and a gradual decrease in exercise tolerance, which occur only when the ventricle begins to fail.

The clinical features vary, depending on the pathologic cause; however, a holosystolic murmur at the apex is a nearly constant feature. If the disease is severe, the apex beat is hyperdynamic and displaced laterally, and an S_3 usually is found when left ventricular dysfunction also is present.

Mitral Valve Prolapse

Chest pain and palpitations are the most prominent symptoms in elderly and young patients, although most patients are asymptomatic. Other symptoms that may represent an arrhythmic etiology are dizziness, syncope, and early fatigue.

The clinical picture includes a midsystolic click and a late systolic or holosystolic murmur characteristic of mitral regurgitation. In some patients, the murmur, click, or both are not appreciated until the patient stands or performs the Valsalva maneuver. An apical S_3-S_4 gallop usually is present at the time of heart failure.

Diagnostic tests:

Test	Results Indicating Disorder	CPT Code
ECG	May be normal with disease Identification of ventricular hypertrophy or strain Nonspecific ST or T wave changes Atrial enlargement	93040–93042
Chest x-ray	May be normal with disease Ventricular prominence Atrial enlargement Calcifications Evidence of heart failure	71010–71030
Echocardiography	Lesions or abnormalities in the valvular area Disturbed valvular flow	93303–93318, 93320–93321, 93662, 93350
Cardiac catheterization	Identification of myocardial damage in anticipation of valvular surgery	93526–93529
Coronary angiography	Identification of myocardial damage in anticipation of valvular surgery	75600–75790

Differential diagnosis: The diagnosis of VHD in elderly persons sometimes is overlooked because the early symptoms are vague and nonspecific. Murmurs in older adults are common and frequently determined to be functional or insignificant. The barrel chest of an older individual may obscure a murmur; with an increased anteroposterior diameter, left ventricular hypertrophy may not be detected.

Murmurs have been associated with conditions other than VHD (i.e., hypertension, anemia, thyroid disease) so this differential must be considered.

Patients with established VHD need to have a specific determination of the causes of valvular involvement.

Treatment:

Aortic Stenosis

Symptoms of aortic stenosis (angina, heart failure, syncope) are associated with substantial valvular obstruction and a risk of sudden death.

Except for prophylaxis against endocarditis, no proven medical therapy exists for aortic stenosis. For patients with elevations in cholesterol, statins may be indicated to limit further reduction of the aortic valve diameter. Aortic valve replacement is associated with a higher mortality (5–15%) in elderly patients than in younger patients. Factors associated with greater operative risk include emergency surgery, left ventricular dysfunction, significant coronary disease, cachexia, additional valve replacement, or concomitant CABG surgery. The proper selection of the type of valve is important in elderly patients. The bioprosthetic valves are advantageous in that their use obviates the need for systemic anticoagulation (which is associated with substantial morbidity and mortality in the elderly). The disadvantage of this valve type is that the tissue degrades, and 30% to 40% of patients require reoperation in 10 years. The mechanical valves are more durable and have better hemodynamic profiles, but these require lifelong anticoagulation therapy.

Aortic balloon valvuloplasty is an alternative treatment method; however, because it is associated with rapid restenosis and significant residual outflow obstruction, it is reserved as a palliative procedure for the symptomatic patient who is not a surgical candidate or as a bridge to surgery.

Aortic Regurgitation

Acute aortic regurgitation warrants surgery if symptoms are more than mild. Chronic aortic regurgitation requires medical treatment of the early signs of heart failure with ACE inhibitors, calcium channel blockers, digitalis, diuretics, or vasodilators. Surgical treatment (aortic valve reconstruction or replacement) is indicated before the ejection fraction decreases to <55%.

Mitral Stenosis

Therapies for the symptomatic patient with mitral stenosis include medical therapy, percutaneous balloon mitral valvuloplasty, commissurotomy, and mitral valve replacement. Patients with symptoms of mild heart failure are managed with diuretics and salt restriction to decrease left atrial pressures. Because atrial fibrillation occurs in most patients with moderate-to-severe stenosis, anticoagulation and rate control (with digitalis, β-blockers, or calcium channel blockers) often are indicated. Because of the high risk associated with anticoagulation in elderly patients, however, a less aggressive approach to therapy may be taken. When the patient has severe symptoms of mitral stenosis, valve replacement is indicated.

Mitral Regurgitation

Medical management of mitral regurgitation includes use of ACE inhibitors, digitalis, diuretics, and vasodilators to reduce the symptoms of heart failure and reduce the regurgitant volume. Mitral valve surgery is considered in asymptomatic and symptomatic patients with progressive disease before signs of irreversible left ventricular dysfunction are present. The mortality associated with mitral valve replacement is 10% to 15% but may be 50% in higher risk patients (i.e., in the presence of severe left ventricular dysfunction, concomitant coronary artery disease requiring revascularization, multivalve surgical procedures, emergency surgery, or advanced age).

Mitral valve repair is associated with a lower operative mortality than mitral valve replacement and is preferred in that preservation of the existing valve architecture allows synchrony of left ventricular contraction. When mitral annular calcification is the cause, medical therapy is prudent because the operative risk is substantially higher in patients with this disease process. Acute mitral regurgitation from papillary muscle rupture or chordal rupture requires patient stabilization followed by surgery, which still carries a high mortality.

Mitral Valve Prolapse

Medical management with β-blockers may stabilize patients; anticoagulation to prevent emboli is warranted. Mitral valve surgery is needed in patients with progressive ventricular dilation.

Follow-up: For patients treated medically for valvular disease, close follow-up to monitor the effectiveness of treatment, adverse effects of medication, and progressiveness of the disease process is indicated. Medication therapy, particularly the use of anticoagulation therapy, requires meticulous attention. Surgically treated patients are monitored for valve function, fluid balance, and anticoagulation. Periodic echocardiographic monitoring is indicated.

Sequelae: Valve replacement risks include thrombus formation, infection, or rupture at the attachment points to the valve ring. Infective endocarditis, which may occur with artificial valves, has a high risk of mortality and requires reoperation. There is a high prevalence of gallstones in patients with prosthetic valves, thought to be due to low-grade intravascular hemolysis.

In patients who are not surgical candidates, the symptoms of heart failure are progressive and disabling. Even in surgical patients, the symptoms of heart failure may recur or persist.

Prevention/prophylaxis: In patients with prosthetic valves, the risk of thromboembolism decreases with an individualized antithrombolytic regimen. The specific therapy is determined based on the comorbid state and the patient's overall status.

Consider prophylactic antibiotic therapy in all patients with valvular disease, especially patients with valve replacement, rheumatic heart disease, aortic regurgitation, or mitral valve prolapse with significant mitral regurgitation murmurs.

Referral: All patients with symptoms of progressive valvular disease must be managed collaboratively with the physician. Many require further collaboration with a cardiologist. The Practice Guidelines for Cardiothoracic Surgery Concerning Valvular Heart Disease include the indications for surgery. In general, these include symptoms that cannot be controlled with medical therapy or indications of a threat to survival (i.e., angina, dyspnea, effort syncope or progressive impairment of ventricular contractility, and infective endocarditis).

Education: Elderly persons constitute 40% to 60% of all cases of endocarditis. Instruct all at-risk patients in the importance of good dental care and antibiotic prophylaxis. Patients are taught to monitor and report febrile illness.

Instruct all patients with valve disease requiring medication therapy to report lack of therapeutic effect or any adverse effects of the drugs. Teach the patient to be aware of drug-food interactions (e.g., green leafy vegetables and anticoagulants). Teach the patient with disabling heart failure about energy-conserving measures. Patients with hemodynamically significant valvular heart disease may need to limit vigorous physical activity. Deterioration may be rapid and symptoms insidious, so patients are taught to report any change in condition.

RESPIRATORY DISORDERS

CHRONIC BRONCHITIS

SIGNAL SYMPTOMS▶ daily chronic cough, increased sputum production, wheezing, dyspnea (seen more with mixed bronchitis and emphysema)

Chronic bronchitis	ICD-9-CM: 491.9
Chronic bronchitis with emphysema	ICD-9-CM: 491.20

Description: Chronic bronchitis is a daily chronic cough with increased sputum production lasting for at least 3 consecutive months in at least 2 consecutive years. The cough is usually worse on wakening. Chronic bronchitis is considered one type of chronic obstructive pulmonary disease (COPD); it frequently occurs concurrently with emphysema.

Etiology: Chronic bronchitis is caused by inflammation and hypertrophy of the bronchial and bronchiolar walls in response to noxious stimuli (tobacco). Hyperplasia and hypertrophy of goblet cells in smaller airways and of mucus glands around cartilaginous airways contribute to mechanical obstruction. Mucociliary clearance is impaired. Inflammatory mediators play a large role in chronic bronchitis, injuring airway epithelial cells; neutrophilic attracting cytokines predominate in COPD.

Occurrence: At high risk are individuals with a long history of cigarette smoking. Chronic bronchitis affects >14,150,000 people in the United States. In 1999, there were 1172 deaths from chronic bronchitis.

Age: Chronic bronchitis affects approximately 29% of the population 65 to 74 years old and 21% >75 years old; it usually presents in the 40s or 50s.

Ethnicity: Higher for whites than African-Americans.

Gender: More common in women than in men.

Contributing factors: Frequent exposure to tobacco smoke either by direct or second-hand smoke inhalation, industrial gases or fumes, dust particles, aerosol sprays, dander, frequent respiratory infections, and repeated allergic responses all contribute to the development of chronic bronchitis.

Signs and symptoms: Changes in appetite or activity tolerance are possible. Symptoms may include chronic cough with copious sputum, wheezing, recurrent respiratory infections, fatigue, and dyspnea on exertion. Signs may include neck vein distention during expiration in the absence of heart failure, increased anteroposterior diameter of thorax, rhonchi and wheezes, prolonged expiration, hyperresonance on percussion, decreased heart and breath sounds, tachypnea, cyanotic skin color, and clubbing of nail beds. As the disease progresses, hypoxemia and pulmonary hypertension may lead to cor pulmonale.

Diagnostic tests:

Test	Results Indicating Disorder	CPT Code
Chest x-ray	Increased vascular markings indicate cardiac hypertrophy	71010–71035
Spirometry with bronchodilator challenge	Improvement in forced expiratory volume after inhaled bronchodilator indicates that bronchodilator therapy may be indicated	94060–94070
PFTs	Early findings: reduced midexpiratory flow rate. Increased total lung capacity, increased residual volume, decreased vital capacity and FEV_1	78596
Pulse oximetry	Oxygen saturation <92% indicates need for arterial blood gases to assess oxygenation and ventilation	94760–94762
Arterial blood gases (late in disease)	Hypoxemia, compensated respiratory acidosis; during acute exacerbations, worsening of acidemia	82803–82810
ECG	Sinus tachycardia, supraventricular arrhythmias	93272
CBC	Normal to polycythemia	85022–85025
Sputum culture in acute exacerbations	*Haemophilus influenzae, Streptococcus pneumoniae, Moraxella catarrhalis*	89350

PFTS, pulmonary function tests; FEV_1, forced expiratory volume in 1 second.

Differential diagnosis:

- Carcinoma of the lung
- Asthma
- Interstitial lung disease
- Congestive heart failure
- Pneumonitis, bronchiectasis
- Chronic rhinitis
- Chronic sinusitis
- Pharyngitis
- Extrinsic compression lesions should be considered when diagnosing chronic bronchitis

Treatment: Treatment is individualized to the patient's condition with the focus on preventing complications and maximizing functional abilities and early recognition and treatment of complications. Symptomatic relief and support through pulmonary rehabilitation is recommended. Although pulmonary rehabilitation does not improve lung function, it does increase exercise tolerance and quality of life. Smoking cessation, if applicable, is a treatment priority.

Pharmacological treatment includes an inhaled anticholinergic muscarinic agent, ipratropium (Atrovent), four times daily. An inhaled β_2-agonist, such as albuterol (Proventil), also is included four times daily, either as needed or regularly. These agents may be prescribed in combination as Combivent, four times daily. The use of a spacing chamber can improve the delivery of a metered dose; metered-dose inhaler and mininebulizer are equally effective. A long-acting β_2-agonist, salmeterol (Serevent), also is prescribed twice daily. For inflammatory flareups or if the bronchodilator is ineffective, a steroid may be added to the regimen. An inhaled steroid, fluticasone (Flovent), twice daily, sometimes is prescribed, particularly if there is a suspected asthmatic component as well. Advair Diskus is a combination of fluticasone and salmeterol for once-daily use. Oral prednisone also is used if inhaled agents are ineffective and the patient is symptomatic. Theophylline still is prescribed by some practitioners but is no longer preferred because of its weak action, poor side-effect profile, and toxicity. Although Cochrane abstracts indicate that mucolytics are helpful in the treatment of chronic bronchitis, research in the United States does not support this conclusion. A new class of pharmacological agents which assist with mucociliary clearance, the P2Y(2) receptor agonists, are currently in clinical trials.

Acute exacerbations are treated with antibiotic therapy, although some sources recommend steroid treatment only. A second-generation β-lactam, such as cefuroxime, is the treatment of choice. Alternatives include a second-generation macrolide or trimethoprim/sulfamethoxazole; some sources suggest a fluoroquinolone owing to increasing antibiotic resistance to the usual agents.

Oxygen therapy should be initiated for a PaO$_2$ of 55 mm Hg at rest. Oxygen therapy is the only drug therapy to change the natural history of COPD for patients with resting hypoxemia (see COPD section).

Follow-up: The degree of dyspnea reflects the effectiveness of treatment. Follow-up visits should be scheduled for 3 to 6 months and as needed. Monitor for signs and symptoms of complications. Further evaluation is individualized to the assessment findings.

Sequelae: Monitor for bronchopulmonary infections, bronchial pneumonia, cor pulmonale, pulmonary hypertension, polycythemia pulmonary embolism, spontaneous pneumothorax, and progression to emphysema.

Prevention/prophylaxis: Prophylactic measures include annual influenza vaccine; pneumococcal vaccine; avoidance of crowds, especially during cold and flu seasons; and avoidance of extreme variations in temperature. A home humidifier may be helpful in thinning secretions but should be avoided if the patient has concurrent asthma. Postural drainage three to four times a day also may aid in mobilizing secretions. Smoking cessation and the avoidance of second-hand smoke is essential in the prevention of chronic bronchitis.

Referral: Refer to a physician or specialist if complications occur with no response to treatment.

Education: Compliance to the treatment regimen is facilitated through the patient's knowledge of the respiratory system, the disease process, precipitating factors of the disease, drug education, proper use of inhalers, and signs and symptoms of complications. Maintenance of hydration allows for clearance of low-viscosity mucus. For patients in a poor nutritional state, the use of liquid oral supplements is recommended. Advise patients to reduce alcohol consumption because alcohol depresses the respiratory drive. Encourage aerobic exercise as tolerated. Patients should be cautioned about using OTC medications such as cough suppressants, narcotics, sleeping pills, antihistamines, and oxygen therapy. Participation in a pulmonary rehabilitation program and support group should be encouraged.

CHRONIC OBSTRUCTIVE PULMONARY DISEASE

SIGNAL SYMPTOMS ▶ dyspnea (emphysema), chronic cough and sputum production (chronic bronchitis)

Chronic obstructive pulmonary disease	ICD-9-CM: 496
Emphysematous	ICD-9-CM: 492.8
With asthma	ICD-9-CM: 493.2
With chronic bronchitis	ICD-9-CM: 491.20

Description: COPD is characterized by progressive obstruction of airflow, which becomes irreversible. COPD may take the form of emphysema, chronic bronchitis, unremitting asthma, or a combination of these. Airflow limitation is usually progressive and associated with an abnormal inflammatory response of the lungs to noxious particles or gases. Although most patients with COPD have a combination of the aforementioned entities, usually one predominates.

Etiology: Emphysema is characterized by obstruction to airflow caused by abnormal airspace enlargement distal to terminal bronchioles. No fibrosis occurs, but the walls of the airspaces are destroyed, possibly because of oxidative changes from protease-antiprotease imbalance. Air becomes trapped, hindering effective oxygen and carbon dioxide exchange.

The clinical diagnosis of chronic bronchitis is based on certain symptom criteria. A chronic, productive cough, typically worse on awakening and lasting for 3 consecutive months in 2 sequential years, is considered diagnostic after other causes of mucus hypersecretion have been ruled out. Inflammation in the lining of the airways results in hyperplasia of goblet cells, edema and inflammation of mucosa, and hypertrophy of mucus glands (see section on Chronic Bronchitis).

Unremitting asthma is a chronic inflammatory airway disorder with hyperactivity of the airway. In older patients, asthma tends to become less reversible, at which point it becomes a chronic obstructive disease.

Smoking is a prominent factor in the development of almost all types of COPD.

Occurrence: Prevalence of COPD in elderly persons has been increasing steadily since 1971; an estimated 17 million diagnosed patients exist in the United States, with almost as many in the asymptomatic to early symptomatic period. It is the fourth major cause of death in the United States. Globally the United States ranks eighth in deaths from COPD.

Age: Because of the natural history of the disease (including a 20- to 40-year preclinical period of damage), the elderly population is most affected. Rates are highest in the >75 age group, followed by the >65 age group.

Ethnicity: Rates of COPD and mortality from COPD are higher among whites than among nonwhites.

Gender: More women than men are diagnosed with and die from COPD.

Contributing factors: Smoking is the primary cause of COPD. Early age at starting, total pack-years, and current smoking practice contribute to COPD mortality. Smoking/oxidative stress/neutrophils gravitate to lungs/inflammation/inflammatory cytokines, CD8 lymphocyte, alveolar macrophage, and proteases. Other contributing factors for COPD include air pollution, occupational exposures, severe viral pneumonia at a young age, passive smoking, airway hyperactivity, possibly viral infection; rarely, a genetic component owing to α_1-antitrypsin deficiency exists. Changes in the weather cause exacerbation of symptoms; environmental allergens and biochemical mediators also play a role in asthmatic COPD.

Signs and symptoms: Symptoms of emphysema include mild exertional dyspnea progressing to difficulty breathing at rest, barrel chest, diminished breath sounds, occasional wheezing, occasional respiratory infections, infrequent cough or sputum production, use of accessory muscles for respiration, and weight loss. Symptoms of chronic bronchitis include frequent productive cough, especially in the morning; frequent infections; wheezing; decreased breath sounds; and cyanosis. Asthma symptoms include periodic dyspnea; wheezing; decreased breath sounds; cough, especially at night; cyanosis; and nocturnal and seasonal exacerbation of symptoms. Because the older COPD patient usually has a combination of more than one type of COPD, symptoms often vary.

A careful history regarding onset and timing of symptoms, changes in activity and exercise patterns, smoking, and occupational background helps to establish diagnosis. Physical examination does not reveal early stages of COPD but does help in establishing a baseline and uncovering comorbidities. Initially the patient may present frequently with sinus or respiratory infections. As the disease progresses, changes in the respiratory pattern (e.g., prolonged expiration, pursed-lip breathing, use of accessory muscles of respiration, hypertrophied sternocleidomastoid muscles) can be seen. Weight loss is seen frequently in the later stages of emphysema, when the patient becomes dyspneic while trying to eat. Right-sided heart failure and cor pulmonale seen in the later stages may present as jugular venous distention, hepatomegaly, or peripheral edema. The patient's color may appear ruddy or dusky, depending on oxygenation. In the early to middle stages, chest auscultation may reveal longer expirations, with wheezing on forced expiration. Later, as the chest hyperinflates, breath sounds become distant, and percussion is hyperresonant. Wheezes sometimes can be heard (most frequently with chronic bronchitis); the presence of crackles suggests possible pulmonary edema or pneumonia. The chest takes on a barrel-like appearance. Hyperinflation restricts diaphragmatic movement. As the cardiovascular system attempts to compensate, tachycardia or a gallop rhythm commonly occurs. Heart sounds are distant.

Diagnostic tests:

Test	Results Indicating Disorder	CPT Code
PFTs	Stage I: mild FEV_1/FVC <70%; FEV_1 ≥80% predicted With or without chronic symptoms (cough, sputum production) Stage II: moderate FEV_1/FVC <70%; 30% ≥ FEV_1; FEV_1 <80% predicted IIA: 50% FEV_1 ≤80% predicted IIB: 30% FEV_1 ≤50% predicted With or without chronic symptoms (cough, sputum, production, dyspnea) Stage III: severe FEV_1/FVC <70%; FEV_1<30% predicted or FEV_1<50% predicted plus respiratory failure or clinical signs of right heart failure (source: GOLD guidelines) Decreased single breath diffusing lung capacity for carbon monoxide	78596
Bronchodilator response with PFT	Baseline FEV_1; after bronchodilator, 15% suggests some reversibility, 20% suggests asthmatic component	94664, 94665
Pulse oximetry	Oxygen saturation <92% indicates need for arterial blood gases to assess oxygenation and ventilation	94760-94762
Arterial blood gases (late in disease)	Hypoxemia, compensated respiratory acidosis; during acute exacerbations, worsening of acidemia	82803-82810
ECG	Sinus tachycardia, supraventricular arrhythmias, right-axis deviation, pulmonary hypertension with ongoing S waves in lateral precordial leads	93272
CBC	Normal to polycythemia	85022-85025
Sputum culture in acute exacerbations	*H. influenzae, S. pneumoniae, M. catarrhalis*	89350
Chest x-ray	Sometimes normal; most useful in advanced disease Hyperinflation with diaphragmatic flattening Hyperlucency of lungs, rapid tapering of vascular shadows Bullae Pulmonary hypertension—prominent hilar shadows, right heart enlargement anteriorly If predominantly basilar findings, consider α_1-antitrypsin deficiency	71010-71035
Exercise test: 6-minute walk	Oxygen desaturation, oxygen uptake, and carbon dioxide production; V_D/V_T	94799

FVC, forced vital capacity; V_D/V_T, dead space-to-tidal volume ratio.

High-resolution computed tomography (CT) also may be employed for diagnosis of COPD.

Differential diagnosis:

- Lung cancer
- Bronchiectasis
- Acute bronchitis
- Occupational lung disease
- Acute viral infection

Treatment: Individualize treatment goals according to the stage of disease, comorbidities, and patient goals. Use collaborative management with a physician specializing in respiratory conditions. Smoking cessation is a primary goal of treatment. The American Lung Association offers smoking cessation classes free or at minimal cost. If the patient is ready to quit, bupropion (Zyban) sustained-release, 150 mg orally daily for 3 days, then twice a day for 7 to 12 weeks, can be prescribed, after you establish its compatibility with the other medications the patient may be taking. Weekly follow-up phone calls for the first few weeks may help maintain the patient's motivation. Alternatively, or in combination with bupropion, nicotine patches and other products are available OTC. Nicotine patches are expensive. Adequate hydration is important. Treat infections early and aggressively to prevent complications or further loss of lung function. The patient should receive yearly influenza vaccine unless contraindications exist. Pneumococcal vaccine also should be given once, with the option to repeat in 5 years if first dose was given before age 65 years.

The use of antibiotic prophylaxis in acute exacerbations of COPD is controversial. Most authorities agree that low-level antibiotic therapy benefits the patient when fever, purulent sputum, or other symptoms of a bacterial infection exist. Prophylactic antibiotics are not recommended. When choosing a suitable agent, keep in mind that typical respiratory organisms include *S. pneumoniae, H. influenzae,* and *M. catarrhalis.* Knowledge of local patterns of antibiotic resistance is important in prescribing. Although recommendations vary, most include macrolides, a β-lactam/β-lactam inhibitor combination, a tetracycline, or a fluoroquinolone. The patient or caregiver should be instructed to call if symptoms worsen after 3 days of antibiotic therapy. Consult with a pulmonary or internal medicine specialist if the patient does not improve.

Inhaled anticholinergics and bronchodilators are the mainstay of pharmacotherapy for COPD; education is needed in administration of metered-dose inhalers. Older patients should use a spacer chamber. An alternative approach is the nebulizer, which is less portable but can be administered with an oral mouthpiece or a mask. For patients with nonasthmatic COPD, the use of an ipratropium metered-dose inhaler can be instituted; the usual dosage is 2 to 4 puffs four times daily. Ipratropium is also available as nebulizer therapy. It is not effective in treating acute bronchospasm; patients should be instructed about this and advised to use their β-agonist inhaler for acute problems or to seek urgent care. Anticholinergics should be used cautiously in patients with narrow-angle glaucoma, prostatic hypertrophy, or bladder neck obstruction, and they are contraindicated in patients who are allergic to atropine. Because of the route of administration (inhalation), side effects are minimal. Combivent, a combination of ipratropium and albuterol in a metered-dose inhaler, is also available. The usual dosage is 1 to 2 puffs four times daily. A new, long-acting anticholinergic, tiotropium, is expected to be available soon, in once-daily dosing. β-Agonist metered-dose inhaler therapy is most effective in treating patients with asthmatic COPD, but it also is used to treat patients with nonasthmatic COPD. Inhaled β-agonists are powerful bronchodilators that usually provide a measure of relief on administration. The most commonly used agent is albuterol (Proventil, Ventolin) metered-dose inhaler, 1 to 2 puffs every 4 to 6 hours as needed or four times daily; albuterol is also available in a nebulizer. Salmeterol xinafoate (Serevent) metered-dose inhaler, 2 puffs twice daily (every 12 hours) is a long-acting inhaled β-agonist used for COPD management. The effects of β-agonists are antagonized by β-blockers. β-Agonists are sympathomimetic agents that cause transient tachycardia, nervousness, and elevation in blood pressure. Use β-agonists cautiously with cardiovascular disease; concurrent therapy with xanthines (e.g., theophylline) or other sympathomimetics (often found in OTC decongestants or cold remedies) exaggerates side effects. Patients should be instructed to seek care if their breathing changes or it does not respond to the prescribed medication regimen.

The use of methylxanthines, such as theophylline and aminophylline, has decreased significantly. They are now considered third-line or fourth-line agents, to be used when inhaled bronchodilators or anticholinergic agents do not control symptoms well. Dosage is individualized, with the timed-release forms being preferred. Significant side effects occur, including increased nervousness or agitation, increased heart rate, and gastrointestinal effects. Also, many drug interactions are associated with the methylxanthines. Frequent drug level measurements are required to monitor for methylxanthine toxicity; subtherapeutic drug levels, especially in older patients, usually are not adjusted because of lack of monitoring. Doses should be reduced in the presence of hepatic or cardiac disease or a history of seizures.

Oral corticosteroids and sometimes inhaled steroids are prescribed for patients with COPD that is refractory to treatment or for patients experiencing an exacerbation. Use of inhaled glucorticosteroids should be reserved for the following patients:

- Symptomatic patients with documented spirometric response to inhaled steroids
- FEV_1 <50% predicted and repeated exacerbations requiring oral steroids or antibiotics or both

Short courses of oral steroids are preferred to a maintenance course whenever possible. If the patient has a history of cor pulmonale, average doses of oral steroids can cause fluid retention and precipitate an episode of right-sided heart failure. Patients with asthmatic COPD may use inhaled corticosteroids instead of oral corticosteroids or after tapering off the use of oral corticosteroids. Because of the potential of these drugs to mask infection, careful monitoring is required. Instruct patients to rinse their mouth and equipment after using the inhaler, to prevent oral candidiasis. Fluticasone propionate (Flovent) is available in three dosage strengths: 40 mg/puff, 110 mg/puff, and 220 mg/puff. Dosage for each is 2 puffs twice daily. Advair Diskus, used for asthma, combines fluticasone and salmeterol in a once-daily dose.

Use the foregoing information as a guideline. In addition to medication management, quality of life and functionality are important issues to consider when treating patients with COPD. Every patient should have an advanced directive. Pulmonary rehabilitation and exercise do not prolong life but enhance functioning and improve quality of life. For the patient with severe COPD, maintaining comfort and any element of functionality is helpful. When dyspnea is unrelieved by medications and interferes with functionality, low-level oxygen therapy may be instituted, either temporarily during and after an acute exacerbation or on a long-term basis. If the patient has Medicare, criteria must be met for long-term therapy to be reimbursable. The duration of dyspnea and activity level of the patient determine type of oxygen delivery. Oxygen is the only therapy shown to prolong life in hypoxemic COPD patients. Criteria for long-term oxygen therapy includes:

- PaO_2 = 55 mm Hg or SaO_2 = 88% with or without hypercapnia
- PO_2 = 55 to 60 mm Hg or SaO_2 = 89% if there is evidence of pulmonary hypertension, polycythemia, or peripheral edema suggesting congestive heart failure

Nutrition is a treatment concern for many older patients with COPD. The exertion of breathing burns extra calories and tires these patients so much that they cannot eat. Medications also may contribute to anorexia. Small, frequent feedings with easily chewed and digested foods are recommended. Supplementation with a liquid nutritional preparation may help. Consultation with a nutritionist may be indicated.

Several surgical options, including lung volume reduction therapy, lung resections, transplants, and laser bullectomy, are available in selected circumstances. Consultation with a pulmonary specialist is advised, with possibility of referral to a thoracic surgeon.

If the patient is at home, supportive services, such as home care nurse, physical therapy, and home health aide, may be instituted after an acute exacerbation of COPD. End-stage COPD patients may be candidates for hospice care, if this is in accord with their wishes.

Follow-up: A newly diagnosed patient should be seen frequently until an optimal treatment plan is in place and disease education has been completed. For stable patients who are maintaining their usual activities of daily living, routine reassessment every 3 to 6 months is advisable, with instructions to the patient or caregiver to schedule an interim visit if there is a change in status, increased symptoms, or an infection. For stable patients with other significant comorbidities, visits every 3 months are advisable.

Patients who are unstable or have had an acute exacerbation need more frequent follow-up visits initially. Collaborative management with these patients is advised strongly; during the immediate postacute period, a pulmonary specialist should manage the patient. Patients who continue to smoke should be counseled at every visit to quit.

Sequelae: COPD can lead to infections, particularly respiratory (pneumonia, recurrent bronchitis, viral infections), cor pulmonale, pulmonary hypertension, malnutrition, acute or chronic respiratory failure, steroid-induced myopathy or Cushing's syndrome, bullous lung disease, polycythemia, and sleep-related hypoxemia. Depression frequently is associated with COPD.

Prevention/prophylaxis: COPD is almost 100% preventable by avoidance of smoking. Perform spirometry to establish a baseline on every patient >40 years old who smokes.

Vaccinations include annual influenza vaccine and pneumococcal vaccine once, except if initial dose was before age 65, repeat in 5 years.

Referral: Collaborative management is advised in all but stable, moderately ill patients. Refer patients to a pulmonary specialist during instability, for hospital and postacute care and for determination of the need for oxygen therapy. Refer patients to a surgeon if the option of surgery is deemed appropriate. Refer patients to physical therapy for reconditioning; occupational therapy also may be helpful in teaching breathing techniques and energy-conserving measures. Postacute COPD patients dwelling in the community should be referred for home care. Also, refer all patients to community resources and support groups.

Education: Teach the patient, family, and caregivers about the disease process and its management; the role of smoking in causing COPD; the possibility of reversibility in the early/moderate stage with smoking cessation; medications; oxygen therapy precautions; and the need to seek care early if infection develops, dyspnea increases, or a change in cognitive status occurs. Advise patients of the need for regular follow-up visits, even if no symptoms are present.

LUNG CANCER

SIGNAL SYMPTOMS ➤ cough dyspnea weight loss anorexia hemoptysis

| Neoplasm, lung primary | ICD-9-CM: 162.9 |
| Neoplasm, secondary | ICD-9-CM: 197.0 |

Description: Lung cancer is a malignant neoplasm of the parenchyma of the lung. Most (82%) lung neoplasms are non–small cell lung cancer (NSCLC), which includes squamous cell carcinoma, adenocarcinoma, and large cell carcinoma. Small cell lung cancer (SCLC) accounts for 18% of lung malignancies and includes the histologic subtypes oat cell, polygonal cell, lymphatic, and spindle cell.

Etiology: Research has shown conclusively that >85% of lung cancer cases are associated with tobacco smoking. The inhalation of other carcinogens, usually through occupational exposure, account for most other cases of lung cancer. Patients with preexisting diseases that involve the lungs, such as COPD, prior lung cancers, sarcoidosis, and scleroderma, are at increased risk for developing lung cancer. Radiation exposure may cause lung cancer. Some research suggests there may be a genetic predisposition to carcinoma of the lung.

Occurrence: Lung cancer is the most common cause of cancer-associated deaths in the United States. It is the second most common cancer among men and women. Annually, >180,000 new cases are diagnosed. Lung cancer is responsible for 32% of cancer deaths in men and 25% of cancer deaths in women. The incidence in women is increasing rapidly.

Age: Lung cancer can occur at any age, but there is a dramatic increase in new diagnosis after age 40 years.

Ethnicity: African-American men <54 years old have a higher incidence than white men. No significant difference in African-American and white women.

Gender: More men have lung cancer than women, but the incidence rate for women is rising.

Contributing factors: The cumulative dose or pack-years for cigarette smoking is related directly to the risk of developing lung cancer. The more cigarettes smoked per day and the longer the individual has smoked, the higher the risk of developing lung cancer. The risk of lung cancer is 30 times higher in smokers than in nonsmokers. Cigar and pipe smokers and passive smokers have double the risk. The risks of developing NSCLC steadily decline for people who quit smoking and approach that of a nonsmoker after 15 years of abstinence. Individuals who have smoked for >20 years probably always will have a slightly increased risk of developing the disease, even after 15 years as a nonsmoker. There is no change in risk of SCLC with smoking cessation; early age at beginning to smoke is a significant risk factor.

Asbestos exposure alone increases the risk of developing pulmonary carcinoma, but when combined with smoking, the risk increases to 100 times that of a nonsmoker. Other inhaled agents implicated in the development of the disease are radon, arsenic, nickel, chromates, halo ethers, alkylating compounds, and polycyclic aromatic hydrocarbons. Radon is a risk factor; air pollution also is thought to contribute to the development of lung cancer. Sarcoidosis carries a threefold increased risk; scleroderma increases risk of bronchoalveolar cancer.

Signs and symptoms: Signs and symptoms of lung cancer are usually present only after the disease has progressed beyond the early stages. Routine screening for the disease with chest x-ray examination is not recommended because it is neither specific nor sensitive. Symptoms suggestive of lung cancer include smoking, a new or changing cough, hoarseness, hemoptysis, anorexia, cachexia, unexplained weight loss, dyspnea, hypoxia, wheezing, unresolving pneumonia, and chest wall pain. Patients initially may present with symptoms related to extrathoracic disease, including tracheal obstruction, esophageal obstruction with dysphagia, laryngeal nerve paralysis, phrenic nerve paralysis with elevated hemidiaphragm, sympathetic nerve paralysis or Horner's syndrome, pleural effusion owing to lymphatic obstruction, Pancoast's syndrome involving the eighth cervical and first and second thoracic nerves, or superior vena cava syndrome from vascular obstruction.

Patients with pericardial and cardiac extension of tumor may have symptoms of arrhythmia, tamponade, or failure. The presenting illness in patients with lung cancer may be paraneoplastic syndromes, including hypercalcemia, hypophosphatemia, hyponatremia with syndrome of inappropriate antidiuretic hormone, and hypercoagulable states. Occasionally, skeletal-connective syndromes, clubbing, and osteoarthropathy are initial symptoms of lung cancer.

Diagnostic tests: After a history and physical examination suggestive of disease, the following tests are recommended:

Test	Results Indicating Disorder	CPT Code
Chest x-ray	Nonspecific abnormalities, including hilar masses, atelectasis, pleural effusions, peripheral masses, and infiltrates	71070–71035
Sputum for cytology	Positive in 80% of centrally located tumors	89350

After the diagnosis of abnormal chest x-ray and referral to a specialist, other tests may be ordered, including blood chemistry, CT scan of the chest and upper abdomen, bronchoscopy, and selected PFTs. A positron-emission tomography scan may be ordered to help with staging. PFTs should include screening spirometry with or without bronchodilators (as needed), diffusing capacity, and resting oxygen saturation. Definitive diagnosis is established by tissue pathology and histology.

Differential diagnosis: Tuberculosis, infectious granuloma, pneumonia, empyema, bronchiectasis, abscess, sarcoidosis, pneumonitis, and asbestosis all can mimic lung cancer.

Treatment: Surgical resection, radiation therapy, and occasionally chemotherapy are indicated for NSCLC; staging of the disease determines the treatments. Chemotherapy and radiation are the treatments of choice for SCLC.

Follow-up: Patients should be seen for follow-up every 2 months after treatment for lung cancer. Every visit includes a chest x-ray. During years 2 to 5, follow-up should be every 3 months with a chest x-ray. Yearly examinations are advised thereafter.

Sequelae: Disability and death are the chief sequelae of lung cancer. The 5-year survival rate is 13% for NSCLC and <10% for SCLC.

Prevention/prophylaxis: Prevention of lung cancer should focus on smoking cessation. Ask about and record the tobacco use status of every patient, advise patients who smoke to quit, and offer smoking cessation treatment at every office visit.

Referral: On suspecting lung cancer, refer the patient to a pulmonary specialist and possibly a cardiothoracic surgeon and an oncologist.

Education: Many smoking cessation programs are available. Examples include the American Academy of Family Physicians Stop Smoking Kit, various pamphlets from the American Cancer Society, and A Healthy Beginning Counseling Kit from the American Lung Association. The primary health-care provider can assess the smoker's motivation to quit and offer motivational intervention based on the four *R*s:

Risks: Review acute, long-term, and environmental risks with the patient. Encourage the patient to identify risks that are most important to him or her.

Rewards: Help the patient to identify potential benefits of quitting.

Repetition: Reinforce risks and rewards identified by the patient on a regular basis.

Relapse prevention: Communicate caring, concern, and encouragement. Let the patient talk about feelings related to quitting smoking. Provide education about the process of smoking cessation. Guide the patient in the use of nicotine replacement therapies, such as gum or a patch. Provide information about support groups and community programs available to help with smoking cessation.

PNEUMONIA

SIGNAL SYMPTOMS ▶ fever or hypothermia, new cough with or without sputum, chest discomfort or dyspnea, fatigue, headache

| Pneumonia | ICD-9-CM: 486 |

Description: Community-acquired pneumonia (CAP), an acute lower respiratory tract infection of the lung parenchyma, can be bacterial or viral. Bacterial pneumonia is the most common type in older adults. CAP refers to pneumonia that begins outside of the hospital or is diagnosed within 48 hours of admission; the patient must not have resided in a long-term care facility for 14 days before symptom onset. Pneumonia also is classified as nosocomial (acquired from a hospital or nursing home).

Etiology: The most common cause of CAP is *S. pneumoniae.* Other common pathogens include *Staphylococcus aureus, H. influenzae,* and other gram-negative and anaerobic bacteria. In patients with COPD, *S. pneumoniae, H. influenzae, M. catarrhalis,* and *Legionella* predominate. Aspiration pneumonia is caused most often by anaerobes and *S. pneumoniae.* Nosocomial infections in older patients are caused by a variety of organisms, including *Klebsiella pneumoniae, S. pneumoniae, S. aureus, H. influenzae, Pseudomonas aeruginosa, Escherichia coli,* anaerobes, *Legionella,* and *Chlamydia.* It is often the norm to have a mixture of organisms.

Occurrence: CAP is not a reportable disease, so occurrence in the ambulatory population is difficult to ascertain. Each year, there are 2 million to 3 million cases of CAP, resulting in approximately 10 million health-care provider visits, >500,000 hospitalizations, and >50,000 deaths. The annual incidence of hospitalizations is 260 in 100,000 and 962 per 100,000 in patients $\geq$65 years old. It is the sixth most common cause of death in the United States.

Age: Pneumonia is the most common cause of death from infectious disease in older patients. Elderly persons are at 5 to 10 times the risk of younger adults for dying of pneumonia. Of cases, 60% occur in patients $\geq$65 years old.

Ethnicity: Not significant.

Gender: More men than women are diagnosed with pneumonia.

Contributing factors: Comorbidities, influenza, chronic pulmonary conditions, smoking, alcoholism, malnutrition, colonization of the oropharynx by gram-negative bacteria, institutional setting, decline in immune function, hospitalization, use of sedating medications, and diminished cough reflex may contribute to development of pneumonia. Swallowing problems from esophageal or neurological conditions or the presence of a feeding tube can lead to aspiration pneumonia. Risk factors for pneumonia-related death include age >65, comorbid disease (e.g., diabetes, renal insufficiency, COPD, congestive heart failure), active malignancy, leukopenia, fever >101°F, immunosuppressed state, pneumonia caused by *S. aureus* or gram-negative rods, aspiration, and airway obstruction. Signs and symptoms associated with pneumonia-related mortality include dyspnea, chills, altered mental status, tachypnea, hypotension, hypothermia, and hyperthermia. Laboratory abnormalities associated with increased mortality are hyponatremia, hyperglycemia, abnormal liver function studies, hypoalbuminemia, azotemia, hypoxemia, and azotemia.

Signs and symptoms: Typical symptoms include fever, chills, cough, and rusty or thick sputum, with associated gastrointestinal upset or anorexia, malaise, and diaphoresis. These characteristic symptoms are frequently absent, particularly in the frail elderly, leading to a lag time before diagnosis. In the older patient, mental status changes (i.e., confusion), new onset or increased frequency of falls, increased respiratory rate, hypotension, anorexia, a marked functional decline, and new onset of urinary incontinence are typical symptoms. Caregivers or family members may report that the patient is not his or her usual self. Physical examination of the chest reveals crackles that do not clear with cough or deep breathing. Increased respiratory rate (>24 breaths/min) is typical. If the patient is not able to deep breathe adequately, crackles may be absent. Dullness to percussion, egophony, and bronchial breath sounds may be present. A fever of 100°F, with tachycardia, may be present. Signs of dehydration may occur. The patient may appear anxious, restless, or withdrawn. Concurrent symptoms of congestive heart failure may appear.

Diagnostic tests:

Test	Results Indicating Disorder	CPT Code
Chest x-ray (gold standard); findings typically lag behind clinical symptoms by 48 hours	Variable: patchy airspace infiltrates, diffuse alveolar or interstitial infiltrates, lobar consolidation. Pleural effusion, empyema, or cavitation may be an incidental finding	71010–71035

Other diagnostic tests usually are reserved for candidates for hospital admission. Sputum for Gram stain is recommended for all patients but is difficult to obtain in practice, particularly in an outpatient setting. For hospitalized patients, CBC and differential, serum creatinine, BUN, glucose, electrolytes, and liver function tests are recommended. If *Legionella* is suspected, a urinary antigen assay test for *Legionella* serogroup 1 should be done. Selected patients may require tuberculosis, human immunodeficiency virus (HIV), and other tests. Sputum for Gram stain and culture and two pretreatment blood cultures should be obtained. In patients with comorbidities affecting oxygenation, pulse oximetry is indicated to evaluate oxygen saturation and need for oxygen therapy.

Differential diagnosis:
- Influenza or parainfluenza
- Adenoviruses
- Fungal agents
- Toxoplasma
- Tuberculosis
- Pulmonary embolism with infarction

- Vasculitis of the pulmonary bed
- Pneumothorax

Treatment: A crucial element in treatment is the choice of setting. For community-dwelling older patients, the presence of a responsible caregiver and a supportive home environment is necessary. Temporary measures to increase support and monitor status of response may be introduced by ordering home health services. If the patient fails to recover or deteriorates despite these interventions, hospitalization should be contemplated. Infectious Diseases Society of America guidelines advocate the use of the PORT (Pneumonia Patient Outcome Research Team) prediction rule as a guideline for determining outpatient treatment versus hospitalization; this can be accessed at http://www.journals.uchicago.edu/CID/journal/issues/v31n2/000441/000441.html. Use of the PORT prediction rule should be tempered by clinical judgment. The American Thoracic Society addresses PORT guidelines but summarizes that candidates for admission are patients who have multiple risk factors for a complicated course (contact: http://www.thoracic.org/adobe/statements/commacq1-25.pdf).

Objective criteria for hospital admission include:

- Inability to take oral medications or fluids
- Acute mental status changes
- Severe acute metabolic, hematologic, or electrolyte abnormalities
- Acute concomitant medical condition (e.g., malignancy, hepatic disease, renal insufficiency, cardiac disease)
- Hypoxemia on room air (PaO_2 <60 mm Hg)
- Multilobar involvement on chest x-ray
- Secondary suppurative infection (e.g., meningitis, endocarditis, empyema)
- Severe vital sign abnormality (systolic blood pressure <90 mm Hg, pulse >125/min, respirations >30/min)

Antimicrobial treatment is usually empirical and is directed at eradicating the most frequently occurring agents in the patient's setting. If diagnostic testing yields a definite organism, treatment is directed toward its elimination. Otherwise, the recommendation for outpatients is administration of a macrolide, doxycycline, or fluoroquinolone with enhanced activity against *S. pneumoniae.* For older patients or patients with significant comorbidities, a fluoroquinolone is often the first choice. This information is intended as a guideline; each provider is responsible for knowing local patterns of drug resistance and reviewing prescribing guidelines.

In addition to antimicrobial treatment measures, supportive and restorative measures are necessary for optimal recovery. Oxygen therapy is based on determinations of arterial blood gases or pulse oximetry during the acute phase. Nutritional supplementation also may be indicated.

Physical therapy measures for strengthening and ambulation may be initiated during the acute recovery period and continued during convalescence or replaced by restorative nursing measures.

Follow-up: Follow-up depends on comorbidities and response to prescribed treatment regimen. Independent community-dwelling older adults or caregivers should be instructed to call if symptoms worsen, if no response occurs after 3 to 5 days of treatment, or if symptoms recur. A follow-up visit after completion of treatment, to assess response and further interventions, is helpful. Patient teaching regarding self-care and increasing functional status can be given at this time, with further visits depending on individual status. Follow-up chest x-ray, if indicated, should be delayed for at least 6 weeks because resolution takes 6 to 12 weeks. Frail elderly persons in a long-term care facility need more frequent and prolonged monitoring after an acute episode of pneumonia.

Sequelae: The older patient with comorbidities is especially prone to complications, including severe deconditioning and decline in activities of daily living level. If nutrition is poor, coexisting lung disease is present, or both, the patient may never return to baseline. Adult respiratory distress syndrome or multiple organ dysfunction syndrome also may occur, resulting in significant morbidity and mortality. Superinfections, recurrence, or opportunistic infections may occur in susceptible patients.

Prevention/prophylaxis: Older patients should have an annual influenza vaccination. If unable to take the influenza vaccine and living in a long-term care facility, the patient may receive amantadine or rimantadine prophylaxis during the peak influenza period. The pneumococcal vaccine is administered once in patients $\geq$65 years old. Antibiotics should be prescribed prudently. Teach patients with comorbidities to avoid contact with persons having known respiratory infections.

Referral: Refer patients with comorbidities to infectious disease, internal medicine, or pulmonary specialists for inpatient management and initial follow-up. Manage patients in long-term care facilities collaboratively, until a return to baseline is achieved. Refer patients to a dietitian for nutritional guidance and to physical therapy for reconditioning, strengthening, and increasing level of activities of daily living. Refer patients to home care services (nursing, physical therapy, home health aide) as needed for in-home support.

Education: Provider education regarding appropriate prescribing of antibiotics is helpful in decreasing drug-resistant organisms. Teach groups of older adults (especially adults with comorbidities) about preventive measures. Educate patient and caregivers in management, including the importance of nutrition and hydration and deep breathing exercises.

PULMONARY EMBOLISM

SIGNAL SYMPTOMS▶   dyspnea, acute onset, chest pain on inspiration, anxiety

| Pulmonary embolism | ICD-9-CM: 415.10 |

Description: Pulmonary embolism is the occlusion of one or more pulmonary vessels by a traveling thrombus originating from a distant site. Although a blood clot is the most common embolism, fat, air, bone marrow, tumor cells, amniotic fluid, and foreign material also can occlude the pulmonary vasculature.

Etiology: Pulmonary embolism usually is caused by a dislodged thrombus from one of the veins of the legs or pelvis (deep vein thrombosis); thrombi distal to the popliteal area are less likely to migrate and cause pulmonary embolism.

Occurrence: Between 600,000 and 700,000 cases are diagnosed each year, with 60,000 deaths annually.

Age: The incidence of pulmonary embolism increases steadily with age with a 1.8% annual incidence in persons age 65 to 69 compared with 3.1% in persons age 85 to 89.

Ethnicity: Not significant.

Gender: Women are affected more frequently than men.

Contributing factors: Risk factors for pulmonary embolism are indicated by Virchow's triad of stasis or prolonged immobility, hypercoagulation, and venous trauma (endothelial injury with inflammation of the vessel lining). Stasis may be occupational or medical (e.g., congestive heart failure, postsurgical paralysis, chronic illness or debilitation, tumor compression). Venous trauma damaging the deep veins of the legs; orthopedic procedures from arthroscopy to hip, knees, or pelvic repair; or trauma from falls, burns, or crush injuries may contribute to thrombus formation and lead to pulmonary embolism. Hypercoagulation is associated with connective tissue diseases, malignant tumors, and stroke. A genetic factor involving inactivated protein C, occurring in about 5% of the population, also predisposes to hypercoagulation. Other risk factors include use of estrogen, advanced age, and obesity. A past history of deep venous thrombosis or pulmonary embolism is associated with recurrence.

Signs and symptoms: Signs and symptoms of pulmonary embolism tend to be nonspecific, so the diagnosis is frequently missed. In the Prospective Investigation of Pulmonary Embolism Diagnosis (PIOPED) study, older patients presented with the same symptoms as younger ones. The problem may occur when these symptoms are attributed to aging or existing comorbidities. Dyspnea (acute onset), anxiety or apprehension, pleuritic chest pain, cough, tachypnea, and accentuation of the pulmonic component of S_2 are frequently present and may be accompanied by diaphoresis, syncope, tachycardia, S_3 gallop, hypoxemia, or hemoptysis. Physical examination usually reveals tachypnea. Auscultation of the lungs may be normal or may show localized wheezing, consolidation, or friction rub. Jugular venous distention and atrial arrhythmia may be present. Examination of the legs, especially of the iliofemoral and popliteal areas, may reveal signs of deep venous thrombosis; the arms, abdomen, and pelvic areas also should be examined for pain, erythema, or palpable vein cords. Although deep venous thrombosis occurs in the calf area of the leg as well, these thrombotic areas account for <5% of pulmonary emboli.

Diagnostic tests:

Test	Results Indicating Disorder	CPT Code
Chest x-ray	Used to rule out other pulmonary pathology; atelectasis, pleural effusion, parenchymal infiltrates common; elevation of hemidiaphragm on affected side. Chest x-ray also is needed to assist in evaluating ventilation-perfusion scan	71010–71035
Lung scan: ventilation-perfusion scan	Normal results rule out pulmonary embolism High-probability results are diagnostic Low-probability results with clinical symptoms indicate need for pulmonary angiography. Further testing also needed in patients with underlying cardiopulmonary disease	78596
Pulmonary angiography (gold standard)	Intraluminal filling defect in >1 projection	75741–75746
Helical CT angiography	Positive for thrombus identification in proximal pulmonary arteries; less helpful in segmental arteries	71260-50-70-75

D-dimer is not recommended because of lack of standardization and because comorbidities commonly seen with aging can affect results.

Differential diagnosis:

- Pneumonia
- MI
- Pericarditis
- Congestive heart failure
- Pleural effusion
- Panic attacks
- Hyperventilation syndrome
- Pneumothorax
- Esophageal rupture

- Gastritis
- Gastric or duodenal ulcer
- Gastroesophageal reflux disease
- Asthma.

Treatment: Anticoagulation is the cornerstone of treatment. Anticoagulation reduces the incidence of fatal pulmonary embolism by approximately 60% to 70%. Parenteral heparin therapy is guided by activated partial thromboplastin time determinations; a weight-based nomogram is recommended for older adults. The activated partial thromboplastin time should be maintained at 1.5 to 2.5 times control. Subtherapeutic dosing in the initial 24 hours can lead to increased clotting. Low-molecular-weight heparin has the same efficacy as unfractionated heparin but does not require coagulation monitoring. It is administered once or twice daily; dosing is based on body weight. Low-molecular-weight heparin is much more costly. Oral anticoagulation with warfarin (Coumadin) is initiated shortly after heparin. Heparin therapy is continued for approximately 5 days after beginning the warfarin to ensure adequate anticoagulation. Prothrombin time is measured to maintain the patient with an international normalized ratio (INR) in the therapeutic range of two to three times control levels. Warfarin is used for long-term maintenance of ≥6 months, with measurements of the INR three times during the initial week of therapy, tapering to twice weekly for 2 weeks, then once weekly or every other week. Dosage is adjusted based on these results. Patients with genetic hypercoagulability or recurrent thrombus may be maintained on anticoagulants for life. If the patient is not a candidate for anticoagulation, placement of a vena cava filter is effective to block emboli before they reach the lungs; findings are inconclusive regarding long-term consequences of filter insertion. Selected patients may be candidates for thrombolytic therapy immediately after pulmonary embolism; studies have shown equal rates of complications from thrombolytic therapy in young and older hemodynamically unstable patients. Absolute contraindications to anticoagulation include active internal bleeding, hemorrhagic stroke, or gastrointestinal bleeding. Risk of hemorrhage in the older patient is increased even when comorbid conditions are controlled for; older women are at a higher risk of hemorrhage than men.

Follow-up: Follow-up visits are on an individualized basis. Anticoagulation usually is continued for a minimum of 6 months after pulmonary embolism. Further therapy is based on risk factors for pulmonary embolism, potential for recurrence, and risks associated with anticoagulation. Close monitoring for control of anticoagulation is essential.

Sequelae: Unrecognized pulmonary embolism can be fatal; many are diagnosed at autopsy. Other complications include alveolar collapse, atelectasis, and pulmonary infarction. The condition tends to recur. Complications from anticoagulation include uncontrolled bleeding and hematoma.

Prevention/prophylaxis: Patients should avoid controllable risk factors for pulmonary embolism. Encourage frequent ambulation, use of antiembolic stockings, safety precautions to avoid injury to lower extremities, evaluation of possible hypercoagulation pathology, and prophylactic anticoagulation after orthopedic and other surgery for high-risk patients; intermittent pneumatic compression also is recommended, unless contraindicated. Prolonged sitting should be avoided.

Referral: Refer patients to internal medicine or emergency medicine for emergent evaluation and initial treatment plan. When stable, patients can be managed on warfarin with INR testing in their usual place of residence.

Education: Teach the patient, family, or caregiver about risk factors and preventive measures, disease pathology, monitoring for signs of recurrence, and need for compliance with anticoagulation therapy. Instruct the patient to use a soft toothbrush and an electric razor and to report bleeding gums, hemoptysis, and any blood in stool or urine. Advise patients to avoid aspirin, to consult with their health-care provider before taking any OTC medications, and to take precautions to avoid bumping or bruising.

PULMONARY TUBERCULOSIS

SIGNAL SYMPTOMS▶   productive, prolonged cough; fatigue; low-grade fever; night sweats; poor appetite; weight loss

Pulmonary tuberculosis	ICD-9CM: 011.90

Description: Pulmonary tuberculosis is a chronic necrotizing infection caused by a slow-growing acid-fast bacillus (AFB), *Mycobacterium tuberculosis*. Tuberculosis is the most important, fatal infection among humans. The primary site for most cases of tuberculosis is the lungs; extrapulmonary tuberculosis, which can affect any organ or tissue, is more common among individuals infected with HIV.

Etiology: The infection spreads by inhalation of airborne particles or droplets produced by persons with active pulmonary or laryngeal tuberculosis during coughing, sneezing, singing, and other expiratory efforts. The development of infection after exposure depends on the exposed person's ability to mount an effective immune response on the cellular level. In the initial 2 to 4 weeks before cellular immunity response occurs, direct pulmonary infection may develop, or lymphohematogenous circulation may lead to miliary, meningeal, or tuberculosis adenitis. When T cells recognize the specific antigen, they become sensitized, engaging the macrophages in destroying or containing the tubercle bacilli. This leads to healing, with no residual or calcified lymph nodes in the pulmonary or tracheobronchial areas. This latent stage is typical of 90% to 95% of infected persons, leaving them at lifelong risk for reactivation. Tuberculin skin testing documents exposure at 2 to 10 weeks after exposure.

Occurrence: Tuberculosis occurs worldwide. An estimated 10 to 15 million individuals in the United States are infected with *M. tuberculosis,* with 3 million deaths annually. An estimated 10% of infected individuals develop active tuberculosis in their lifetime. In 2001, an estimated 15,989 cases were reported in the United States, for a case rate of 5.6 per 100,000. This is a decline of 2% from 2000 and a 40% decrease from 1992, when the number of cases peaked in the United States. In adults >65 years old, there was a 50% decline in the case rate, from 19.1 to 9.1. In 2001, the case rate in long-term care facilities was 2.8. The case rate among foreign-born persons is at least eight times higher than among individuals born in the United States.

Age: Children and adolescents are more likely to have primary disease; adults and elderly are more likely to have recrudescent disease.

Ethnicity: Persons born in geographic areas where tuberculosis is more prevalent, including Asia, Africa, and Latin America, are at higher risk. Native Americans are at higher risk because of environmental factors (crowding, poor health, poor nutrition).

Gender: Tuberculosis occurs in men more frequently than in women.

Contributing factors: Contributing factors include:

- HIV infection
- Substance abuse (especially intravenous drug use)
- Recent infection with *M. tuberculosis* (<2 years ago)
- Chest x-ray findings suspicious of previous tuberculosis with no treatment or ineffective treatment
- Diabetes mellitus
- Silicosis
- Prolonged corticosteroid therapy
- Other immunosuppressive therapy
- Cancer of the head and neck
- Hematologic and reticuloendothelial diseases
- End-stage renal disease
- Intestinal bypass or gastrectomy
- Chronic malabsorption syndromes
- Low body weight (<10% ideal body weight)

Other factors associated with increased risk include homelessness, residence in a congregate setting (nursing home, boarding home, prison, mental health facility), low socioeconomic status, and health-care work in a high risk area.

Signs and symptoms: Typical presentation includes cough, hemoptysis, weight loss, anorexia, adenopathy, fever, night sweats, decreased activity level, and pleuritic pain. In the average population, the onset is gradual and may go undetected for some time. In the older patient, these findings are not usually present, or they are so subtle and so intermingled with other chronic illness symptoms as to be undistinguishable. Weight loss, dyspnea, or anorexia may be the only symptoms. Typical simulations include pneumonia, bronchitis, or congestive heart failure with pleural effusion. Extrapulmonary tuberculosis may manifest with symptoms typical to the site involved (e.g., urinary incontinence or frequency and urgency for bladder tuberculosis).

Physical examination may be unrevealing: Nonspecific signs such as fever or weight loss may be the only findings. In some persons, a positive tuberculin test reaction is the only manifestation. Chest examination may show post-tussive apical rales. If pleural effusion is present, percussion in the area may be dull.

Diagnostic tests: Current recommendations call for targeted testing of at-risk individuals. The standard intradermal test to screen for exposure to tuberculosis or to detect an active case of tuberculosis is the Mantoux test, with intermediate purified protein derivative (PPD) 5 units. The test is technique specific; if administered too deeply, without producing the required bleb, it is invalid and must be repeated at another site. Interpretation of the result is also subject to error; the area of induration or hardness, not erythema, must be measured with a millimeter ruler 48 to 72 hours after the agent is administered. The results show the ability of the person tested to mount a delayed-type hypersensitivity response to prior infection. Appropriate measurement parameters for reactive and nonreactive results are as follows:

Test	Results Indicating Exposure	Selected Population	CPT Code
PPD tuberculin skin test	5 mm	HIV-positive persons Recent contacts of tuberculosis case Persons with fibrotic changes on chest x-ray consistent with old healed tuberculosis Patients with organ transplants and other immunosuppressed patients	86580, 86585
	10 mm	Recent arrivals from high-prevalence countries Injection drug users Residents and employees of high-risk congregate settings Mycobacteriology laboratory workers Persons with clinical conditions that place them at high risk Children <4 years old Children/adolescents exposed to high-risk adults	
	15 mm	Persons with no known risk factors for tuberculosis	

When reporting or recording results, specify reactive or nonreactive and the millimeter measurement for induration. Many patients have an impaired delayed-type hypersensitivity response to the tuberculin testing; a negative reaction does not exclude disease. This absence of a response is known as anergy and is found in immunosuppressed individuals, including HIV-positive persons, persons on immunosuppressive drugs or corticosteroid therapy, persons with sarcoidosis, persons with Hodgkin's disease, and persons with recent vaccination with bacille Calmette-Guérin. Anergy testing is no longer recommended as part of a routine tuberculosis screening program for HIV-positive individuals (contact: http://www.cdc.gov/epo/mmwr/preview/mmwrhtml/00049386.htm; accessed November 1, 2002). Two-step testing is recommended initially for adults who will be retested periodically, such as health-care workers and long-term congregate living residents. The PPD is administered; if negative, a second PPD is given 1 to 3 weeks later. If the second PPD is positive, it probably represents a boosted response to a prior infection or bacille Calmette-Guérin vaccine, not a seroconversion, and should be addressed accordingly. If the second PPD is negative, the person is considered uninfected, and any subsequent positive PPD indicates a new infection.

Test	Results Indicating Disorder	CPT Code
Chest x-ray, posterior anterior view Note: Abnormalities are suggestive of but not diagnostic for tuberculosis; this test may be used to rule out pulmonary tuberculosis in a person with a positive tuberculin test and no symptoms of disease	*Active disease:* Abnormalities seen in apical or posterior segments of upper lobe or superior segments of lower lobe. In HIV-positive or immunosuppressed persons, lesions may appear anywhere in lungs and may differ in size, shape, density, and cavitation	71020 71021 (with apical lordotic)
In select cases, other views, such as apical lordotic, may be indicated.	*Latent or old healed lesions:* Dense pulmonary nodules in hilar or upper lobes, with or without cavitation. Have "hard," sharply demarcated margins. Smaller, nodular or fibrotic lesions in upper lobes and a positive tuberculin test indicate latent infection and should be treated accordingly. Calcified granulomas usually do not progress to active tuberculosis	
Sputum for AFB	Detection of AFB in stained smears is suggestive but not diagnostic; may be other mycobacteria. Negative smear does not rule out tuberculosis	89350
Sputum culture should be done on all specimens regardless of AFB result	Positive culture for *M. tuberculosis* is diagnostic. Drug sensitivity testing should be done on all initial cultures	94664 (induced sputum)

Differential diagnosis: Pneumonia, lymphoma, fungal infections, congestive heart failure, pleural effusion, and lung cancer can mimic tuberculosis.

Treatment: Before treatment, obtain baseline values for liver function, bilirubin, CBC, BUN, creatinine, and serum uric acid; if ethambutol (EMB) is used, baseline visual acuity should be measured. The goal of treatment is safety and efficacy in the shortest time period. For newly diagnosed, active tuberculosis, initial treatment consists of combined therapy using four first-line drugs: isoniazid (INH), rifampin (RIF), pyrazinamide (PZA), and EMB, until culture results are complete. Follow-up cultures should be done, usually monthly until negative, to determine response to treatment. If culture is not negative after 3 months, suspect drug resistance or noncompliance and re-evaluate. After culture is negative, obtain one further culture at treatment completion; for drug-resistant tuberculosis, different culture guidelines apply. Several treatment options are available. The most commonly used is presented here (for further information, consult with the Centers for Disease Control and Prevention [CDC]).

Note: HIV-positive individuals require specific modifications in therapy and CDC guidelines should be consulted. Multidrug-resistant tuberculosis also requires different regimens; see CDC guidelines.

Daily for 2 months:

INH, 5 mg/kg (300 mg maximum)

RIF, 10 mg/kg (600 mg maximum)

PZA, 15 to 20 mg/kg (2 g maximum)

EMB, 15 to 25 mg/kg (1 g maximum)

Then daily for 4 months:

INH and RIF (see preceding dosage schedule)

In lieu of daily therapy for 4 months, the same agents (INH, RIF) can be used as follows:

INH, 15 mg/kg (900 mg maximum) two or three times weekly by directly observed therapy (DOT)

RIF, 10 mg/kg (600 mg maximum) two or three times weekly by DOT

The basis for treatment is availability of two drugs to which the bacterium is susceptible. Prolonged treatment is needed. Compliance is key to successful control of disease.

Follow-up: See culture guidelines earlier. Follow-up chest x-ray examination may be done at therapy termination to evaluate response. Periodic liver enzymes are necessary, especially if the patient is taking INH, to monitor for effects on hepatotoxicity. For the frail elderly adult in a long-term care facility, more frequent monitoring for adverse effects of treatment, including anorexia, polyneuropathy, or development of medication-induced hepatitis, is warranted. DOT is the norm in these settings, so compliance is less of a concern. Refer community-dwelling elderly to the local or state health department for follow-up, monitoring of medication compliance and side effects, patient and family education, and testing of close contacts. Tuberculosis is a reportable disease.

Many agencies charged with monitoring and control have outreach services, such as home visits. Emphasize to patients that compliance is crucial to successful control. If no follow-up visitation is available through the monitoring agency, see the patient for monthly follow-up visits in the office.

Sequelae: Possible complications include development of drug-resistant organisms, particularly if a patient is noncompliant with the prescribed treatment. Secondary infection of cavitary lesions and development of treatment-associated hepatitis or polyneuropathy are possible. If treatment is ineffective, spread of disease to other close contacts can occur.

Prevention/prophylaxis: For older patients residing in long-term care facilities, PPD testing before admission to the facility is required unless there is documented evidence of a positive test result in the past. Two-step testing (described earlier) is recommended initially. Annual retesting is recommended. Patients with a positive PPD reaction need a chest x-ray to evaluate for active or latent disease. Staff members are required to have tuberculin skin testing at initial employment and annually.

When targeted testing reveals a positive tuberculin skin reaction but no evidence of active tuberculosis, it is often referred to as *latent tuberculosis infection*. The person has been exposed to and infected with *M. tuberculosis* but does not have active disease and cannot infect others.

The decision to institute chemoprophylaxis is a clinical judgment, based on a comparison of individual factors with the risk of developing tuberculosis (see under Contributing Factors) versus the risk of INH toxicity. Chemoprophylaxis is with INH, 300 mg orally daily for 6 months in an otherwise healthy person; 9 months is considered optimal if compliance is not an issue. Alternatively, INH, 15 mg/kg orally twice weekly by DOT, may be substituted. For HIV-positive persons or close contacts of patients with drug-resistant tuberculosis, see CDC recommendations. A shorter course of RIF and PZA previously recommended has been associated with fatal and severe liver injuries and so is no longer recommended.

Referral: Patients may be referred to a government-associated community agency such as the health department or to an infectious disease or pulmonary specialist for initial evaluation and management recommendations. Refer patients with concurrent positive HIV status or confirmed acquired immunodeficiency syndrome (AIDS) to specialized treatment services or collaborate in management with specialists in this area. Refer patients with severe anorexia or malnutrition to a dietitian.

Education: Teach patient, caregivers, close contacts, and paraprofessional providers about the nature of the disease, its mode of transmission, screening and control measures, and follow-up required. Teach the patient or caregiver about medications, drug actions and possible side effects, length of treatment, and need for compliance.

RESTRICTIVE LUNG DISEASE

SIGNAL SYMPTOMS rapid, shallow respirations; dyspnea; decreased activity tolerance; easy fatigability; nonproductive, irritating cough provoked by deep breathing or exertion

Pulmonary fibrosis, interstitial	ICD-9-CM: 515
Black lung disease	ICD-9-CM: 500
Silicosis	ICD-9-CM: 502

Description: Restrictive lung disease refers to a heterogeneous group of disorders that share a common abnormal ventilatory function. Restricted breathing is characterized by small tidal volume and rapid rate. The hallmark restrictive pattern is a decrease in lung volumes, principally total lung capacity and vital capacity.

Etiology: Restrictive lung diseases, which have a variety of etiologies, are divided into subgroups based on the location of the pathology:

Restrictive/parenchymal/interstitial: In addition to a decrease in total lung capacity and vital capacity, residual volume is decreased.
Forced expiratory flow rates are maintained.
- Sarcoidosis
- Idiopathic pulmonary fibrosis
- Pneumoconiosis
- Occupational lung disease
- Drug/radiation-induced interstitial lung disease

Restrictive/extraparenchymal: Abnormalities can be predominantly in inspiration or in inspiration and expiration.
Neuromuscular:
- Diaphragmatic weakness/paralysis
- Myasthenia gravis*
- Muscular dystrophies*
- Cervical spine injuries*
- Guillain-Barré syndrome*
Chest wall:
- Kyphoscoliosis
- Obesity
- Ankylosing spondylitis*

Occurrence: The incidence of restrictive lung disease is undeterminable because several distinct entities are involved. Occupational lung diseases are common in farmers and in people who work with silica, asbestos, beryllium, or cotton.

* Limitations may be inspiratory and expiratory

Age: Occupationally induced disease is seen predominantly in the older population; other restrictive lung diseases may occur at any age.

Ethnicity: Not significant.

Gender: The incidence is higher in men than women for occupational types of restrictive lung disease.

Contributing factors: Risk factors vary with etiology, including exposure to occupational dust, abnormalities in skeletal structure, genetics, and autoimmune disorders.

Signs and symptoms: Patients have a gradual onset of dyspnea, initially occurring only with exertion and progressing to dyspnea at rest. The breathing pattern is rapid and shallow. A nonproductive cough may be present. A careful history may disclose prior occupational risk factors. Use of tobacco also should be ascertained; it is common for patients to have a mixed pattern of obstructive and restrictive disease. Physical findings may reveal skeletal abnormalities, such as kyphoscoliosis, limiting lung expansion. The initial presentation of breathing problems often occurs after an acute respiratory viral infection.

Physical assessment of the lung initially may be unremarkable. With progression of the disease, inspiratory crackles ("Velcro") typically are heard at the bases. Cyanosis and clubbing of fingers and toes may occur. In the end stages, signs of right-sided heart failure, including cor pulmonale, appear.

Diagnostic tests: Because of the diverse nature of the conditions leading to restrictive lung disease, it is challenging to address diagnostic testing and results. Many results are specific to the causative condition.

Test	Results Indicating Disorder	CPT Code
PFT	Normal FEV_1/FVC ratio but decreased FVC and FEV_1; decreased total lung capacity, residual volume, and functional residual capacity. Residual volume-to-total lung capacity ratio is normal to low. Most have a gas exchange problem with marked decrease in single breath diffusing lung capacity for carbon monoxide	78596
Chest x-ray	Increased interstitial markings, especially in lower fields. Hilar and mediastinal lymphadenopathy in sarcoidosis, some lymphomas, and silicosis. Pleural effusion and thickening with collagen-vascular disease, lymphoma, and asbestosis	71010–71035
High-resolution CT	In idiopathic pulmonary fibrosis, patchy, peripheral bibasilar reticular abnormalities in the subpleural area; with advanced disease, subpleural fibrosis and honeycomb pattern are present	76380 71250 (CT of lung) 71260 (with contrast)

In the late stages, arterial blood gases help to identify the degree of hypoxemia and carbon dioxide retention.

Differential diagnosis:

- Infectious or neoplastic diseases
- COPD
- Congestive heart failure can mimic restrictive lung disease

Treatment: Therapy depends on the cause of disease and the disease progression. Occupational exposures should be avoided. Corticosteroid therapy with prednisone, 1 mg/kg per day initially, is indicated for most interstitial diseases, tapering after 8 to 12 weeks to maintenance. Cytotoxic agents, including azathioprine (Imuran) and cyclophosphamide (Cytoxan), are given concurrently with prednisone. In the end stage, administer supplemental oxygen for supportive care. Lung transplantation may be considered in selected cases. Research indicates that idiopathic pulmonary fibrosis is related more to fibroblastic proliferation than inflammation. Two antifibrotic agents, pirfenidone and Interferon-gamma-1b are in clinical trials. Etanercept, a soluble tumor necrosis factor-α receptor antagonist licensed for use in the treatment of rheumatoid arthritis, also looks hopeful.

Follow-up: Follow-up visits are scheduled as indicated by symptoms and comorbidities. Periodic chest x-rays or PFTs may help to chart diseases course and to evaluate response to treatment.

Sequelae: Use of corticosteroids or immunosuppressives may result in increased risk of infection. Pulmonary hypertension and right-sided heart failure may occur. Restrictive lung diseases are chronic.

Prevention/prophylaxis: Give patients pneumococcal pneumonia and influenza vaccine. Advise patients to avoid known exposures, tobacco use, and persons with acute, infectious upper respiratory illness.

Referrals: Initially refer patients to pulmonary specialist for bronchoscopy and possible biopsy; thereafter, collaborative management is appropriate. If immunosuppressives are used, refer the patient for initial recommendations and periodic re-evaluation.

Education: Teach the patient about chronic disease management, regular self-care habits, and early intervention in acute illness.

UPPER RESPIRATORY TRACT INFECTION

SIGNAL SYMPTOMS nasal congestion, rhinorrhea/mucopurulent discharge, sore throat, cough, headache, malaise

| Upper respiratory tract infection (URI) | ICD-9-CM: 465.9 |

Description: URI, most frequently the common cold, usually is caused by a virus and results in inflammation of the nasal passages. Most URIs are self-limiting and accompanied only by minor somatic complaints.

Etiology: URIs usually are caused by a virus such as rhinovirus; influenza A, B, and C viruses; parainfluenza viruses; respiratory syncytial viruses; coronaviruses; adenoviruses; and enteric cytopathogenic human orphan (ECHO) viruses. Additionally, *Mycobacterium avium* and *Pneumocystis carinii* have been found in older patients who are not immunosuppressed. In 40% of cases, no agent can be identified. The usual mode of transmission is hand-to-hand from contaminated nasal secretions. The incubation period is 1 to 3 days, with the usual URI lasting 6 to 10 days.

Occurrence: URIs are the most common cause of short-term disability in the United States; there are >62 million cases of the common cold annually. Acute URIs are the most frequent reason for seeking a healthcare provider in the United States; 75% of all antibiotic prescriptions in a given year are for acute URIs.

Age: URIs occur much more frequently in children than in adults.

Ethnicity: Noncontributory.

Gender: URIs occur equally in men and women.

Contributing factors: Risk factors for developing URIs include exposure to infected individuals and contact between nose or conjunctiva and contaminated fingers. Older persons with diabetes get more frequent URIs than the general population.

Signs and symptoms: The most common signs and symptoms include nasal obstruction and stuffiness (80–100% of patients), sneezing (50–70%), and scratchy throat (50%). Other signs and symptoms include cough (40%), hoarseness (30%), malaise (20–25%), headache (25%), and fever >100°F (<1%). Physical examination may reveal mucopurulent nasal drainage, nasopharyngeal mucosal swelling, and lymphadenopathy.

Diagnostic tests: No diagnostic tests are indicated for the nonspecific URIs. Diagnosis is clinical based on symptoms. If symptoms persist >10 days, a CBC may be ordered to rule out other causes. A throat culture or rapid strep test is used if streptococcal pharyngitis is suspected.

Differential diagnosis:

- Symptoms of influenza
- Chronic rhinitis
- Sinusitis
- Epstein-Barr virus
- Mumps and rubeola mimic URIs

The use of medications such as nasal sprays (when use is continuous), antihypertensives, hormones, psychotropic drugs, aspirin, and nonsteroidal anti-inflammatory drugs can cause symptoms similar to those of URIs.

Treatment: URIs usually are managed on an outpatient basis. Patients with significant COPD or cardiac disease should be evaluated on an indi-

vidual basis. URIs are treated with rest, increased fluid intake, and symptom relief measures such as humidified air (not recommended for asthma patients). OTC medications may be taken for pain, fever, congestion, or cough relief. Topical nasal and oral decongestants are available, with topical decongestants preferred owing to fewer systemic side effects. The nasal decongestant of choice is oxymetazoline; use of nasal decongestants for >3 days may result in rebound vasocongestion and is not recommended. The oral decongestant of choice is pseudoephedrine. Nasal and oral decongestants are associated with elevated blood pressure and should be used cautiously in the elderly. When a cough is nonproductive or prevents normal rest and activities, it may be treated with a cough suppressant that contains dextromethorphan or codeine. There is no evidence that guiafenesin is any more effective than increasing fluids. Rinsing with mouthwashes, sucking on lozenges or hard candy, gargling with warm saline, and using products with local anesthetics such as benzocaine or phenol may provide subjective relief of sore throat pain. The use of antihistamines, vitamin C (ascorbic acid), and expectorants is controversial. *Antibiotics are not indicated* (see under Education). One randomized controlled study found that zinc intranasal gel decreased duration of symptoms. There is insufficient evidence to recommend Echinacea products for treating or preventing URIs owing to the number and variability of Echinacea products. One randomized controlled study of antihistamines showed a small reduction in sneezing and runny nose on the first 2 days of a URI; side effects were dry mouth and drowsiness.
Follow-up: See the patient if symptoms last >6 to 10 days or if the patient develops fever associated with systemic symptoms, difficulty breathing, or purulent nasal drainage.
Sequelae: Possible complications include lower respiratory tract infection, sinusitis, and aggravation of asthma symptoms; in older individuals with comorbidities, URI may contribute to exacerbation of other symptoms (e.g., COPD, hyperglycemia, congestive heart failure) or may lead to pneumonia.
Prevention/prophylaxis: Advise the patient to perform frequent proper hand washing, avoid touching the face, and avoid contact with infected people. Pneumococcal and influenza vaccinations are recommended for all older adults.
Referral: Usually neither referral nor consultation is necessary if the patient has an uncomplicated URI.
Education:

Provider Education*

Diagnosis of nonspecific URI or acute rhinopharyngitis denotes an infection that is typically viral and in which sinus, pharyngeal, and lower airway symptoms may be present but not prominent.

* Adapted from CDC Principles of Judicious Antibiotic Use. Contxt: http://www.cdc.gov/drugresistance/community/.Accessed November 18, 2002.

Antibiotic treatment of adults with nonspecific URI does not improve illness resolution and is not recommended. There are no studies specifically testing the impact of antibiotic treatment on complications of acute URIs in adults. Life-threatening complications of URIs are rare.

Purulent nasal or pharyngeal secretions (commonly seen in patients with uncomplicated URIs) do not predict bacterial infection and do not benefit from antibiotic treatment.

Patient Education

Explain the disease process, signs and symptoms, and treatment (including side effects of medications). Discuss prevention strategies and when to contact a health-care provider. Educate patients and families about dangers of antibiotic resistance owing to inappropriate prescribing.

REFERENCES

Arrhythmias

Aronow, WS: Treatment of ventricular arrhythmias in older adults. J Am Geriatr Soc 43:688, 1995.

Arrhythmias and conduction disorders. In Abrams, WB, et al (eds): The Merck Manual of Geriatrics, ed 2. Merck Research Laboratories, Whitehouse Station, NJ, 1995.

Chung, M, and Klein, A: Atrial fibrillation. In Rubenstein, E, and Federman, DD (eds): Scientific American Medicine, 1978–1998. Scientific American Medicine, New York, 1997.

Fenton, JM. The clinician's approach to evaluating patients with dysrhythmias. AACN Clinical Issues 12:72, 2001.

Furberg, CT, et al: Prevalence of atrial fibrillation in elderly subjects (The Cardiovascular Health Study). Am J Cardiol 74:236, 1994.

Greenberg, HM, et al: Interactions of ischaemia and encainide/flecainide treatment: A proposed mechanism for the increased mortality in CAST I. Br Heart J 74:631, 1995.

Horowitz, LN, and Lynch, RA: Managing geriatric arrhythmias: I. General considerations. Geriatrics 46:31, 1991.

Kamath, S, and Yh Lip, G: Managing cardiac arrhythmias. Practitioner 244:559, 2000.

Langberg, JJ, LeLurgio, DB: Ventricular arrhythmias. In Rubenstein, E, and Federman, DD (eds): Scientific American Medicine, 1978–1998. Scientific American Medicine, New York, 1997.

Lynch, RA, and Horowitz, LN: Managing geriatric arrhythmias: II. Drug selection and use. Geriatrics 46:41, 1991.

Murgatroyd, FD, et al: Cardiac arrhythmias in the elderly. In Camm, AJ, and Martin, A (eds): Geriatric Cardiology: Principles and Practices. John Wiley & Sons, New York, 1994.

Ravikishore, AG, and Camm, AJ: Dangerous and treatable cardiac arrhythmias in elderly people. In Sinclair, AJ, and Woodhouse, KW (eds): Acute Medical Illness in Old Age. Chapman & Hall, London, 1995.

Rippe, JM, and Albert, JS: Arrhythmias. In: Manual of Cardiovascular Diagnosis and Therapy. Little, Brown, Boston, 1985.

Spratt, KA, et al: Disturbances in cardiac rhythm. In Messerli, FH (ed): Cardiovascular Disease in the Elderly, ed 3. Kluwer Academic Publishers, Boston, 1993.

Tchou, PJ, and Trohman, RG: Supraventricular tachycardia. In Rubenstein, E, and Federman, DD (eds): Scientific American Medicine, 1978–1998. Scientific American Medicine, New York, 1997.

Tresch, DD: Evaluation and management of cardiac arrhythmias in the elderly. Med Clin North Am 85:527, 2001.

Heart Failure

American Heart Association: Heart and stroke statistics update. 2001. Contact: http://www.americanheart.org/statistics.

Aronow, WS: The ELITE study. Drugs Aging 12:423, 1998.

Braunwald, E: Heart failure. In Harrison's Principles of Internal Medicine, ed 13. McGraw-Hill, New York, 1994.

Cannon, L, and Marshall, J: Cardiac disease in the elderly population. Clin Geriatr Med 9:3, 1993.

Carelock, J, and Clark, A. Heart failure: Pathophysiological mechanicsm. Am J Nurs 101:26, 2001.

Chen, YT, et al: Risk factors for heart failure in the elderly: A prospective community-based study. Am J Med 106:605, 1999.

Cleland, JGF, et al: What is the optimal medical management of ischemic heart failure? Prog Cardiovasc Dis 43:433, 2001.

Colucci, WS, and Braunwald, E: Pathophysiology of heart failure. In Braunwald, E, et al (eds): Heart Disease: A Textbook of Cardiovascular Medicine, ed 6. WB Saunders, Philadelphia, 2001, p 534.

Dec, GW, and Hutler, AM: Congestive heart failure. In Rubenstein, E, and Federman, DD (eds): Scientific American Medicine, 1978–1998. Scientific American Medicine, New York, 1997.

Diller, P, and Smucker, D: Management of heart failure. Primary Care September:651, 2000.

Dracup, K, et al: Rethinking heart failure. Am J Nurs 95:7, 1995.

Gottdiener, JS, et al: Predictors of CHF in the elderly: The Cardiovascular Study. J Am Coll Cardiol 35:1628, 2000.

Guerra-Garcia, H, et al: Congestive heart failure: Treatment modifications in the elderly. Consultant 34:4, 1994.

Heart failure: Evaluation and care of patients with left-ventricular systolic dysfunction. AHCPR Clinical Practice Guideline, Agency on Health Care Policy and Research, US Department of Health and Human Services, Rockville, MD, 1994.

Luchi, R, et al: Congestive heart failure in the elderly. J Am Geriatr Soc 39:8, 1991.

Massie, B, and Wolfe, C: Heart failure. In Messerli, F (ed): Cardiovascular Disease in the Elderly, ed 3. Kluwer Academic Publishers, Boston, 1993.

Pitt, B, et al: Effect of losartin compared with captopril on mortality in patients with symptomatic heart failure: Randomized trial—the Losartan Heart Failure Survival Study ELITE II. Lancet 355:1582, 2000.

Rich, MW: Epidemiology, pathophysiology and etiology of congestive heart failure in older adults. J Am Geriatr Soc 45:968, 1997.

The Heart Outcomes Prevention Evaluation Study Investigators: Effects of an angiotension-converting-enzyme inhibitor, ramipril, on cardiovascular events in high risk patients. N Engl J Med 342:145, 2000.

Tresch, DD: Clinical manifestations, diagnostic assessment, and etiology of heart failure in elderly patients. Clin Geriatr Med 16:445, 2000.

Hypertension

Cushman, W, and Black, HR: Hypertension in the elderly. Cardiol Clin 17:79, 1999.

Gifford, R: Managing hypertension in the elderly: Dispelling the myths. Cleve Clin J Med 62:29, 1995.

Joint National Committee: The Sixth Report of the Joint National Committee on Detection, Evaluation, and Treatment of High Blood Pressure. Arch Intern Med 157:2413, 1997.

Kaplan, N: Hypertension in the elderly. Annu Rev Med 45:27, 1995.

Kaplan, N: Southwestern Internal Medicine Conference: The promises and perils of treating the elderly hypertensive. Am J Med Sci 305:183, 1993.

Kochar, M: Hypertension in elderly patients. Postgrad Med 91:393, 1992.

National High Blood Pressure Education Program Working Group: National High Blood Pressure Working Group report on hypertension in the elderly. Hypertension 23:275, 1994.

Oparil, S, and Calhoun, DA: High blood pressure. In Rubenstein, E, and Federman, DD (eds): Scientific American Medicine, 1978–1998. Scientific American Medicine, New York, 1997.

Rippe, JM, and Alpert, JS: Hypertension. In: Manual of Cardiovascular Diagnosis and Therapy. Little, Brown, Boston, 1985.

Sadowski, AV, and Redeker, NS: The hypertensive elder: A review for the primary care provider. Nurse Practitioner 21:99, 1996.

Thakkar, RB, and Oparil, S: What do international guidelines say about therapy? J Hypertens 19(Suppl 3):S23, 2001.

Vardan, S, and Mookherjee, S: Perspectives on isolated systolic hypertension in elderly patients. Arch Fam Med 9:319, 2000.

Weinburger, M: Hypertension in the elderly. Hosp Pract 103:103, 1992.

Ischemic Heart Disease

Cohn, PF: Treatment of chronic myocardial ischemia: Rationale and treatment options. Cardiovasc Drugs Ther 12:217, 1998.

Elder, A, and Fox, K: Ischaemic heart disease in the elderly. In Martin, A, and Camm, AJ (eds): Geriatric Cardiology: Principles and Practice. John Wiley & Sons, New York, 1994.

Fazar, E, et al: Angina pectoris and silent ischemia in the elderly: A management update. Geriatrics 47:24, 1992.

Frishman, W: Treatment of myocardial ischemia and myocardial infarction in the elderly. South Med J 86:S29, 1993.

Howard, BV, et al: Rising tide of vascular disease in American Indians: The Strong Heart Study. Circulation 99:2389, 1999.

Howell, J, and Hedges, J: Differential diagnosis of chest discomfort and general approach to myocardial ischemia decision making. Am J Emerg Med 9:571, 1991.

Hutler, AM: Ischemic heart disease: Angina pectoris. In Rubenstein, E, and Federman, DD (eds): Scientific American Medicine, 1978–1998. Scientific American Medicine, New York, 1997.

Liao, Y, et al: Mortality from coronary heart disease and cardiovascular disease among US Hispanics: Finding from the National Interview Survey. J Am Coll Cardiol 30:1200, 1997.

Limacher, M: Clinical features of coronary heart disease in the elderly. In Lowenthal, D (ed): Cardiovascular Clinics. FA Davis, Philadelphia, 1992, p 63.

Pepine, C, and Pepine, A: Intervention therapy for coronary artery disease in the elderly. In Lowenthal, D (ed): Cardiovascular Clinics. FA Davis, Philadelphia, 1992, p 175.

Salley, R, and Robinson, C: Ischemic heart disease in the elderly: The role of coronary angioplasty and coronary artery bypass grafting. South Med J 86:S15, 1993.

Segal, B: Managing angina in the elderly: An update. Geriatrics 44:55, 1989.

Tresch, D, and Alla, HR: Diagnosis and management of myocardial ischemia (angina) in the elderly patient. Am J Geriatr Cardiol 10:337, 2001.

Myocardial Infarction

Almeda, FQ, et al: The contemporary management of acute myocardial infarction. Crit Care Clin 17:411, 2001.

American Heart Association: Heart and Stroke Statistical Update. 2000. Contact: http://www.americanheart.org.

Cannon, L, and Marshall, J: Cardiac disease in the elderly population. Clin Geriatr Med 9:3, 1993.

Carnevali, D, and Patrick, M: Nursing Management for the Elderly, ed 3. JB Lippincott, Philadelphia, 1993.

Chorzempa, A, and Tabloski, P: Post myocardial infarction treatment in the older adult. Nurse Practitioner 26:36, 2001.

Devlin, W, et al: Comparison of outcomes in patients with myocardial infarction aged >75 years with that in younger patients. Am J Cardiol 75:573, 1995.

Friesinger, GC, and Ryan, TJ: Coronary heart disease: Stable and unstable syndromes. Cardiol Clin 17:93, 1999.

Fulmer, T, and Walker, M (eds): Critical Care Nursing of the Elderly. Springer, New York, 1991.

Herlitz, J, et al: Optimal treatment after acute myocardial infarction in the elderly. Drugs Aging 6:3, 1995.

Pasternak, RC, and Braumwald, E: Acute myocardial infarction. In Isselbacker, KJ, et al (eds): Harrison's Principles of Internal Medicine, ed 13. McGraw-Hill, New York, 1994.

Pollard, TJ: The acute myocardial infarction. Prim Care 27:631, 2000.

Ryan, TJ, et al: Update. ACC/AHA Guidelines for the Management of Patients with Acute Myocardial Infarction: Executive Summary and Recommendations. Circulation 100:1016, 1999.

Sinclair, D: Myocardial infarction: Considerations for geriatric patients. Can Fam Physician 40:1172, 1994.

Sokolyk, S, and Tresch, D: Treatment of myocardial infarction in elderly patients. Compr Ther 20:10, 1994.

Suarez, G, et al: Prediction on admission of in-hospital mortality in patients older than 70 years with acute myocardial infarction. Chest 108:1, 1995.

The Heart Outcomes Prevention Evaluation Study Investigators: Effects of an angiotension-converting-enzyme inhibitor, ramipril on cardiovascular events in high risk patients. N Engl J Med. 342:145, 2000.

Thompson, L, et al: Geriatric acute myocardial infarction: A challenge to recognition, prompt diagnosis, and appropriate care. Crit Care Nurs Clin North Am 4:2, 1992.

Tresch, DD: Management of the older patient with acute myocardial infarction. J Am Geriatr Soc 46:1157, 1998.

Valvular Heart Disease

Banning, AP: Valvular disease: The GP's key role. Practitioner 243:740, 1999.

Bonow, RO, et al: Guidelines for the management of patients with valvular heart disease: Executive summary. A report of the American College of Cardiology/American Heart Association Task Force on Practice Guidelines (Committee on the Management of Patients with Valvular Heart Disease). Circulation 98:1949, 1998.

Boon, NA, and Bloomfield, P: Medical management of valvular heart disease. Heart 87:395, 2002.

Booth, DC, and Demaria, AN: Valvular heart disease in the elderly. In Messerli, FH (ed): Cardiovascular Disease in the Elderly, ed 3. Kluwer Academic Publishers, Boston, 1993.

Currie, PJ: Valvular heart disease: A correctable cause of congestive heart failure. Postgrad Med 89:123, 1991.

Griffin, BP: Valvular heart disease. In Rubenstein, E, and Federman, DD (eds): Scientific American Medicine, 1978–1998. Scientific American, New York, 1998.

Hara, JH: Valvular heart disease. Prim Care 27:725, 2000.

Hinchmann, DA, and Otto, CM: Valvular disease in the elderly. Cardiol Clin 17:137, 1999.

Kaiser, G: Practice guidelines in cardiothoracic surgery. Ann Thorac Surg 59:1264, 1995.

Marzo, KP, and Herling, IM: Valvular disease in the elderly. In Fran, KL, and Brest, AN (eds): Cardiovascular Clinics. FA Davis, Philadelphia, 1993, p 175.

McEwan, JR, and Oakley, CM: Valve disease in the elderly. In Martin, A, and Camm, AJ (eds): Geriatric Cardiology: Principles and Practices. John Wiley & Sons, New York, 1994.

Shipton, B, and Wahba, H: Valvular heart disease: Review and update. Am Fam Physician 63:2201, 2001.

Tresch, DD: Atypical presentations of cardiovascular disorders in the elderly. Geriatrics 42:31, 1987.

Valvular heart disease. In Abrams, WB, et al (eds): The Merck Manual of Geriatrics, ed 2. Merck Research Laboratories, Whitehouse Station, NJ, 1995.

Chronic Bronchitis

Chang, JT, et al: COPD in the elderly: A reversible cause of functional impairment. Chest 108:736, 1995.

Guthrie, R: Community-acquired lower respiratory tract infections: Etiology and treatment. Chest 120:2021, 2001.

Hirschmann, JV: Do bacteria cause exacerbations of COPD? Chest 118:193, 2001.

Hunter, MH: COPD: management of acute exacerbations and chronic stable disease. Am Fam Physician 64:603, 2001.

Kellerman, DJ: P2Y(2) receptor agonists: A new class of medication targeted at improved mucociliary clearance. Chest 121(5 Suppl):201S, 2002.

Mannino, DM: COPD: Epidemiology, prevalence, morbidity and mortality, and disease heterogeneity. Chest 121, 2002.

Muro, S: Expression of IL-15 in inflammatory pulmonary diseases. J Allergy Clin Immunol 108:970, 2001.

Murray, JF, and Nadel, JA: Abnormalities of the mucociliary transport system. In: Textbook of Respiratory Medicine, ed 3. WB Saunders, Philadelphia, 2000.

Nichol, KL, et al: Relation between influenza vaccination and outpatient visits, hospitalization, and mortality in elderly persons with chronic lung disease. Ann Intern Med 130:397, 1999.

Petty, TL: COPD in perspective. Chest 121(5 Suppl):116S, 2002.

Poole, PJ, and Black, PN: Oral mucolytic drugs for exacerbations of chronic obstructive pulmonary disease: systematic review. BMJ 322:1271, 2001.

Postma, DS, and Kerstjens, HAM: Evidence-based healthcare: A scientific approach to health policy. Evidence-Based Clinical Practice 5, 2001.

Rodarte, JR: Chronic bronchitis and emphysema. In Goldman, L, and Bennett, JC (eds): Cecil Textbook of Medicine, ed 21. WB Saunders, Philadelphia, 2000.

Schols, AMWJ, et al: Plasma leptin is related to proinflammatory status and dietary intake in patients with chronic obstructive pulmonary disease. Am J Respir Crit Care Med 160:1220, 1999.

Sethi, S, et al: Airway inflammation and etiology of acute exacerbations of chronic bronchitis. Chest 118:1557, 2000.

Stockley, RA: Communications to the editor. Chest 120:4, 2001.

Tagaya, E, et al: Effect of a short course of clarithromycin therapy on sputum production in patients with chronic airway hypersecretion. Chest 122:213, 2002.

Watanakunakorn, C: Communications to the editor. Chest 118:6, 2000.

Wouters, EF: Systemic effects in COPD. Chest 121(5 Suppl):127S, 2002.

Chronic Obstructive Pulmonary Disease

Adams, SG: Antibiotics are associated with lower relapse rates in outpatients with acute exacerbations of COPD. Chest 117:1345, 2000.

Celli, BR: The importance of spirometry in COPD and asthma: effect on approach to management. Chest 117(2 Suppl):15S, 2000.

Crapo, RO: Single-breath carbon monoxide diffusing capacity. Clin Chest Med 22:637, 2001.

Dudgeon, D: Managing dyspnea and cough. Hematol Oncol Clin North Am 16:557, 2002.

Enright, PL: Controversies in the use of spirometry for early recognition and diagnosis of chronic obstructive pulmonary disease in cigarette smokers. Clin Chest Med 21:645, 2000.

Ferguson, GT: Office spirometry for lung health assessment in adults: A consensus statement from the National Lung Health Education Program. Chest 117:1146, 2000.

Ferguson, GT: Update on pharmacologic therapy for chronic obstructive pulmonary disease. Clin Chest Med 21:723, 2000.

Friedman, M: Exacerbations of COPD: prevention and treatment. Journal of COPD Management 1, 2000.

Hunter, MH: COPD: management of acute exacerbations and chronic stable disease. Am Fam Physician 64:603, 2001.

Lau, AC: Hospital re-admission in patients with acute exacerbation of chronic obstructive pulmonary disease. Respir Med 95:876, 2001

Mannino, DM: COPD: epidemiology, prevalence, morbidity and mortality, and disease heterogeneity. Chest 121(5 Suppl):121S, 2002.

Mannino, DM, et al: National Center for Health Statistics Chronic Obstructive Pulmonary Disease Surveillance—United States, 1971–2000. 2000. Contact:

http://www.cdc.gov/mmwr/preview/mmwrhtml/ss5106a1.htm.   Accessed November 19, 2002.

McCrory, DC: Management of acute exacerbations of COPD: a summary and appraisal of published evidence. Chest 119:1190, 2001.

McEvoy, CE: Corticosteroids in chronic obstructive pulmonary disease. Clinical benefits and risks. Clin Chest Med 21:739, 2000.

Meyers, BF: Lung transplantation: a decade of experience. Ann Surg 230:362, 1999.

Petty, TL: COPD in perspective. Chest 121(5 Suppl):116S, 2002.

Petty, TL: Simple Spirometry for Frontline Practitioners. Laennec Publishing, Fairfield, N.J., 1998.

Petty, TL: (2001). Simple office spirometry. Clinics in Chest Medicine, 22(4), 845-59.

Rennard, SI: COPD in 2001: a major challenge for medicine, the pharmaceutical industry, and society. Chest 121(5 Suppl):113S, 2002.

Schapira, RM, and Reinke, LF: Chronic obstructive pulmonary disease. In Noble, J (ed) Textbook of Primary Care Medicine, ed 3. Mosby, St. Louis, 2001, p 677.

Schulman, LL: Lung transplantation for chronic obstructive pulmonary disease. Clin Chest Med 21:849, 2000.

Sullivan, SD: The economic burden of COPD. Chest 117(2 Suppl):5S, 2000.

Tierney, LM, et al (eds): Current Medical Diagnosis and Treatment 2001. Lange Medical Books/McGraw-Hill, New York, 2001, p 283.

U.S. Department of Health and Human Services, Public Health Service, National Institutes of Health, National Heart, Lung, and Blood Institute: Global Initiative for Chronic Obstructive Lung Disease: Pocket Guide to COPD Diagnosis, Management, and Prevention. NIH Publication No. 2701B, 2001.

Weisman, IM: Clinical exercise testing. Clin Chest Med 22:679, 2002.

Wouters, EF: Systemic effects in COPD. Chest 121(5 Suppl):127S, 2002.

Lung Cancer

BTS guidelines: guidelines on the selection of patients with lung cancer for surgery. Thorax 56:89, 2001.

Chesnutt, MS, and Prendergast, TJ: Bronchogenic carcinoma. In Tierney, LM, et al (eds): Current Medical Diagnosis and Treatment 2001. Lange Medical Books/McGraw-Hill, New York, 2001, p 309.

Deslauriers, J: Clinical and surgical staging of non-small cell lung cancer. Chest 117(4 Suppl 1):96S, 2000.

Dolan, S, and Funahashi, A: Neoplasms of the lung. In Noble, J (ed) Textbook of Primary Care Medicine, ed 3. Mosby, St. Louis, 2001, p 749.

Dyspnea. Mechanisms, assessment, and management: a consensus statement. American Thoracic Society. Am J Respir Crit Care Med 159:321, 1999.

ESMO Minimum Clinical Recommendations for diagnosis, treatment and follow-up of small-cell lung cancer (SCLC). Ann Oncol 12:1051, 2001.

ESMO Minimum Clinical Recommendations for diagnosis, treatment and follow-up of non-small-cell lung cancer (NSCLC). Ann Oncol 12:1049, 2001.

Fujita, A: Combination chemotherapy in patients with malignant pleural effusions from non-small cell lung cancer: Cisplatin, ifosfamide, and irinotecan with recombinant human granulocyte colony-stimulating factor support. Chest 119:340, 2001.

Hagge, RJ: Positron emission tomography: brain tumors and lung cancer. Radiol Clin North Am 39:871, 2001.

Miller, BA, et al (eds): Racial/Ethnic Patterns of Cancer in the United States 1988–1992. NIH Pub. No. 96-4104. National Cancer Institute, Bethesda, Md., 1996.

Mountain, CF: Staging classification of lung cancer. A critical evaluation. Clin Chest Med 23:103, 2002.

Neville, A: Lung cancer. Clin Evidence 6:1181, 2001.

Prager, D, et al: Bronchogenic carcinoma. In Murray JF, and Nadel, JA (eds): Textbook of Respiratory Medicine, ed 3. WB Saunders, Philadelphia, 2000, p 1415.

Younes, RN: Follow-up in lung cancer: how often and for what purpose? Chest 115:1494, 1999.

Pneumonia

American College of Emergency Physicians. Clinical policy for the management and risk stratification of community-acquired pneumonia in adults in the emergency department. Ann Emerg Med 38:107, 2001.

Amsden, GW: Pneumococcal macrolide resistance: Myth or reality? J Antimicrob Chemother 44:1, 1999.

Atlas, SJ, et al: Safely increasing the proportion of patients with community-acquired pneumonia treated as outpatients: An interventional trial. Arch Intern Med 158:1350, 1998.

Bartlett, JG, et al: Practice guidelines for the management of community-acquired pneumonia in adults. Clin Infect Dis 31, 2000.

Bentley, DW: Practice guideline for evaluation of fever and infection in long-term care facilities. Clin Infect Dis 31:640, 2000.

Chesnutt, MS, et al (eds): Current Medical Diagnosis and Treatment 2001. Lange Medical Books/McGraw-Hill, New York, 2001, p 291.

Feikin, DR, et al: Mortality from invasive pneumococcal pneumonia in an era of antibiotic resistance, 1995–1997. Am J Public Health 90:223, 2000.

Gonzales, R, et al: Decreasing antibiotic use in ambulatory practice: Impact of a multidimensional intervention on the treatment of uncomplicated acute bronchitis in adults. JAMA 28:1512, 1999.

Lipchik, RJ: Pneumonia. In Noble, J (ed): Textbook of Primary Care Medicine, ed 3. Mosby, St. Louis, 2001, p 662.

Marrie, TJ, et al: A controlled trial of a critical pathway for treatment of community-acquired pneumonia. JAMA 283:749, 2000.

Niederman, MS: Guidelines for the management of adults with community-acquired pneumonia. Diagnosis, assessment of severity, antimicrobial therapy, and prevention. Am J Respir Crit Care Med 163:1730, 2001.

Syrjala, H, et al: High-resolution computed tomography for the diagnosis of community-acquired pneumonia. Clin Infect Dis 27:358, 1998.

Wipf, JE, et al: Diagnosing pneumonia by physical examination: Relevant or relic? Arch Intern Med 159:1082, 1999.

Pulmonary Embolism

Agnelli, G, et al: Benefits of extending anticoagulant therapy for idiopathic deep vein thrombosis are not maintained once treatment is discontinued. Med J Aust 175:88, 2001.

Almoosa, K: Is thrombolytic therapy effective for pulmonary embolism. Am Fam Physician 65:1097, 2002.

Arcasoy, SM, and Kreit, JW: Thrombolytic therapy of pulmonary embolism: A comprehensive review of current evidence. Chest 115, 1999.

Chesnutt, MS, and Prendergast, TJ: Pulmonary thromboembolism. In Tierney, LM, et al (eds): Current Medical Diagnosis and Treatment 2001. Lange Medical Books/McGraw-Hill, New York, 2001, p 321.

Clinical policy: critical issues in the evaluation and management of patients presenting with syncope. Ann Emerg Med 37:771, 2001.

Douketis, JD, et al: Elevated cardiac troponin levels in patients with submassive pulmonary embolism. Arch Intern Med 162:79, 2002.

Dyspnea. Mechanisms, assessment, and management: a consensus statement. American Thoracic Society. Am J Respir Care 1999. Accessed on NIH/NLM MEDLINE, November 25, 2002.

Elliot, CG, et al: Chest radiographs in acute pulmonary embolism: Results from the International Cooperative Pulmonary Embolism Registry. Chest 118:33, 2000.

Fuster, V, et al: ACC/AHA/ESC guidelines for the management of patients with atrial fibrillation. A report of the American College of Cardiology/American Heart Association Task Force on Practice Guidelines and the European Society of Cardiology Committee for Practice Guidelines on diagnosis and management of acute pulmonary embolism. Task Force on Pulmonary Embolism, European Society of Cardiology. Eur Heart J 16:1301, 2000.

Guidelines and Policy Conferences (Committee to develop guidelines for the management of patients with atrial fibrillation) developed in collaboration with the North American Society of Pacing and Electrophysiology. Eur Heart J 22:1852, 2000.

Goldhaber, SZ: Acute pulmonary embolism: Clinical outcomes in the International Cooperative Pulmonary Embolism Registry (ICOPER). Lancet 353:1386, 1999.

Huisman, MV: Recurrent venous thromboembolism: Diagnosis and management. Curr Opin Pulm Med 6:330, 2000.

Kelly, J: Role of D-dimers in diagnosis of venous thromboembolism. Lancet 359:456, 2002.

Kyrle, PA: High plasma levels of factor VIII and the risk of recurrent venous thromboembolism. N Engl J Med 343:457, 2000.

Lipchik, RJ, and Presberg, KW: Venous thromboembolism and pulmonary hypertensive diseases. In Noble, J (ed): Textbook of Primary Care Medicine, ed 3. Mosby, St. Louis, 2001, p 729.

Masotti, L, et al: Pulmonary embolism in the elderly: Clinical, instrumental and laboratory aspects. Gerontology 46:205, 2000.

Prevention of pulmonary embolism and deep vein thrombosis with low dose aspirin: Pulmonary Embolism Prevention (PEP) trial. Lancet 355:1295, 2000.

Stein, PD: The role of newer diagnostic techniques in the diagnosis of pulmonary embolism. Curr Opin Pulm Med 5:212, 1999.

Tapson, VF: The diagnostic approach to acute venous thromboembolism. Clinical practice guideline. American Thoracic Society. Am J Respir Crit Care Med 160:1043, 1999.

The use of oral anticoagulants (warfarin) in older people. AGS Clinical Practices Committee. American Geriatric Society. J Am Geriatr Soc 48:224, 2000.

van Den Belt, AG, et al: Fixed dose subcutaneous low molecular weight heparins versus adjusted dose unfractionated heparin for venous thromboembolism. Cochrane Database System Review 2:CD001100, 2000.

van Der Heijden, JF: Vitamin K antagonists or low-molecular-weight heparin for the long term treatment of symptomatic venous thromboembolism. Cochrane Database System Review 4:CD002001, 2002.

Vanscoy, GJ: Outpatient management of venous thromboembolism. J Thromb Thrombol 7:109, 1999.

Wakefield, TW: Current status of pulmonary embolism and venous thrombosis prophylaxis. Semin Vasc Surg 13:171, 2000.

White, RH: A population-based study of the effectiveness of inferior vena cava filter use among patients with venous thromboembolism. Arch Intern Med 160:2033, 2000.

Pulmonary Tuberculosis

American Family Physician: Clinical guidelines: American Thoracic Society adopts diagnostic standards for tuberculosis. Am Fam Physician 63:979, 2001.

Ashkin, D: Won't get fooled again by tuberculosis. Chest 116:856, 1999.

Byrd, RP: Nutrition and pulmonary tuberculosis. Clin Infect Dis 35:634, 2002.

Cegielski, JP, et al.: The global tuberculosis situation: progress and problems in the 20th century, prospects for the 21st century. Infect Dis Clin North Am 16:1, 2002.

Centers for Disease Control and Prevention: Anergy skin testing and preventive therapy for HIV-infected persons: revised recommendations. MMWR CDC Surveill Summ 46 (No. RR15):1, 1997. Retrieved November 1, 2002 from http://www.cdc.gov/epo/mmwr/preview/mmwrhtml/00049386.htm

Centers for Disease Control and Prevention, Division of Tuberculosis Elimination: Surveillance reports: reported tuberculosis in the United States 2001. Retrieved October 20, 2002 from http://www.cdc.gov/nchstp/tb/surv/surv2001/default.htm

Centers for Disease Control and Prevention, Division of Tuberculosis Elimination: Core curriculum on tuberculosis: what the clinician should know, 4th ed, 2000. Retrieved October 20, 2002 from http://www.cdc.gov/nchstp/tb/pubs/corecurr/default.htm

Centers for Disease Control and Prevention: Public health dispatch: Update: fatal and severe liver injuries associated with rifampin and pyrazinamide treatment for latent tuberculosis infection. MMWR 51: 998, 2002. Retrieved November 10, 2002 from http://www.cdc.gov/mmwr/preview/mmwrhtml/mm5144a4.htm

Gubser, VL: Healthy People 2000: Tuberculosis and the elderly: a community health perspective. Journal of Gerontol Nurs 24:36, 1998.

Horsburgh CR, et al.: Practice guidelines for the treatment of tuberculosis. Clin Infect Dis 31:633, 2000. Retrieved November 1, 2002 from http://www.journals.uchicago.edu/CID/journal/issues/v31n3/000549/000549.html

Jerant, AF: Identification and management of tuberculosis. Am Fam Physician 61:2667, 2000.

Kamholz, SL: Treatment challenges: multi-drug resistant tuberculosis. Program and abstracts of CHEST 2001: 67th Annual Scientific Assembly of the

American College of Chest Physicians; November 4–8, 2001: Philadelphia. Retrieved October 21, 2002 from http://www.medscape.com/viewarticle/412928.

Medinger, A: Death associated with rifampin and pyrazinamide 2-month treatment of latent mycobacterium tuberculosis. Chest 121:1710, 2002.

Perez-Guzman, C: Does aging modify pulmonary tuberculosis? A meta-analytical review. Chest 116:961, 1999.

Reuben, DB, et al.: Geriatrics at Your Fingertips: 2001 Edition. Excerpta Medica, Inc. for the American Geriatrics Society, Belle Meade, NJ, 2001, p 67.

Rosenzweig, D: Tuberculosis and nontuberculous mycobacterial diseases. In Noble, J. (ed): Textbook of Primary Care Medicine. ed 3. Mosby, St. Louis, 2001, p 669.

Schaeffer-Pautz A: A chest wall mass in a 73-year-old man. Chest 120:2051, 2001.

Schluger NW: Challenges of treating latent tuberculosis infection. Chest 121:1733, 2002.

Wisnivesky JP, et al.: Diagnosis and management of tuberculosis in the elderly patient. Clin Geriatr 9:58, 2001.

Wisnivesky, JP, et al.: Evaluation of clinical parameters to predict *Mycobacterium tuberculosis* in inpatients. Arch Intern Med 160:2471, 2002.

Restrictive Lung Disease

Alhamad, EH: Pulmonary function tests in interstitial lung disease: what role do they have? Clin Chest Med 22:715, 2001.

Balmes, JR: Occupational respiratory diseases. Prim Care Clin Office Pract 27, 2000.

Becker, JW: Evaluation of patients with chronic respiratory symptoms. Immunol Allergy Clin N Am 19:1, 1999.

Chang, JA: Assessment of health-related quality of life in patients with interstitial lung disease. Chest 116:1175, 1999.

Efferen, LS: Research yields better classifications for idiopathic interstitial pneumonias. 2002. Contact: http://www.medscape.com/viewarticle/412925. Accessed November 21, 2002.

Epler, GR: Bronchiolitis obliterans organizing pneumonia. Arch Intern Med 161:158, 2001.

Hansell, DM: High-resolution computed tomography in the evaluation of fibrosing alveolitis. Clin Chest Med 20:739, 1999.

Idiopathic Pulmonary Fibrosis (IPF): Highlights from the 98th International Conference of the American Thoracic Society. Contact: http://www.medscape.com/viewarticle/436464_3. Accessed November 21, 2002.

Meek, PM, et al: Dyspnea. Mechanisms, assessment, and management: a consensus statement. American Thoracic Society. Am J Respir Crit Care Med 159:321, 1999.

Pride, NB: Tests of forced expiration and inspiration. Clin Chest Med 22:599, 2001.

Schlueter, DP: Interstitial lung diseases. In Noble, J (ed): Textbook of Primary Care Medicine, ed 3. Mosby, St. Louis, 2001, p 688.

Stam, H: Evaluation of diffusing capacity in patients with a restrictive lung disease. Chest 117:752, 2000.

Tierney, LM, et al: Current Medical Diagnosis and Treatment 2001. Lange Medical Books/McGraw-Hill, New York, 2001.

Britton, J: Interferon gamma-1b therapy for cryptogenic fibrosing alveolitis. Thorax 55(Suppl 1):S37, 2000.

Upper Respiratory Infection

Adam, P, et al: A clinical trial of hypertonic saline nasal spray in subjects with the common cold or rhinosinusitis. Arch Fam Med 7:39, 1998.

Glasziou, P, and Del Mar, C: Upper respiratory tract infection: Effects of treatments. Clin Evidence 6:1200, 2001.

Gonzales, R, et al: Principles of appropriate antibiotic use for treatment of non-specific upper respiratory tract infections in adults: Background. Special report: CDC principles of judicious antibiotic use. Ann Emerg Med 37, 2001.

Hickner, JM, et al: Principles of appropriate antibiotic use for acute rhinosinusitis in adults: Background. Ann Intern Med 134:498, 2001.

Hueston, WJ, et al: Criteria used by clinicians to differentiate sinusitis from viral upper respiratory tract infections. J Fam Pract 46:487, 1998.

McKee, MD, et al: Antibiotic use for the treatment of upper respiratory infections in a diverse community. J Fam Pract 48:993, 1999.

National Center for Health Statistics: Fast stats A to Z. 2002. Contact: http://www.cdc.gov/nchs/fastats/colds.htm. Accessed November 17, 2002.

Prasad, AS: Duration of symptoms and plasma cytokine levels in patients with the common cold treated with zinc acetate: A randomized, double-blind, placebo-controlled trial. Ann Intern Med 133:245, 2000.

Ressel, G: Principles of appropriate antibiotic use: Part III. Acute rhinosinusitis. Centers for Disease Control and Prevention. Am Fam Physician 64:685, 2001.

Tierney, LM, et al (eds): Current Medical Diagnosis and Treatment 2001. Lange Medical Books/McGraw-Hill, New York, 2001, p 231.

Update on Antibiotic Resistance. 2002. Contact: http://www.cdc.gov/drugresistance/community/. AccessedNovember 18, 2002.

Chapter *6*
ABDOMINAL DISORDERS

ACUTE RENAL FAILURE

SIGNAL SYMPTOMS▶ oliguria, anuria, mental confusion, somnolence, xerostomia

Acute renal failure (ARF)	ICD-9 CM: 584.9

Description: ARF is a rapid reduction of renal function, associated with azotemia, with or without oliguria. ARF is classified into three categories: *prerenal*, stemming from poor renal perfusion; *postrenal*, caused by obstruction; and *intrinsic*, caused by injury to the kidney (e.g., from glomerulonephritis or tubular necrosis). The most common type of ARF is prerenal failure and acute tubular necrosis.

Etiology: ARF occurs when the amount of blood flow to the kidneys is decreased or the renal tubules are damaged from a toxin or ischemia, resulting in an abrupt decline in renal function. Intravascular volume depletion, prolonged ischemic damage to the kidney, and any obstruction to the flow in urine can cause ARF. This reduction in the glomerular filtration rate (GFR) is evidenced by a rise in the plasma creatinine level.

Occurrence: An estimated 5% of patients admitted to the hospital develop ARF; this percentage increases with the acuity of the patient's condition and the length of hospitalization.

Age: ARF can occur in patients of all ages. Considering the high percentage of hospitalized older adults who experience congestive heart failure, sepsis, or surgical procedures with associated volume depletion, development of ARF is possible in all critically ill or older surgical patients. Mortality secondary to ARF increases with age.

Ethnicity: No known prevalence exists among ethnic groups.

Gender: ARF occurs equally in men and women.

Contributing factors: Heatstroke, dehydration, vomiting, diarrhea, congestive heart failure, hemorrhage, excessive diuresis, pancreatic disease, cirrhosis, burns, trauma, peritonitis, and early sepsis are precursors to prerenal ARF. Surgical patients are susceptible to ARF because of volume depletion. Intrinsic cases of ARF result from patient exposure to nephrotoxic drugs (angiotensin-converting enzyme [ACE] inhibitors, certain nonsteroidal anti-inflammatory drugs [NSAIDs], aminoglycosides, acyclovir, some cephalosporins, and trimethoprim-sulfamethoxazole), tubular necrosis, interstitial nephritis, and chronic disease such as polyarteritis or systemic lupus erythematosus. Obstructions caused by bladder, pelvic, or retroperitoneal tumors; calculi; benign prostatic hyperplasia; and a neurogenic bladder may contribute to postrenal ARF. Older adults who take anticholinergic drugs are prone to develop postrenal azotemia.

Signs and symptoms: The signs and symptoms of ARF depend on the disease category of ARF. A thorough history is important to discern all causes of ARF; multiple causes may be identified in an individual patient. The patient may complain of anorexia, headache, fatigue, vomiting, diarrhea, muscle cramps, somnolence, weakness, back pain, foul-smelling concentrated urine, oliguria, or xerostomia. Patients also may report shortness of breath. Family members or patients may report seizure disorders or mental confusion or both. Delirium and dehydration may be the first indications of ARF in a frail older adult. All causes of altered renal perfusion, trauma, infection, and obstruction should be explored.

Physical examination may reveal ecchymosis, hypertension, petechiae, crackles, rash, tachycardia, and tachypnea. Patients also may present with myoclonus, pericardial or pleural rub, peripheral edema, and rales. Examine for signs of volume depletion and infection. Palpate the kidneys for tenderness and the bladder for enlargement. Rectal and vaginal examinations are appropriate when obstruction is suspected.

Diagnostic tests: Urine is analyzed for sediment, osmolarity, and urine sodium and creatinine levels. In prerenal and postrenal ARF, the sediment is usually normal, but sometimes hyaline casts are present. Tubular epithelial cells, cellular casts, and debris are common findings in acute tubular necrosis. In prerenal disease, the ratio of blood urea nitrogen (BUN) to plasma creatinine is usually >20:1, whereas in acute tubular necrosis the ratio is <15:1. Laboratory findings in ARF consist of hyponatremia, hyperkalemia, hypocalcemia, azotemia, and decreased creatinine clearance. Renal ultrasonography or computed tomography (CT) should detect a normal-sized or slightly enlarged kidney in ARF.

Test	Results Indicating Disorder	CPT Code
Urinalysis	Prerenal and postrenal hyaline casts may be present	81000–81009
BUN	Prerenal >20:1 Intrinsic >15:1	84520
CBC	Anemia, infection	85022–85025
Creatinine	Elevated	82565
Serum electrolytes	Hyponatremia Hyperkalemia Hypocalcemia Azotemia	84295 84132 82310
CT scan	Normal or slightly enlarged kidney	72160
Renal ultrasound	Normal or slightly enlarged kidney. A false-negative ultrasound can occur if the obstruction is early or retroperitoneal fibrosis is detected	76770–76778

CBC, complete blood count.

Differential diagnosis:

- Glomerulonephritis
- Systemic vasculitis
- Urinary tract obstruction
- Pyelonephritis

Treatment: Patients with ARF require hospitalization and often intensive care. Treatment measures are aimed at reversing correctable causes of ARF. For patients with intrinsic ARF, therapy is directed toward hyponatremia, hyperkalemia, medication dosage, anemia, or metabolic acidosis. The nephrologist may consider hemodialysis, peritoneal dialysis, and hemofiltration in severe cases. Volume-depleted patients are restored with saline. The use of loop diuretics in critically ill oliguric patients is not recommended. For patients with elevated serum phosphorus levels, give oral phosphate-binding agents, such as aluminum-containing or calcium carbonate antacids, to maintain the serum phosphorus level at <5.5 mg/dL. Order a low-protein diet with 0.5 g/kg of body weight per day of protein to prevent a rise in the BUN level. Use urinary catheters cautiously in older adults because a high prevalence of infection is associated with catheterization.

Follow-up: Management of the patient recovering from ARF depends on the initial cause of the kidney dysfunction, if the reversible cause was corrected, and if any sequelae occurred. Dietary management may require interdisciplinary consultation, including physician specialists, a nutritionist, nursing staff, the patient, and family members. For patients who recover from a reversible cause of ARF, monitor serum creatinine level and calculate creatinine clearance every 3 months until renal function stabilizes. All medications need to be reviewed and dosages adjusted according to the GFR and the serum concentrations of the medications.

Sequelae: Volume overload resulting in pulmonary edema, hypertensive crisis, hyperkalemia, anemia, infections, cardiac disease, hemorrhage including upper gastrointestinal bleeding, and death are possible complications of ARF. Infection is the primary cause of death in patients with ARF, and cardiopulmonary disorders are the second most common cause of death from ARF.

Prevention/prophylaxis: ARF can be avoided in some instances when nephrotoxic medications are indicated for medical therapy. Monitor renal function, adjust medication dosages accordingly, and try alternative medications if the potential exists for developing ARF. For surgical patients, ARF often can be prevented if fluid balance, blood volume, and blood pressure are monitored.

Referral: All patients with ARF require hospitalization. Referral to a specialist is highly recommended; these patients often have concomitant problems that a specialist would manage in the acute care setting. Postrenal ARF may require collaboration with a nephrologist, urologist, and radiologist.

Education: For the reversible causes of ARF, teach patients to avoid dehydration and excessive heat, to avoid taking any over-the-counter (OTC) medications before contacting their health-care provider, and, if applicable to their case, to recognize the signs and symptoms of congestive heart failure.

BLADDER CANCER

SIGNAL SYMPTOMS▶ painless hematuria, urinary frequency or urgency, mild suprapubic pain; often asymptomatic

Primary	ICD-9 CM: 188.9
Secondary	ICD-9 CM: 198.1
Carcinoma in situ (CIS)	ICD-9 CM: 233.7
Benign	ICD-9 CM: 223.3
Uncertain behavior	ICD-9 CM: 236.7
Unspecified	ICD-9 CM: 239.4

Description: Of bladder cancers, 90% are transitional urothelial cell cancer, 8% are squamous cell cancer, and the rest are adenocarcinoma. In bladder cancer, the posterior and lateral walls of the bladder are involved more frequently than the superior wall. Bladder cancer can be categorized as *superficial, invasive,* and *metastatic.* Superficial, or early, bladder cancer occurs when the lesion is located on the surface of the mucosa or when the tumor penetrates the mucosa and submucosa only. Invasive bladder cancer develops when lesions pervade the bladder muscularis or the perivesical fat. Metastatic bladder cancer is characterized by lymph node, visceral, or bone tissue involvement.

Etiology: Occupational exposures to aniline dye, leather processing, paint, rubber, and possibly tobacco tars, because of suspected chemical carcinogens, have been linked to the development of bladder cancer. Squamous cell bladder cancer has been linked to chronic infection with *Schistosoma haematobium*.

Occurrence: In the United States each year, >50,000 new cases of bladder cancer are diagnosed, and >12,000 deaths can be attributed to bladder cancer.

Age: The average age of onset is in the late 60s.

Ethnicity: *S. haematobium* infection is prevalent in Africa and the Middle East. The incidence of bladder cancer increases among people from the industrialized areas of the northeastern United States because of their higher exposure to carcinogens.

Gender: Bladder cancer is four times more common in men than in women.

Contributing factors: History of smoking increases the risk of bladder cancer. Pelvic irradiation, certain drugs (e.g., cyclophosphamide), and abnormal tryptophan metabolism contribute to the development of bladder cancer. Excessive coffee consumption, use of some artificial sweeteners (e.g., saccharin sodium and cyclamate sodium), and overuse of phenacetin-containing analgesics have been suggested risk factors. Occupational exposure to dyes, rubber, and leather has been shown to increase the risk of developing bladder cancer. There also has been an association between developing bladder cancer and working as a hairdresser, machinist, printer, painter, or truck driver. Exfoliation of cancer cells by cystoscopy, brushing, or transurethral biopsy or resection may spread bladder cancer cells to other sites within the bladder that may be irritated from instrumentation. Some association has been shown with developing bladder cancer and a long history of indwelling catheters and urinary calculi.

Signs and symptoms: Gross, painless hematuria, pyuria, burning, and frequency are common in the presentation of bladder cancer. Symptoms of advanced cancer may include pelvic or flank pain and lower extremity edema resulting from lymphatic or venous blockage. Patients also may complain of abdominal pain, anorexia, and bone pain.

The clinician should palpate and percuss for evidence of any kidney enlargement and perform a prostate examination on men and pelvic examination on women. Additionally, the examination should be directed toward searching for possible sites of metastasis in the lungs, liver, bone, and lymph nodes.

Diagnostic tests:

Test	Results Indicating Disorder	CPT Code
CBC	Possible microcytic anemia or infection	85031
Renal function test	Rule out renal parenchymal disease	80069
Urinalysis	>5 red blood cells	81000–81099
Cystoscopy with bladder barbotage and biopsy	Diagnostic of bladder cancer	52000, 52004, 52354
IVP	Rule out ureteral obstruction	74400–74415
CT scan of abdomen, pelvis	Lymphadenopathy	74160, 72193
Chest x-ray	Rule out metastasis	71010–71035

IVP, intravenous pyelogram.

Differential diagnosis:

- Neurogenic bladder
- Nephrolithiasis
- Urinary tract infection
- Benign prostatic hypertrophy
- Other genitourinary cancers

Treatment: Management of bladder cancer depends on the stage of the disease. Initially, surgical intervention to remove the bladder tumors is warranted. Some patients may require a cystectomy with a urostomy, continent urostomy, or replacement bladder. For patients with multiple recurrent superficial bladder tumors, the urologist may request collaboration with an oncologist for chemotherapy after surgery. Advanced disease generally requires surgery, radiation, and chemotherapy with combination agents. The patient's age and health status at the time of diagnosis must be considered in the management of bladder cancer.

Follow-up: Patients with superficial low-grade bladder cancer require a cystoscopy at designated intervals, although the value of repeated testing has been questioned. The need for supplemental nutritional support, pain management, prevention of complications such as skin breakdown, and an advanced directive should be discussed during future follow-up care. Patients with a urostomy may need assistance from an ostomy nurse.

Sequelae: Metastasis to other parts of the body can occur. Survival of the untreated patient may be <2 years.

Prevention/prophylaxis: Encourage patients who smoke to quit and all patients to decrease exposure to harmful chemicals.

Referral: Refer patients with clinically significant hematuria to a urologist. An oncologist also may be involved in the patient's management of the disease. Patient and family support is important at this time; information pertaining to hospice services should be provided. Patients with a urostomy may seek support from a local chapter of a urostomy association (UOA) at 1-800-826-0826 or www.uoa.org.

Education: Older adults with bladder cancer may need to be educated about palliative support measures when the disease becomes terminal.

BOWEL OBSTRUCTION

SIGNAL SYMPTOMS abdominal distention with cramping, absent or minimal peristalsis, obstipation

Bowel obstruction ICD-9 CM: 560.9

Description: Absent or minimal peristalsis and abdominal distention with cramping are signs of bowel obstruction. A bowel obstruction is an intestinal blockage classified as a mechanical obstruction or as an adynamic ileus, acute or chronic, simple or strangulated. Bowel obstructions occur in the small intestine and in the colon.

Etiology: A mechanical bowel obstruction results when there is a complete or partial blockage of the lumen of the bowel by a lesion. A simple mechanical obstruction occurs without insult to the vascular or neurological system. Strangulation of the bowel in older adults happens when there is a twisting of the bowel, resulting in ischemia of the bowel wall. The bowel may become edematous and infarcted, leading to perforation and gangrene. An adynamic ileus may result from metabolic disturbances such as hypokalemia or when injury or illness causes reduced blood supply to the bowel. In the case of functional or paralytic obstruction, gut motility is impaired.

Occurrence: An estimated 20% of all hospital admissions for acute abdominal conditions are for suspected bowel obstruction.

Age: Bowel obstruction from all causes except intussusception is more prevalent in older adults.

Ethnicity: No prevalence is known among ethnic groups.

Gender: Bowel obstruction occurs equally in men and women.

Contributing factors: Patients with recent history of surgery, vertebral fractures, lower lobe pneumonia, fractured ribs, severe trauma, hypokalemia, and myocardial infarctions are at risk for developing an adynamic ileus. Neoplasms, hernias, inflammatory disease, diverticulitis, mesenteric ischemia, stricture formation, volvulus (especially of the sigmoid colon), gallstones, and fecal impactions can cause a mechanical bowel obstruction. Patients with a history of abdominal surgery may develop adhesions that can cause a small bowel obstruction.

Signs and symptoms: Clinical presentation of bowel obstruction depends on the site and the cause of the obstruction. In adynamic ileus, patients may report hiccups, vomiting, and abdominal distention with cramping. Pain is usually continuous rather than colicky. Obstipation may or may not occur. Fever may be present. Auscultation generally reveals absent or minimal peristalsis. Diffuse minimal abdominal tenderness may be elicited. Presentation of a mechanical small bowel obstruction includes abdominal cramps located in the epigastrium or around the umbilicus, with associated pain that can be more severe the higher the obstruction. Profuse vomiting occurs early with a small bowel obstruction. The vomitus first may consist of mucus and bile in a high small bowel obstruction. With a lower ileal obstruction, the vomitus becomes feculent. Diarrhea may occur in partial small bowel obstruction. Obstipation exists with complete obstruction. The patient may have a low-grade fever.

Inspect the abdomen for evidence of surgical scars and external hernias. Borborygmi may be heard on auscultation; however, late in the presentation of a strangulated bowel, peristalsis may be minimal or absent. Abdominal distention is found; the abdomen may not be tender, in the case of a strangulated bowel. With mechanical obstruction of the large bowel, symptoms are similar to a small bowel obstruction but appear more gradually. The patient complains of persistent constipation leading to abdominal distention. Vomiting may be absent, if the ileocecal valve is functioning. Physical examination reveals loud borborygmi, no abdominal tenderness, and an empty rectal vault. Patients with a strangulating bowel may exhibit signs of shock late in the presentation of the obstruction.

Diagnostic tests: White blood cells (WBCs) may be slightly elevated to 15,000/mm^3; a shift to the left may occur without an elevation of the WBCs in older adults. Hematocrit may be elevated in dehydrated patients. A urinalysis may reveal an increase in specific gravity owing to the excess fluid loss. Serum electrolytes are ordered to determine degree of dehydration and plan for intravenous replacement. A rise in the BUN could indicate blood in the intestine or dehydration or both. The serum amylase level may be moderately elevated. Positive test result for occult blood in the stool suggests bowel strangulation or carcinoma of the bowel. Chest x-ray and supine and upright plain abdominal films determine presence of air-fluid levels, external hernias, or marked dilation of the bowel. If possible, the chest x-ray should be obtained after the nasogastric tube has been inserted. Colonoscopy is performed to determine the site of the obstruction. Barium enema is also diagnostic for bowel obstruction. Oral barium is contraindicated in patients with a suspected colonic obstruction because a hardened mass of the barium can form above the obstruction.

Test	Results Indicating Disorder	CPT Code
WBC count	15,000/mm^3	85048
Hematocrit	May be elevated	85022–85025
Urinalysis	Increase in specific gravity	81000–81099
Serum electrolytes	Dehydration	80051
BUN	Blood in intestine Dehydration	84520

Serum amylase
FOBT
Chest x-ray
Abdominal x-ray
Colonoscopy
Barium enema
	Moderately elevated
	Bowel strangulation,
	   carcinoma
	Air/fluid levels
	External hernias, marked
	   dilation of bowel
	Determine size of obstruction
	Narrow twisted part of the lumen
		82150
		82270
		71010–71035
		74000–74022
		45380
		74270–74280

FOBT, fecal occult blood test.

Differential diagnosis:

- Acute appendicitis
- Cholecystitis
- Pancreatitis
- Diverticulitis

Treatment: Initial treatment of a bowel obstruction consists of hospitalization for nasogastric suctioning, urinary catheter to monitor output, and fluid and electrolyte replacement with intravenous fluids. Decompression can be achieved by insertion of a small lubricated rectal tube. The surgeon may order prophylactic intravenous antibiotics. For an acute mechanical obstruction, surgery is indicated to correct the underlying cause (e.g., repair a hernia, lyse adhesions, correct a volvulus, or remove a gallstone or high fecal impaction). For patients with adynamic ileus, nasogastric suctioning and intravenous fluids may be all that is necessary to relieve the obstruction; for other patients with an ileus, colonoscopic decompression may be required. Terminally ill patients with bowel obstruction should receive palliative care, including pain relief and intravenous hydration.

Follow-up: Postoperative care of the patient with a surgically corrected bowel obstruction includes monitoring for return of bowel function, maintaining fluid and electrolyte balance with intravenous alimentation, and observing for signs of sepsis. After discharge from the hospital, the patient should return within 2 weeks for surveillance. Patients being treated nonsurgically also should be monitored accordingly; observe for signs of recurrence of the bowel obstruction. If an ileus persists >1 week, an underlying mechanical obstruction should be ruled out, and a laparotomy may be necessary.

Sequelae: After correction of a bowel obstruction, slow return of bowel function is an early complication. The possibility of ensuing bowel obstructions and sepsis needs to be monitored in all patients. For patients who are not surgical candidates, complications such as perforation and peritonitis should be considered.

Prevention/prophylaxis: Caregivers must understand the importance of avoiding fecal impactions in patients at risk for this condition.

Referral: Recommend a surgical consultation for patients with susceptible bowel obstruction.

Education: Inform older adults with diagnosed untreated internal and external hernias of the possible complication of bowel obstruction.

CHOLECYSTITIS

SIGNAL SYMPTOMS pain that may radiate to back, especially right after eating fatty foods

Acute	ICD-9 CM: 575.0
Chronic	ICD-9 CM: 575.1

Description: Cholecystitis, an acute or chronic inflammation of the gallbladder, results from an obstruction of the cystic duct.

Etiology: The pathologic origin of gallstones is unknown. Cholecystitis occurs when a gallstone obstructs the cystic duct usually except in cases involving trauma, recent surgery, or sepsis. Most gallstones are a result of cholesterol accumulation.

Occurrence: Approximately 10% of the U.S. population of adults $\geq$40 years old have gallstones; 90% of cases of cholecystitis are associated with gallstones. Each year in the United States, >500,000 people undergo a cholecystectomy after cholecystitis.

Age: Presentation commonly is in the 50s and 60s.

Ethnicity: A high prevalence for cholecystitis exists in older Native Americans and whites; the disease is less prevalent in African-Americans. The prevalence of gallbladder disease is highest in the Pima Indians of Arizona.

Gender: Twice as many women as men have cholecystitis.

Contributing factors: Nonmodifiable risk factors for cholecystitis include female gender and family history of gallbladder disease. Obesity is a known predisposing factor to cholecystitis. Diabetes, inflammatory bowel disease, chronic hemolysis, pancreatic insufficiency, and hyperlipidemia predispose patients to gallstone development. The consumption of a large, fatty meal may result in cholecystitis. Gallstone formation may be attributed to use of exogenous estrogens prescribed for postmenopausal hormone replacement and clofibrate used to treat hyperlipidemia. Gallbladder stasis, a precursor to gallstone formation, occurs with extended total parenteral nutrition. Patients who experience rapid weight loss are at high risk for the development of gallstones.

Signs and symptoms: One type of presentation of acute cholecystitis includes nausea, vomiting, malaise, fever (which may be low grade), and abdominal pain that radiates around the sides to the back as in biliary colic; another type is associated with an acute change in mental status as the only outward sign. Physical examination may reveal right upper quadrant subcostal tenderness and pain on inspiration (Murphy's sign). In a patient who has reported symptoms for days, rebound tenderness may suggest perforation. Abdominal tenderness may be absent, however. Jaundice is present in <50% of patients.

Diagnostic tests:

Test	Results Indicating Disorder	CPT Code
WBC count	12,000–15,000/mm^3 with peripheral leukocytosis	85048
Serum amylase	Elevated	82150
Serum bilirubin	Elevated	82247
Alkaline phosphatase	Elevated	84075
Real-time ultrasound	Gallstones, thickening of gallbladder wall, obstruction of common bile duct, dilation of biliary tract	76700–76705
HIDA scan	Obstruction of the cystic or common hepatic duct	78223

Differential diagnosis:

- Perforated peptic ulcer in older adults
- Appendicitis
- Liver abscess
- Diverticulitis
- Hepatitis
- Acute pyelonephritis
- Gastrointestinal carcinoma
- Acute pancreatitis
- Myocardial ischemia
- Herpes zoster
- Pneumonia
- Gastritis

Treatment: Patients with acute cholecystitis require hospitalization. Nasogastric suctioning, intravenous fluids with electrolytes, and intramuscular analgesics for severe pain are ordered. In older adults with suspected infection, intravenous antibiotics should be given, adjusting the dosage for creatinine clearance. Effective single-agent antibiotics, such as ampicillin, cephalosporins, and penicillins, are recommended except in cases of extremely debilitated patients. Patients with signs of gram-negative sepsis may require combination antibiotic treatment. Laparoscopic or open cholecystectomy should be considered when the patient stabilizes. When surgery is contraindicated in patients with acute calculus cholecystitis, treatment with an ursodeoxycholic acid may be considered if an adequately functioning gallbladder is present and gallstones are determined to be composed of cholesterol. Additional medical management for patients not deemed surgical candidates includes lithotripsy with bile salts.

Follow-up: Postoperative management includes monitoring for impending infection, adverse drug reactions and interactions, and changes in functional and mental status. For the frail older adult who is not a surgical candidate, observation for complications is crucial. Ultrasound of the gallbladder at 6-month intervals is recommended. For older women still prone to cholelithiasis after surgery, dosages of estrogen preparations may need to be reduced if applicable.

Sequelae: Complications of acute cholecystitis may result from severe inflammation with necrosis to the gallbladder; abscess formation and localized perforation stone formation may occur subsequently in the bile ducts. The mortality rate for patients with perforation is about 30%. Frail older adults, especially those who are diabetic, are at high risk for complications from cholecystitis.

Prevention/prophylaxis: The importance of resting and avoiding risk factors after acute cholecystitis or an exacerbation of chronic cholecystitis needs to be emphasized.

Referral: A surgical consultation is necessary if acute cholecystitis is suspected. A gastroenterologist should be consulted for the frail older adult who is not a surgical candidate.

Education: Encourage patients with chronic cholecystitis and patients for whom surgery is contraindicated to report early signs and symptoms of an acute attack, to prevent complications.

CHRONIC RENAL FAILURE

SIGNAL SYMPTOMS ▶ anorexia, fatigue, pruritus

| Chronic renal failure (CRF) | ICD-9 CM: 585 |

Description: CRF can result from any long-term cause of renal dysfunction. In older adults, renal disease is often secondary to other age-related conditions. CRF is characterized by a decrease in the GFR.

Etiology: CRF involves progressive, irreversible damage to both kidneys.

There are many causes of CRF, including diabetic nephropathy, hypertensive disease, glomerulonephritis, and cystic kidney disease. In about 6% of cases, the cause is unknown.

Occurrence: CRF is diagnosed in >40,000 patients per year in the United States. It is estimated that >19 million adults in the United States or 11% of the population have chronic kidney disease.

Age: CRF can occur at any age; the incidence increases with age.

Ethnicity: African-Americans are 3.9 times more likely to have end-stage renal disease (ESRD) and 6.7 times more likely to have hypertensive ESRD. Also at great risk for developing CRF are Native Americans, Southeast Asians, and Hispanics (especially Mexican-Americans) because of the high prevalence of diabetes and heart disease among these minority populations.

Gender: The overall incidence of ESRD is higher in men than in women; certain causes of ESRD are more common in women, however, such as type 2 diabetes, scleroderma, and systemic lupus erythematosus.

Contributing factors: Identified risk factors for CRF include age, race, sex, and family history of disease. History of ARF and reduced kidney mass contribute directly to the development of CRF. Patients with chronic glomerulonephritis, diabetes, hypertension and atherosclerotic vascular disease, autoimmune diseases, multiple myeloma, amyloidosis, systemic infections, and Wegener's granulomatosis are susceptible to CRF, with diabetes mellitus accounting for 40% of all new cases of CRF. Patients who have been exposed to medications or procedures associated with kidney function decline also are at risk.

Signs and symptoms: An older adult may complain of anorexia, fatigue, urinary urgency, dysuria, nocturia, and weakness in the early stages of CRF. As the disease progresses, the patient usually reports nausea, vomiting, stomatitis, an unpleasant or metallic taste in the mouth, muscle cramps and twitches, dyspnea, orthopnea, and depression. Caregivers may report a decrease in attentiveness of the patient.

Assessment should include assessment for jugular venous distention, peripheral edema, and evidence of bruits. Abdominal findings may include flank tenderness and a palpable bladder. Physical examination may reveal hypertension and peripheral neuropathies with sensory and motor deficits. In late-stage disease, confusion, breathlessness, and intractable hiccups are observed. Xerosis with pruritus occurs; the skin turns a yellow-brown. Uremic frost is formed from crystallized urea during the later stages of renal failure.

Diagnostic tests: The National Kidney Foundation Guidelines for Chronic Kidney Disease (2002) recommends that clinicians calculate the GFR for each patient with chronic renal failure using the serum creatinine level and two equations, modification of diet in renal disease and the Cockcroft-Gault equations.

Test	Results Indicating Disorder	CPT Code
Urinalysis	Proteinuria and urinary sediment, microhematuria	81000–81099
BUN	Increased	84520
CBC	Normochromic anemia Normocytic anemia	85031
Ultrasound of kidneys	Size, presence of obstruction	76770, 76778
Serum electrolytes	Decreased calcium and phosphorus, sodium normal or slightly reduced	80051
Serum creatinine	Increased	84295

Differential diagnosis:

- Urinary tract obstruction
- Vasculitis
- Kidney infection

Treatment: A nephrologist should be consulted initially for patients with a serum creatinine <2.0 mg/dL or GFR of <50 mL/min and for patients with moderate proteinuria (National Guideline Clearinghouse, 2001). Underlying factors that contribute to CRF (e.g., diabetes, heart failure, hypertension, nephrotoxins, hypercalcemia, electrolyte disorders, anemia, metabolic acidosis, infection) must be treated specifically. When uremia develops, dietary protein restriction in older adults is often unnecessary because the average daily intake is often <65 g of protein and 4 to 5 g of salt. Water restriction is unnecessary, unless the patient is in congestive heart failure, has uncontrolled hypertension, or has experienced oliguria. A multivitamin (Nephro-Vite) should be included as part of the daily regimen. For patients who develop nephropathy from analgesic abuse or long-term NSAID use, discontinue the offending medication. ACE inhibitors are the treatment of choice for patients with CRF to prevent the development of glomerulosclerosis. Give enalapril, 5 mg daily for nonhypertensive patients and 20 mg for patients with hypertension. Angiotensin receptor blockers, such as eprosartan mesylate, also can be used for this purpose in patients who cannot tolerate ACE inhibitors. Renal function and potassium levels need to be monitored with drug therapy to avoid hyperkalemia.

If iron-deficiency anemia is detected, give Hemocyte tablets once daily. Patients with anemia associated with CRF can be prescribed darbepoetin alfa parenterally. Patients with hypokalemia require potassium supplementation; monitor potassium blood levels to determine dosage. A nephrologist should manage CFR patients with complex underlying disorders, including patients with polycystic kidney disease with a urinary tract infection, patients with glomerulonephritis, or patients with human immunodeficiency virus (HIV)–associated nephropathy and hepatitis C virus–related kidney disease. Patients with renovascular disease, urinary tract obstruction, or multiple myeloma also require the expertise of a nephrologist to determine treatment, including the need for dialysis or hospitalization.

Follow-up: When the patient is stabilized, monitor CBC, blood chemistries, urine, and blood pressure. Beginning biweekly, review with the patient diet, fluid intake, and medication usage (including OTC drugs). Dosages of any renally excreted medications that the patient must take should be reduced. The GFR should be calculated annually for patients with chronic kidney disease; increase the frequency of calculating the GFR if patients have a GFR <60 mL/min/1.73^2 or are considered high risk for an exacerbation of CRF. Patients are considered to be in renal failure when the GFR is <15 mL/min/1.73^2.

Sequelae: Anemia and pruritus are common complications of CRF. Congestive heart failure also may result from CRF. Patients with pruritus and xerosis should use skin moisturizers; antihistamines are contraindicated because of their sedative effect and potential for central nervous system adverse reactions. For untreated patients with a creatinine level of >10 mg/dL, uremia occurs, and death is imminent within 3 and 5 months.

Prevention/prophylaxis: The use of NSAIDs in the elderly with known history of renal failure should be avoided unless absolutely required.

Referral: When the patient begins to show evidence of deterioration despite supportive treatment, refer him or her to a nephrologist. At this time, discuss the options for vascular or peritoneal access for dialysis. For the patient who is not a candidate for aggressive treatment, provide information about local hospice services to the patient and the family.

Education: Inform patients of the importance of obtaining consent from the health-care provider before taking any OTC medications. During hot weather, instruct patients to avoid strenuous activities and to increase fluid intake to avoid dehydration and hyperthermia. Emphasize strict blood glucose control and blood pressure management. Encourage weight loss and smoking cessation. Have patients report immediately any acute symptoms, such as fever, vomiting, and diarrhea, to the health-care provider.

CIRRHOSIS OF THE LIVER

SIGNAL SYMPTOMS jaundice, fatigue, spider angiomas, palmar erythema, nodular liver

Cirrhosis of the liver	ICD-9 CM: 571.1

Description: Cirrhosis occurs when there is chronic insult to the liver, resulting in fibrous and nodular regeneration of the existing hepatocytes.
Etiology: Chronic alcoholism is the most common cause of cirrhosis in

the United States. The cause of primary biliary cirrhosis, a chronic inflammatory disease of the liver in which the intrahepatic bile duct is destroyed, is unknown.

Occurrence: A prevalent disease in older adults, cirrhosis of the liver accounts for >30,000 deaths annually in the general population.

Age: Cirrhosis, which has an increase in onset in older adults, is one of the top 10 leading causes of death for patients age 55 to 74. Onset of primary biliary cirrhosis is usually before age 65.

Ethnicity: No known prevalence exists among groups.

Gender: Cirrhosis of the liver is equally prevalent in men and women with chronic alcoholism.

Contributing factors: Chronic alcohol consumption, combined with a poor nutritional intake, contributes to cirrhosis.

Signs and symptoms: Patients report anorexia, fatigue, pruritus, jaundice, and easy bruising of the skin. An assessment tool, such as the AUDIT (Alcohol Use Disorders Identification Test), is recommended to discern alcohol-related problems. It allows the practitioner to explore the patient's history of chronic alcohol use and the status of functional impairment.

Physical examination may reveal evidence of xanthomata; palmar erythema; spider angiomas; clubbing of fingers; and in men decreased body hair, gynecomastia, and testicular atrophy. Palpation of the liver may reveal a firm, nodular liver.

Diagnostic tests: CBC with indices may reveal a macrocytic anemia caused by nutritional deficiencies of vitamin B_{12} and folic acid. A decreased serum albumin level and prolonged prothrombin time occur in cirrhosis. The serum aspartate aminotransferase (AST) level is elevated; the alanine aminotransferase (ALT) level is usually above normal but not to the degree of the AST. A percutaneous liver biopsy can establish the diagnosis of cirrhosis.

Test	Results Indicating Disorder	CPT Code
CBC with indices	May reveal macrocytic anemia	85021–85027
Serum albumin	Decreased	82040
Prothrombin time	Usually prolonged	85610–85611
AST	Elevated	84450
ALT	Above normal	84460
Lactate dehydrogenase	Elevated in metastatic disease	83615–83625

Differential diagnosis:
- Liver cancer
- Alcoholic hepatitis

Treatment: Cessation of all alcohol intake is imperative. Nutritional support includes at least 1 g protein/kg body weight and 2000 to 3000 kcal/day, unless contraindicated by the presence of hepatic encephalopathy or coma. Multiple vitamin supplements should be prescribed; it is recommended, however, that a multiple vitamin without iron be recommended unless iron-deficiency anemia is present.

Follow-up: Surveillance of the older adult with cirrhosis depends on the stability of the patient and the presence of complications. Stable older adults should have repeat liver function tests 6 months to 1 year after initial diagnosis. Unstable patients may need to be monitored monthly. Complications of cirrhosis, listed in under Sequelae, require additional medical therapy. On return visits, observation and testing for changes in mental status and depression may be indicated.

Sequelae: Complications from cirrhosis include ascites, portal hypertension, variceal bleeding, renal failure, and hepatic encephalopathy and hepatocellular carcinoma (which is the leading cause of death for patients with cirrhosis). Alcoholic hepatitis may occur with cirrhosis.

Prevention/prophylaxis: Cessation of alcohol consumption is crucial to the prognosis of cirrhosis. Avoidance of hepatotoxic medications, especially NSAIDs, is recommended for patients with cirrhosis. All patients with cirrhosis should be given the hepatitis A and B vaccine, unless they are shown to be immune to the diseases. The polyvalent pneumococcal vaccine and annual influenza vaccines also are recommended for these patients. Preventive strategies for patients with cirrhosis need to focus on the prevention of complications such as endoscopic screenings and secondary prophylaxis.

Referral: A gastroenterologist should be consulted when varices are suspected and variceal bleeding occurs. An esophagogastroduodenoscopy is performed to manage complicated patients.

Education: Instruct patients to eliminate all alcohol consumption. Recommend an alcohol treatment program, and provide the telephone number for the nearest chapter of Alcoholics Anonymous. An additional organization that may be beneficial to the alcoholic patient is Secular Rational Recovery Systems (530-621-4374). Patients should be requested not to self-medicate with OTC medications, including herbal products. Patients with cirrhosis should eat small frequent meals of a balanced diet containing 1 to 1.5 mg protein/kg per day unless contraindicated by advanced disease. For patients with end-stage liver disease, palliative care measures should be initiated.

COLORECTAL CANCER

SIGNAL SYMPTOMS▶   new-onset constipation or diarrhea, bloating, incomplete bowel evacuation, tenesmus

Colorectal cancer   ICD-9 CM: 153.9

Description: Adenocarcinomas are the most common type of cancer of the large intestine; less common are carcinoid tumors, squamous cell carcinoma, and melanoma. Many colorectal cancers develop from adenomatous polyps of the colon and rectum, which occur most frequently in the sigmoid and rectum. The invasion of cancer of the colon and rectum occurs by direct extension through the bowel wall, hematogenous metastases, perineural extension, metastases to the regional lymph nodes, and intraluminal metastases.

Etiology: The etiology of colorectal cancer is unknown, but the high-calorie, high-fat Western diet has been implicated in its development. Increased exposure to chemical carcinogens also has been indicated as contributing to the development of colorectal cancer.

Occurrence: Colorectal cancer is the second most common malignancy in the United States, and it is associated with a 50% mortality rate. Each year, >150,000 new cases occur, and >50,000 people in the United States die annually.

Age: The incidence of colorectal cancer increases with age; 90% of the cases of colorectal cancer occur in people ≥50 years old, with a peak incidence in the 70s.

Ethnicity: Seventh-Day Adventists and Mormons, because of their dietary habits and overall lifestyle, tend to have a lower rate of colorectal cancer than the general population. There is a higher risk of developing colorectal cancer in the Ashkenazi Jewish population than in the U.S. general population. African-Americans and Hispanics often present with colorectal cancer in later stages of development and have a 50% greater risk for dying of colorectal cancer than whites.

Gender: Colorectal cancer occurs equally in men and women. Women who have had a cholecystectomy may be at greater risk for this type of cancer.

Contributing factors: A family history of colorectal cancer (especially first-degree relatives who developed colorectal cancer at an early age), multiple polyps, Gardner's syndrome, Lurcat's syndrome, and a long history of ulcerative colitis have been linked to the development of colorectal cancer. Patients with a family or personal history of gynecologic cancer and patients diagnosed with Barrett's esophagus have an increased risk of developing colorectal cancer. Reported history of a ureterosigmoidostomy and prior infection with *Streptococcus bovis* have been implicated. A lower incidence of colorectal cancer has been found in patients who regularly take calcium supplementation. Regular intake of low-dose aspirin has been shown to have protective measures against the development of colorectal cancer. There has been some indication that high dietary intake of fats, meats, and beer may contribute to the development of colorectal cancer.

Signs and symptoms: A new onset of constipation or diarrhea may suggest colorectal cancer. Patients may report a change in bowel habits, including change in color, shape, and consistency of the bowel movement. Associated abdominal pain, bloating, and vomiting and rectal bleeding (hematochezia or melena or both) may occur. The patient with rectal cancer may have the sensation of incomplete evacuation. Low back pain or leg pain also may be reported.

 Clinical Pearl: The patient who has been having intestinal bleeding may experience a change in mental status and weakness from anemia.

An abdominal or rectal mass may be palpated. A benign polyp tends to feel soft and pliable, whereas a cancerous mass is generally hard and irregular. An anoscopy may reveal polyps or frank bleeding.

Diagnostic tests:

Test	Results Indicating Disorder	CPT Code
FOBT	Positive for blood	82270
CBC	Evaluate for anemia	85031
Serum albumin	Elevated	82040
Alkaline phosphatase	Elevated	84075–84080
Colonoscopy with biopsy	Diagnosis of colon cancer	45380
Liver function test	Elevation can indicate liver metastases	80076
CEA	Predicts stage of cancer preoperatively	82378

CEA, carcinoembryonic antigen.

Differential diagnosis:
- Diverticulitis
- Weight loss
- Blood in the stool
- Mass in the colon
- Prostatic carcinoma
- Sarcoma
- Inflammatory bowel disease
- Hemorrhoids
- Benign colonic polyps
- Peptic ulcer disease
- Functional bowel disorders

Treatment: The extent of treatment for colorectal cancer depends on how invasive the cancer is in the colon and surrounding sites and the condition of the patient at the time of diagnosis. The prognosis of colorectal cancer is predicted using the Dukes staging method. Patients should be referred to a surgeon for consideration of a radical resection; presence of metastatic disease does not rule out surgery. The chemotherapeutic agent 5-fluorouracil combined with levamisole is an effective adjuvant therapy after a surgical resection of stage III colorectal cancer, even in older adults.

Follow-up: After curative surgery, the following are essential:

- Close monitoring for symptoms of fatigue, weight loss, and change in bowel habits
- Physical examination, especially of the chest and abdomen
- CBC to rule out anemia
- Liver function tests and chest x-ray examination to detect indications of metastatic disease

Given the high recurrence rate of colorectal cancer, patients who have had a colonic resection should have a colonoscopy 6 months after surgery to detect cancerous lesions at the site of the anastomosis and new developments in other sections of the colon; colonoscopy can take place 24 to 36 months if no polyps are detected and every 6 months if polyps are found. CEA levels should be evaluated every 6 months for the first 2 years after the operation; decreasing levels indicate tumor regression (provided that a CEA level was obtained before surgery). Periodic chest x-rays are indicated for evaluation of metastasis to the lungs. Initial follow-up after radical resection for patients with a temporary or permanent colostomy should include counseling, a review of ostomy care, and community resource information. Determine the patient's nutritional status, current weight, and possible need for nutritional supplements. To evaluate for liver metastasis at follow-up examinations, assess the abdomen for fullness and hepatomegaly with irregular liver borders. Evaluate for jaundice.

Sequelae: Complications of colorectal cancer include obstruction and perforation. Postresection recurrence of colorectal cancer is common. Bowel adhesions and fibrosis also may occur. The liver, lungs, and bone are two sites known for metastasis after colorectal cancer.

Prevention/prophylaxis: The American Cancer Society recommends that beginning at age 50 all asymptomatic individuals with no risk factors should have an annual FOBT. A sigmoidoscopy for men and women >65 years old is recommended every 3 to 5 years. Prolonged prophylactic use of aspirin and calcium supplementation may reduce the risk of colon cancer.

Referral: A gastroenterologist should be consulted for colonoscopy with biopsy of the lesion. A surgical consultation should be initiated after diagnosis, for consideration of radical resection. If adjuvant chemotherapy is indicated, an oncologist also is consulted. Depending on the outcome of the surgery, consultation with an endostomal therapist may be necessary. The patient and the family should be given information about local hospice services, as needed.

Education: Teach older adults about the importance of routine surveillance for rectal bleeding and to report change in bowel habits.

CYSTITIS

SIGNAL SYMPTOMS dysuria, frequency, suprapubic tenderness, mental status changes

Cystitis	ICD-9 CM: 595.2, 595.0

Description: Cystitis is an infection of the wall of the bladder, resulting from an ascending infection from the urethra in 95% of cases. Bacteriuria is the main clinical manifestation of cystitis.

Etiology: The susceptibility to urinary tract infections increases in old age because the host defenses of the body, needed to prevent phagocytic bacteria from coming in contact with the bladder mucosa, are diminished or impaired. The most common organism identified in the development of cystitis in older adults is *Escherichia coli,* followed by *Klebsiella* and *Proteus.*

Occurrence: Cystitis is prevalent in older adults, with a 10% to 30% rate of infection.

Age: The incidence of cystitis increases with age, especially for men and all institutionalized older adults.

Ethnicity: No known prevalence exists among ethnic groups.

Gender: Cystitis is more prevalent in older women than in older men; the incidence of cystitis increases with age in older men, related to benign prostatic hypertrophy and prostatitis.

Contributing factors: Predisposing factors to the development of cystitis include indwelling catheters, urethral or condom catheters, neurogenic bladder, analgesic nephropathy, sexual intercourse, functional disability, incontinence, cognitive impairment, diabetes, sickle cell disease, ureteral obstruction, uterine or bladder prolapse, benign prostatic hyperplasia, prostatitis, urethral strictures, bowel incontinence, estrogen deficiencies, ureteral weakness and increase in vaginal pH in women, prior antibiotic therapy, and a history of vesicoureteral reflux or history of renal calculi. Frail older adults in institutionalized settings are also at risk because of lack of adequate fluids and immobility.

Signs and symptoms:

Clinical Pearl: Mental confusion, anorexia, malaise, and incontinence may be the first symptoms of cystitis in an older patient, especially for patients with indwelling catheters or a neurogenic bladder.

Patients may report urgency, frequency, and dysuria. Gross hematuria is more common in younger women than in older adults with cystitis.

Question patients about their sexual history, including use of spermicide. Women may report pelvic pain or vaginal or cervical discharge that may indicate an ascending infection. If fever, flank pain, and other systemic symptoms are reported, consider obstruction when ordering diagnostic tests.

Physical examination may reveal fever, tachypnea, and tachycardia. Suprapubic tenderness may be elicited on palpation. Percussion for costovertebral angle tenderness may be positive with reported flank pain. Vaginal examination in women should rule out discharge or erythema. In men, the prostate gland should be examined gently to assess for enlargement, bogginess, and tenderness.

Diagnostic tests: A dipstick urinalysis for nitrate and leukocyte esterase shows a positive leukocyte esterase and positive nitrate with a gram-negative organism. A microscopic urinalysis in symptomatic bacteriuria shows pyuria and bacteria. Organisms causing urinary tract infections are usually aerobes, such as *E. coli, Klebsiella, Enterobacter,* staphylococci, *Pseudomonas,* and *Proteus.* Gram stain of unspun urine detecting one or more bacteria per oil-immersion field is associated with a colony count of $>10^5$/mL. Additional testing may be necessary if obstruction is suspected.

Test	Results Indicating Disorder	CPT Code
Urinalysis with Gram stain and culture	Asymptomatic $\geq 10^5$ cfu/mL on two consecutive cultures Acute lower tract symptoms $\geq 10^3$ cfu/mL of uropathogen Aspirated indwelling catheter $\geq 10^3$ cfu/mL	81000–81009
Blood cultures (septic)	Urosepsis	87040

cfu, colony-forming units.

Differential diagnosis:

- Urethritis
- Prostatitis
- Pyelonephritis
- Vaginitis

Treatment: Older women with symptomatic uncomplicated bacteriuria should be treated with oral trimethoprim-sulfamethoxazole, 160 mg/800 mg every 12 hours; ciprofloxacin, 250 to 500 mg every 12 hours; levofloxacin, 250 to 500 mg daily; or gatifloxacin, 200 to 400 mg daily for 3 to 7 days. If a woman has been symptomatic >1 week or has functional abnormalities of the urinary tract, a regimen of 7 to 10 days of antibiotics is recommended. Older men with uncomplicated cystitis require medication for 10 to 14 days. Longer treatments, for 4 to 6 weeks, may be necessary to sterilize the urinary tract in older men after an infection.

Monitor renal function before dosing medications. Patients with catheter-associated bacteriuria may require a two-drug combination owing to polymicrobial infection; duration of antibiotic therapy for these patients should be 10 to 14 days. Second-generation or third-generation cephalosporins may be prescribed if there has been known resistance or the patient cannot tolerate the first-line medications.

Follow-up: Repeat cultures 3 to 5 weeks after completion of the medication regimen. Relapse occurs when the same organism is found in the culture specimen shortly after cessation of treatment. Reinfection, a reintroduction of the organism from the fecal reservoir, occurs in 10% to 25% of all cases of cystitis. Change in treatment is warranted if the organisms are resistant to the original treatment.

Sequelae: Untreated symptomatic cystitis can lead to pyelonephritis, sepsis, shock, and death.

Prevention/prophylaxis: Prophylactic use of antibiotics by patients with indwelling catheters is not recommended. For older adults who require frequent instrumentation of the lower genitourinary tract or who have frequent cystitis, give trimethoprim-sulfamethoxazole, 80 mg/400 mg, 1 tablet nightly.

Referral: In complicated cystitis that has progressed to pyelonephritis or urosepsis, consultation with a specialist is recommended for hospitalization.

Education: Inform all patients receiving antimicrobial therapy for cystitis of the necessity of drinking at least 8 oz. of water with each tablet. Encourage patients with recurrent cystitis to drink cranberry juice as part of their daily routine.

DIVERTICULITIS

SIGNAL SYMPTOMS▶ impaired cognitive status, lower quadrant pain

Diverticulitis	ICD-9 CM: 562.11

Description: Diverticulitis is an inflammatory condition that involves perforation of one or more colonic diverticula, which are herniations of the mucosa through the muscularis of the colon. It usually occurs in the sigmoid or descending colon. Inflammation of the diverticulum begins at the apex when the narrow opening of the lumen is exposed to fecal residue. Mucosal erosion within the diverticulum also can occur, leading to diverticulitis.

Etiology: Diverticula are common in older adults. Age-related changes in the elastic matrix of the colon and the resulting sluggish fecal mass are thought to cause increased intraluminal pressure of the colon. Diverticular disease is rare in societies that consume high-fiber diets. It is thought that a low-fiber diet produces less bulky stool and increased intracolonic pressure. Diverticulitis is thought to develop when one or more diverticula are perforated. Approximately 85% of all cases of diverticulitis involve the left colon and sigmoid. Because this perforation is usually a localized process, free intraperitoneal air or diffuse peritoneal signs are usually not evident; their presence would indicate a more severe case and the possible need for surgical consultation.

Occurrence: An estimated 70% of older adults develop diverticulosis by age 85, with the prevalence rising to 80% for adults in their 90s. Approximately 20% to 30% of the population with diverticulosis go on to develop symptoms of diverticulitis, which is usually most severe in older adults.

Age: Diverticulitis is found most commonly in older adults, most commonly in the 60s to 80s.

Ethnicity: Diverticulitis is found almost exclusively in Westernized countries or populations that have begun to consume a refined Western diet. People of Asian descent are more likely to have *right-sided* diverticulitis.

Gender: Diverticulitis occurs equally in men and women.

Contributing factors: Chronic constipation and the need to strain to defecate contribute to diverticulitis. These two conditions lead to colonic wall weakness and raise the intraluminal pressure. Long-term use of NSAIDs increases the incidence of diverticulitis. The development of diverticulitis also has been associated with chronic cigarette smoking, adult polycystic kidney disease, and use of immunosuppressant drugs.

Signs and symptoms: Clinical presentation of diverticulitis in an older adult may be suppressed despite the presence of severe disease. Mental confusion may be the first overt indication of diverticulitis in an older adult with known diverticular disease. History of left lower quadrant pain aggravated by movement and fever may be present. Pain also may be reported in the flank, back, or right side of the abdomen. Patients may describe the pain as dull, aching, and intermittent. A sensation of "bloating" may be the initial complaint offered. Associated complaints of nausea and vomiting suggest obstruction. Constipation or diarrhea, abdominal cramping without the abdominal pain, and fever also may occur. Joint pain may be reported. If the bowel is inflamed adjacent to the bladder, the presentation may mimic a urinary tract infection. Acutely ill patients with a moderate-to-severe episode of diverticulitis may present with lethargy, reflecting signs of fluid depletion and sepsis.

Bowel sounds may be normal in mild disease; however, bowel sounds become hypoactive until there is an obstruction, when a tinkling sound may be heard. Hyperresonance may reflect intestinal obstruction. Localized tenderness is usually present in the left lower quadrant. Rebound tenderness and guarding are signs of peritonitis. A mass palpated in the left lower quadrant may indicate an abscess. Occult rectal bleeding occurs in about 25% of patients with diverticulitis. Tenderness may be elicited during the rectal examination. Patients in acute distress may have pyrexia, tachycardia, and impending signs of hypovolemia.

Diagnostic tests:

Test	Results Indicating Disorder	CPT Code
CBC with differential	Low hemoglobin may show shift to the left	85007, 85009
Westergren erythrocyte sedimentation rate	Elevated to >30 mm/hr	85652
Abdominal x-rays	Supine and upright films can detect air-fluid levels, signs of bowel obstruction, or free air showing ruptured diverticulum	74000–74022
Chest x-rays	May depict pneumoperitoneum in perforated diverticulitis	71010–71035
Ultrasound of abdomen	Rule out ovarian cyst in women	76770
Helical CT scan	An extraluminal mass compressing or displacing the bowel Rule out abscess	74160

Sigmoidoscopy, colonoscopy, and barium enema are usually *avoided* during acute diverticulitis because these tests may cause further perforation or leakage of bowel contents. These tests may be performed several weeks after the resolution of the acute episode.

Differential diagnosis:

- Acute appendicitis—suspect if right lower quadrant symptoms or nonresolution with medical therapy
- Inflammatory bowel disease
- Complicated peptic ulcer disease—suspect if pneumoperitoneum or peritonitis
- Ischemic colitis—suspect if high-risk patient, bloody diarrhea, or thumbprinting
- Pseudomembranous colitis—suspect if antibiotic use or diarrhea
- Vascular ectasia—consider leaking abdominal aortic aneurysm
- Carcinoma of the colon—suspect if weight loss or bleeding
- Urologic disorders, such as infection or ureteric colic
- Gynecologic carcinomas or abscesses

Treatment: For mild cases, and the use of broad spectrum antibiotics such as, ciprofloxacin 250 to 500mg every 12 hours *or* levofloxacin 500mg once a day, plus metronidazole 250-500mg three times a day for 7-10 days. An alternative choice is amoxicillin and clavulanate potassium 875 mg bid for 7-10 days. It is important to follow-up with the patient within 72 hours and inquire about pain, ability to tolerate fluids, and if the patient has become febrile. Ensure before recommending outpatient treatment that there is reliable support system available. Patients treated at home should be able to tolerate oral fluids and lack peritoneal signs.

 Clinical Pearl: Hospitalization should be considered for older adults with diverticulitis, owing to the uncertainty of the severity of the disease because of possibly subdued presentation and comorbid diseases.

Acute treatment for hospitalized patients consists of bed rest; restriction of any fluids by mouth; nasogastric suction if nausea, vomiting, or other indication of obstruction is present; and intravenous fluids and electrolytes. It is recommended to try a single-agent parenteral antibiotic for adequate coverage of bowel flora for the treatment of severe diverticulitis, such as ciprofloxacin, 250 to 500 mg intravenously twice daily, with metronidazole, 250 to 500 mg intravenously three times daily. Pay special attention to the patient's renal function and creatinine clearance level.

Follow-up: Older adults with mild cases treated at home with prescribed therapy should expect improvement by the third day. Hospitalized patients require daily monitoring for persistent signs and symptoms of diverticulitis, laboratory values, and response to treatment. Surgical consultation may be necessary if the patient does not respond to treatment and continues to have an elevated WBC count, fever, rebound tenderness, pain, and tachycardia; approximately 25% of patients with diverticulitis require surgical intervention.

Sequelae: Complications include bowel perforation, peritonitis, abscess, fistula, hemorrhage, and bowel obstruction. Of patients with diverticulitis, >50% eventually have bowel obstruction.

Prevention/prophylaxis: Recognition of early signs and symptoms of diverticulitis helps prevent severe cases.

Referral: Severe episodes of diverticulitis require consultation with a gastroenterologist for hospitalization. Repeated episodes may require surgical consultation for an elective sigmoid resection.

Education: Provide information on a high-fiber diet or fiber supplementation or both. Teach patients to increase their fluid intake unless otherwise cautioned, especially when taking fiber supplements. Diverticulitis recurs in approximately one third of all patients who receive medical management only.

ESOPHAGITIS

SIGNAL SYMPTOMS▶ dysphagia, regurgitation, pyrosis

Esophagitis	ICD-9 CM: 530.11

Description: Esophagitis is an inflammation of the lining of the esophagus.

Etiology: Patients may develop esophagitis if they:

- Ingest medications improperly
- Ingest caustic chemicals
- Have chronic conditions such as scleroderma
- Are exposed to local radiation treatments

A bacterial, viral, or fungal infection can cause esophagitis. *Candida albicans* is the most common fungal infection. The herpes simplex I virus also can cause esophagitis, as does cytomegalovirus. Bacterial esophagitis is rare but can coincide with a fungal or viral infection, making it difficult to diagnose. In gastroesophageal reflux disease (GERD), esophagitis is a common complication.

Occurrence: The exact incidence of esophagitis is unknown.

Age: Esophagitis can occur at all ages.

Ethnicity: No known prevalence exists among ethnic groups.

Gender: Esophagitis occurs equally in men and women.

Contributing factors: In older adults, normal aging changes such as decreased gastric motility and delayed gastric emptying can contribute to the development of esophagitis. Immunosuppressed patients are susceptible to viral, bacterial, and fungal infections. Swallowing certain medications, such as aspirin, tetracycline, ferrous sulfate, NSAIDs, and potassium chloride, without sufficient fluids and not remaining upright for at least 5 minutes after the medication is taken can cause esophagitis. Substances that can weaken the lower the esophageal sphincter (coffee, peppermint, alcohol, spicy foods, citric fruits, nifedipine, verapamil, and progesterone) can contribute to esophagitis.

Signs and symptoms: A history of dysphagia and pain on swallowing is common. Associated pyrosis, regurgitation, coughing, wheezing, and progressive hoarseness may occur. A fever may be present in patients with an infectious process. Patients should be questioned about medication usage, smoking, and intake of substances that weaken the lower the esophageal sphincter; sleeping habits; and use of any tight or restrictive clothing.

Physical examination usually produces no positive findings. Oral thrush may be found in patients with *Candida albicans*. Palpate for any upper abdominal masses or tenderness. Perform a rectal examination to detect any frank bleeding.

Diagnostic tests: If suspicion was aroused on the physical examination, stool should be checked using the guaiac test to determine if there has been any intestinal bleeding. Laboratory studies are not required when antacids, position change, or both relieve pyrosis. For older adults who complain of persistent dysphagia or odynophagia with or without fever, a barium swallow or an endoscopy (with brush and biopsy if structural mucosal damage is suspected) or both are ordered.

Test	Results Indicating Disorder	CPT Code
Barium swallow	Stricture, cancer, PUD	83015
Endoscopy	Esophagitis, cancer, PUD	43239

PUD, peptic ulcer disease.

Differential diagnosis:

- Esophageal stricture (upper gastrointestinal sinus)
- Esophageal carcinoma
- Cholecystitis
- PUD

Treatment: For infectious esophagitis, temporary symptomatic relief can be obtained with sucralfate slurry, 1 g/10 mL orally four times daily. Viscous lidocaine (2%), 15 mL orally every 4 hours as needed to swish and swallow, can be used for short-term temporary relief, unless contraindicated by potential drug interactions or history of cardiac or hepatic disease. For mild cases of *C. albicans* infection, nystatin oral suspension, 400,000 to 600,000 units four times daily spaced evenly over 24 hours, is prescribed. Ketoconazole should not be given at the same time as antacids or H_2 blockers. For severe cases of herpes simplex virus–induced esophagitis, intravenous acyclovir may be given, adjusting the dosage for the patient's weight and creatinine clearance. Esophagitis from radiation can be treated with viscous lidocaine. For erosive esophagitis, use esomeprazole magnesium, 20 to 40 mg daily, or pantoprazole sodium, 40 mg for 4 to 8 weeks.

Follow-up: Patients should report progress at least 1 week after treatment. An endoscopy may be repeated if the patient is still symptomatic but compliant after the initial treatment. Yearly endoscopy is recommended thereafter for patients with severe cases of esophagitis.

Sequelae: Ulceration and bleeding, if reflux esophagitis is present, can occur after esophagitis; Barrett's esophagus with possible adenocarcinoma may be a long-term complication.

Prevention/prophylaxis: Because of the high recurrence rate of esophagitis, patients should be instructed to follow all nonpharmacological measures unless otherwise instructed. Maintenance therapy for esophagitis may be prescribed for an extended time.

Referral: A gastroenterologist should be consulted for the endoscopy and for patients with severe or nonresponsive esophagitis.

Education: Patients with reflux esophagitis should be instructed to raise the head of the bed 4 to 6 inches with shock blocks. Factors that increase abdominal pressure, such as wearing tight restrictive clothing, should be avoided. The patient should avoid smoking and ingestion of fatty foods, coffee, chocolate, peppermints, citric juices, alcohol, and large quantities of fluids with meals. Remind patients not to break or crush extended-release or delayed-release tablets. Teach the patient the importance of swallowing medications with an adequate amount of fluids.

GASTRIC CANCER

SIGNAL SYMPTOMS▶ vague sense of fullness, dyspepsia, weight loss, palpable abdominal mass

| Esophagus | ICD-9 CM: 150.9 |
| Stomach | ICD-9 CM: 151.9 |

Description: Gastric cancer generally is classified as early or advanced carcinoma. Gastric cancer usually begins in the distal portion of the stomach and spreads via the lymph or circulatory system.

Etiology: The etiology of gastric cancer is unknown; however, several dietary risk factors are associated with the incidence of stomach cancer. Adenocarcinoma accounts for 95% of all gastric malignancies. Early gastric cancers generally are confined to the mucosa or submucosa; advanced gastric carcinomas penetrate the muscularis propria with lymph node involvement.

Occurrence: Each year in the United States, >20,000 new cases of gastric carcinoma are diagnosed, 90% of which are adenocarcinomas.

Age: The average age at onset of gastric cancer is 55. Of patients with gastric cancer, >65% are >50 years old.

Ethnicity: A high incidence of gastric cancer has been found in Native Americans, African-Americans, Asians, Hispanics, and Scandinavians.

Gender: Gastric cancer is found predominantly in men with a ratio of 3:2.

Contributing factors: Identified risk factors for the development of gastric cancer include:

- Chronic *Helicobacter pylori* infection (associated with ingestion of spoiled food products)
- Tobacco abuse
- Regular alcohol consumption
- Prolonged ingestion of food products that are high in salt and nitrates
- Long-term, extensive exposure to heavy metals, rubber, and asbestos.

Gastric ulcers and adenomatous polyps are known precursors to gastric cancer. Patients with a history of atrophic gastritis resulting from pernicious anemia and who have had a partial gastrectomy are at risk for developing gastric cancer.

Signs and symptoms: Early detection of gastric cancer is often difficult because of the absence of clinical presentation. In more advanced disease, patients may have a vague sensation of fullness after a meal that is relieved by belching, nausea, anorexia (often to meat), dyspepsia, nonspecific complaints of abdominal pain of varying intensities, and constipation. Epigastric discomfort is present in >75% of patients, and the presentation may be similar to that of a gastric ulcer.

Weight loss and pallor, if the patient is anemic, may be the only signs noted during physical examination. A palpable mass in the abdomen may be felt in an advanced carcinoma. Patients with metastatic disease often have enlargement of the left supraclavicular lymph nodes or ascites or both.

Diagnostic tests: Testing should include:

- CBC with indices to determine presence of anemia
- FOBT to detect bleeding in the intestinal tract
- Endoscopy with a biopsy
- Cytologic examination
- Abdominal CT scan if metastatic disease is suspected

Test	Results Indicating Disorder	CPT Code
CBC with indices	Anemia	85021–85027
FOBT	Positive	82270
Endoscopy with biopsy	Cancer	43239
Abdominal CT scan	Evaluate for metastatic disease	74150

Differential diagnosis:

- Chronic gastritis
- Irritable bowel syndrome (IBS)
- Gastric ulcers
- Reflux esophagitis

Treatment: A partial or complete gastric resection with adjacent lymph nodes is the treatment of choice for gastric cancer. Extensive cancer or metastases negate the need for surgery. Chemotherapeutic agents (most commonly, 5-fluorouracil) have been used alone or in combination with other treatments.

Follow-up: For the patient who has had a gastric resection, continued surveillance every few months is necessary to check for weight loss, bleeding, and obstruction. Laboratory evaluation of CBC, routine liver tests, and measurement of serum CEA should occur at 3- to 6-month intervals for the first year after surgery. An annual endoscopy is recommended for the next 5 years.

Sequelae: Malnutrition, hemorrhage, obstruction, possibly evasive cancer, and metastases are complications from gastric cancer.

Prevention/prophylaxis: Patients should eliminate the use of food products that contain nitrates and are highly salted.

Referral: A gastroenterologist should be consulted for the endoscopy and complicated management problems, including annual follow-up endoscopy. For patients with advanced disease, referral to a local hospice should be made.

Education: After partial and complete gastrectomy, teach patients about the importance of adequate nutrition. Consuming six small meals a day may be necessary instead of the usual three. Supplementation with vitamins, especially vitamin B_{12}, and minerals, such as calcium and iron, should be prescribed. Patients may prefer taking nutritional supplements in place of one or more of the meals each day.

GASTRITIS

SIGNAL SYMPTOMS anorexia, nausea and vomiting, epigastric pain or discomfort with tenderness

Acute gastritis	ICD-9 CM: 535.0
Alcoholic gastritis	ICD-9 CM: 535.30
Nervous gastritis	ICD-9 CM: 306.4
Irritant gastritis	ICD-9 CM: 535.40

Description: Gastritis is an inflammation of the mucosal lining of the stomach.

Etiology: Gastritis represents a group of disorders characterized by inflammation of the stomach lining; each disorder has distinct clinical attributes, pathogeneses, and histologic features. Gastritis may be caused by infectious agents such as *H. pylori* or streptococci, autoimmune reactions, food or drug allergies, parasitic disease, physiologic stressors, normal aging changes, and prior gastric surgery.

Gastritis is divided first into *erosive* and *nonerosive* types; a possible inflammatory process within each group may be categorized as acute or chronic. Chronic gastritis can be classified further as nonatrophic, atrophic, and specific types related to precipitating factors, such as chemical or radiation gastritis. Chronic nonspecific gastritis results from ongoing injury to the gastric mucosa causing chronic inflammation and gastric atrophy.

Occurrence: Exact incidence of gastritis is unknown.

Age: Although gastritis occurs in all ages, it is a common occurrence in older adults.

Ethnicity: No known prevalence exists among ethnic groups.

Gender: Gastritis occurs equally in men and women.

Contributing factors: Many factors can precipitate the development of gastritis. Acute gastritis can be caused by physiologic stressors, hypovolemic shock, aspirin, NSAIDs, alcohol, radiation, gastric lymphoma, Crohn's disease, and *H. pylori* and other bacterial and viral infections. Stress, trauma, burns, and viral and fungal infections can cause acute gastritis. Chronic gastritis can develop because of gastric atrophy, *H. pylori* infection, bile and pancreatic secretions, and pernicious anemia. Most patients who have had a previous gastrectomy develop gastritis.

Signs and symptoms: Anorexia, nausea (with or without vomiting), and epigastric distress aggravated by eating are common with gastritis. Halitosis may be noted. Patients may report a bloating sensation.

Physical examination may be unremarkable in cases of chronic gastritis. Palpate for abdominal masses and liver tenderness. Perform a rectal examination to test for occult blood. Any unexplained weight loss should be noted. Gastrointestinal bleeding may be exhibited by coffee-ground vomitus, melena, hematochezia, or the passing of bright red blood in a nasogastric tube. Any patient suspected of gastrointestinal bleeding should be examined for changes in mental status; coolness of the extremities; and pallor of the nail beds, mucus membranes, and conjunctivae. Assessment should include watching for any changes in cardiac output, such as decreasing blood pressure and increased heart rate.

Diagnostic tests: Diagnostic studies include CBC with indices to detect blood loss and anemia, stool guaiac test, and gastroscopy with a biopsy, which is the definitive diagnostic test for gastritis.

Test	Results Indicating Disorder	CPT Code
CBC	Rule out anemia	85031
Vitamin B_{12} (for patients with atrophic gastritis)	Deficiency of vitamin B_{12}	82607–82608
C-14 urea breath test for *H. pylori*	Testing for presence of *H. pylori*	78267–78268
C-13 urea breath test for *H. pylori*	Testing for presence of *H. pylori*	83013–83014
FOBT	Rule out blood loss	82270
Gastroscopy with biopsy	Definitive diagnostic test	43239

Differential diagnosis:

- PUD
- Gastric carcinomas

Treatment: The treatment options approved by the Food and Drug Administration (FDA) for *H. pylori*–induced peptic ulcers are as follows:

Patients with acute gastritis should avoid offensive agents, such as alcohol, NSAIDs, and aspirin.

H_2 blockers, such as famotidine, ranitidine, or nizatidine, can be given for 6 to 8 weeks. An oral dose of ranitidine, 300 mg, or nizatidine, 300 mg, daily at bedtime can be ordered. The dosage of the H_2 blockers may have to be reduced, however, depending on the creatinine clearance:

If the creatinine clearance is <50 mL/min, reduce the dosage for ranitidine to 150 mg four times daily.

If the creatinine clearance is 20 to 50 mL/min, reduce the dosage for nizatidine to 150 mg daily.

If the creatinine clearance is less than 20 mL/min, reduce the dosage for nizatidine to 150 mg every other day.

Acute hemorrhagic gastritis requires hospitalization for intravenous fluids, nasogastric aspiration, transfusion of blood products as necessary, and monitoring of vital signs.

For eradication of *H. pylori,* the following therapeutic regimens are FDA approved*:

Lansoprazole, 30 mg twice daily, plus amoxicillin, 1 g twice daily, plus clarithromycin, 500 mg three times daily $\times 10$ (or 14) days; *or*

Omeprazole, 20 mg twice daily, plus clarithromycin, 500 mg twice daily, plus amoxicillin, 1 g twice daily $\times$ 10 days (Prevpac); *or*

Omeprazole, 40 mg daily, plus clarithromycin, 500 mg three times daily $\times$ 2 weeks, then omeprazole, 20 mg daily $\times$ 2 weeks; *or*

Lansoprazole, 30 mg three times daily, plus amoxicillin, 1 g twice daily $\times$ 2 weeks (only for persons allergic or intolerant to clarithromycin); *or*

Ranitidine bismuth citrate (RBC), 400 mg twice daily, plus clarithromycin, 500 mg three times daily $\times$ 2 weeks, then RBC, 400 mg twice daily $\times$ 2 weeks; *or*

RBC, 400 mg twice daily, plus clarithromycin, 500 mg twice daily $\times$ 2 weeks, then RBC, 400 mg twice daily $\times$ 2 weeks; *or*

Bismuth subsalicylate (Pepto-Bismol), 525 mg four times daily (after meals and at bedtime), plus metronidazole, 250 mg four times daily, plus tetracycline, 500 mg four times daily $\times$ 2 weeks (Helidac), plus H_2 receptor antagonist therapy as directed $\times$ 4 weeks.

Follow-up: A repeat endoscopy is advised after 6 weeks for patients who had severe gastritis or who continue to have symptoms despite treatment. Obtain a CBC, and check stool for occult blood at subsequent office visits every 3 to 6 months after the diagnosis of gastritis. At each follow-up appointment, review all drugs, including OTC medications.

Sequelae: Acute hemorrhagic gastritis has a high mortality rate in older adults. Patients with untreated chronic gastritis associated with pernicious anemia develop neurological complications.

Prevention/prophylaxis: Alternative anti-inflammatory or non-narcotic analgesics should be considered in the treatment of pain or inflammation in older adults with a history of gastritis. Critically ill older adults need to be monitored for signs and symptoms of hypovolemic shock secondary to acute gastric bleeding.

Referral: Older patients with acute hemorrhagic gastritis require hospitalization, probably with intensive care unit admission. Consultation with

* Source: www.cdc.gov/ulcer/md.htm.

a gastroenterologist for endoscopy and management of complicated cases of gastritis is recommended.

Education: Advise patients to report any black, tar-like stools or frank bleeding to the health-care practitioner immediately. All alcohol, caffeine, salicylates, tobacco, and NSAID product use should be discontinued.

GASTROESOPHAGEAL REFLUX DISORDER

SIGNAL SYMPTOMS regurgitation, pyrosis, hoarseness, chronic cough

| Gastroesophageal reflux disorder | ICD-9 CM: 530.81 |

Description: GERD is a common disorder characterized by various symptoms ranging from mild heartburn to more severe physical complaints, caused by the reflux of gastric contents into the esophagus. These symptoms may or may not occur in patients who present with respiratory symptoms.

Etiology: The presentation of GERD is a complex problem than involves reduction in the tone of the lower esophageal sphincter, episodic relaxation of the lower esophageal sphincter at inappropriate times, decreased secondary peristalsis, and faulty mucosal resistance to caustic fluids.

Occurrence: GERD affects >30% of the U.S. population.

Age: Approximately 70% of elderly experience symptoms daily.

Ethnicity: Severe esophagitis is more common in whites than in non-whites.

Gender: The ratio of men to women with GERD is equal. Severe esophagitis is more common in men than in women (2:1). Barrett's esophagus is more common in men than in women (10:1).

Contributing factors: Intrinsic factors that contribute to the development of GERD include lower esophageal sphincter incompetence, hiatal hernia, and esophageal motility disorders. Substances that weaken the lower esophageal sphincter (coffee, peppermint, alcohol, spicy foods, citric fruits, nifedipine, verapamil, and progesterone) can contribute to esophagitis and relaxation of the lower esophageal sphincter. Smoking, alcohol, obesity, and certain dietary products may contribute to the development of the symptoms of GERD.

Signs and symptoms: Patients should be questioned about medication usage, smoking, and intake of substances that can weaken the lower esophageal sphincter; sleeping habits; and use of any tight or restrictive clothing. Review the patient's dietary habits and elicit if there are food products that the patient regularly ingests that aggravate symptoms of GERD. Question the patient about history of heartburn, pyrosis, regurgitation, nausea, atypical chest pain, hoarseness, cough, choking, pharyngeal tightness, globus sensation, persistent clearing of the throat, odynophagia, weight loss, and asthma. Review the medications the patient is taking to determine if any medications reduce the lower esophageal pressure (e.g., anticholinergics, calcium channel blockers, nitrates, theophylline, morphine, or meperidine) or decrease the lower esophageal sphincter pressure (e.g., hormonal products). Additionally review if the patient is taking medications that irritate the esophageal mucosa, such as NSAIDs, potassium, tetracycline, or quinidine.

Physical examination usually produces no positive findings. Conduct a thorough examination of the oral cavity and a respiratory examination. Palpate for any upper abdominal masses or tenderness. Perform a rectal examination to detect any frank bleeding.

Diagnostic tests: If suspicion was aroused on the physical examination, stool should be checked using the guaiac test to determine if there has been any intestinal bleeding. Laboratory studies are not required when antacids, position change, or both relieve pyrosis. For older adults who complain of persistent dysphagia or odynophagia with or without fever, barium swallow or an endoscopy (with brush and biopsy if structural mucosal damage is suspected) or both are ordered. Any patient presenting with head and neck symptoms of GERD should be considered for a laryngoscopy.

Test	Results Indicating Disorder	CPT Code
Barium swallow	Stricture, cancer, PUD	83015
Endoscopy	Esophagitis, cancer, PUD	43239
Indirect laryngoscopy Direct laryngoscopy	Erythema of the arytenoid, interarytenoid area, or laryngeal surface of the epiglottis; indicates laryngopharyngeal reflux	31505– 31513 31515– 31571

Differential diagnosis:

- Esophageal stricture (upper gastrointestinal sinus)
- Esophageal carcinoma
- Cholecystitis
- PUD

Treatment: The goals for the treatment of GERD include eliminate symptoms, heal esophagitis, manage or prevent complications, and maintain remission. Important to the management of GERD are the nonpharmacological measures that patients need to incorporate along with the medication regimen; these include avoidance of smoking, alcohol, and food products such as chocolate, mints, spicy or acidic foods, and caffeine. Pharmacological recommendations as follows:

Proton-Pump Inhibitors

Drug	Initial Oral Dosage	Maximum Dose
Esomeprazole	20 mg daily × 4 wk	—
Lansoprazole	15 mg daily × 8 wk	60 mg/day
Omeprazole	20 mg daily × 4–8 wk	40 mg/day
Pantoprazole	40 mg daily × 8 wk	—
Rabeprazole	20 mg daily × 8 wk; 20 mg daily maintenance, if needed	—

H₂ Antagonists (for Less Severe GERD)

Drug	Initial Oral Dosage	Maximum Dose
Famotidine	20 mg twice daily × 6 wk	1.5-2 × initial dose
Nizatidine	150 mg twice daily	1.5-2 × initial dose
Ranitidine	150 mg twice daily	1.5-2 × initial dose

The dosage of the H_2 blockers may be reduced, depending on creatinine clearance, as follows:

If the creatinine clearance is <50 mL/min, the dosage for ranitidine is reduced to 150 mg daily.

If the creatinine clearance is 20 to 50 mL/min, the dosage for nizatidine is reduced to 150 mg daily.

If the creatinine clearance is <20 mL/min, the dosage for nizatidine is reduced to 150 mg every other day.

Follow-up: Review lifestyle changes and the impact modifications have had on the patient's symptoms of GERD. Evaluate compliancy with medication regimen.

Sequelae: Ulceration and bleeding, if reflux esophagitis is present, can occur after esophagitis; Barrett's esophagus with possible adenocarcinoma may be a long-term complication.

Prevention/prophylaxis: Prevention of GERD should be aimed at eliminating or at best modifying the extrinsic factors that contribute to the development of the condition. Patients should be encouraged to make lifestyle adjustments and avoid potentially harmful medications to prevent further complications.

Referral: A gastroenterologist should be consulted for the endoscopy and for patients with severe or nonresponsive reflux disease, dysphagia, odynophagia, unexplained weight loss, or evidence of hemorrhage. When a patient presents with laryngopharyngeal reflux, he or she should be referred for an indirect or direct laryngoscopy. If a patient presents with dysphagia, odynophagia, unexplained weight loss, or gastrointestinal bleeding or if a patient did not respond to initial therapy they should be referred to a gastroenterologist.

Education: Patients with reflux esophagitis should be instructed to raise the head of the bed 4 to 6 inches with shock blocks. Factors that increase abdominal pressure, such as wearing tight restrictive clothing, should be avoided. The patient should avoid smoking and ingestion of fatty foods, coffee, chocolate, peppermints, citric juices, alcohol, and large quantities of fluids with meals. Remind patients not to break or crush extended-release or delayed-release tablets. Patients should avoid eating a meal for at least 3 hours before becoming recumbent. Teach the patient the importance of swallowing medications with an adequate amount of fluids. An oral proton-pump inhibitor needs to be ingested 60 minutes before a meal.

GASTROENTERITIS

SIGNAL SYMPTOMS▶ sudden onset of diarrhea, abdominal pain with distention, flatulence, vomiting

Gastroenteritis	ICD-9 CM: 558.9

Description: Gastroenteritis is an infectious response of the gastrointestinal tract to various microorganisms that can be viral, bacterial, or parasitic in origin.

Etiology: Gastroenteritis is caused by exposure to:

- Viruses such as Norwalk virus, Norwalk-like virus, and astrovirus
- Bacteria such as *Salmonella, Campylobacter, Shigella, E. coli,* and *Vibrio cholerae*
- Parasites such as *Giardia lamblia*

Occurrence: Exact incidence of infectious gastroenteritis is unknown because of underreporting of symptoms. Approximately 30% to 40% of gastroenteritis diarrhea in the United States is thought to be viral in origin, with >55% of the adult population exposed to a common enteric calicivirus.

Age: Gastroenteritis occurs at all ages, but its incidence and the mortality rate from infectious diarrhea are higher in older adults. Epidemic cases of gastroenteritis occur in nursing home populations.

Ethnicity: No known prevalence exists among ethnic groups.

Gender: Gastroenteritis is equally prevalent in both sexes, although diarrhea is more common in women.

Contributing factors: Specific to the older adult population, age-related factors such as decreased motility, mucosal atrophy, and decreased gastric acidity inhibit natural defense mechanisms against infectious agents. The use of H_2 blockers, antacids, anticholin-ergic drugs, and narcotics increases the potential for developing gastroenteritis. Gastroenteritis also can be caused by emotional stress, viral or bacterial infection, food intolerance, and organic (shellfish, certain mushrooms) or inorganic (sodium nitrate) poisons. Travel to another country with a change in surroundings or to an area of poor sanitation standards and facilities can contribute to the development of gastroenteritis. Nursing home populations are susceptible to epidemics because of contact with health-care workers who may not use proper hand-washing techniques. Fecal-to-oral contact has been identified as a mode of transmission of organisms.

Signs and symptoms: History of possible fecal-to-oral contact; exposure to other patients with gastroenteritis; and ingestion of certain food products such as mayonnaise, custards, fried rice, vegetables, beef, poultry, bean sprouts, or raw seafood should be explored. Try to estimate approximately the length of time that elapsed since the patient ingested the food product suspected of contamination. Travel to a foreign country or region that may have contaminated water should be recorded, as should any previous history of diarrhea and related symptoms and the duration of the current episode. A sudden onset of diarrhea, abdominal pain with distention, flatulence, and vomiting may be reported. Associated anorexia, headache, fatigue, dizziness, and myalgias are also symptoms of gastroenteritis. Fever may or may not occur in the older adult; mental confusion may result from dehydration. The stool's color, odor, amount, and frequency should be described, and the presence of any blood or mucus in the stool should be discerned. Patient use of prescription drugs, OTC medications, and home remedies needs to be included in the history.

In the physical examination, the skin is checked for signs of rashes or dehydration, and the lymph nodes are assessed for lymphadenopathy. Abdominal examination may reveal distention, hyperactive bowel sounds, and tenderness. Perform a rectal examination to note any bleeding and color of the stool and to check for an impaction.

Diagnostic tests: CBC with differential should be ordered. WBC shift to the left may suggest an infection, and a decreased hemoglobin value indicates anemia from probable blood loss. Serum electrolyte evaluation shows an increased sodium level in dehydrated patients and decreased potassium resulting from the diarrhea. Elevated serum creatinine and BUN levels also occur in dehydration. Stool samples for blood, ova and parasite, leukocytes, and bacteria are ordered to try to identify the microorganism. A stool culture positive for blood is found in bacterial infections and in inflammatory processes; the culture and sensitivity report may show *Salmonella, Campylobacter, Shigella,* and *V. cholerae.* Consider sigmoidoscopy for patients with bloody diarrhea.

Test	Results Indicating Disorder	CPT Code
CBC with differential	WBC shift to the left suggests infection	85007, 85009
	Decreased hemoglobin	85031
Serum electrolytes	Increased sodium in dehydrated patients	80051
	Decreased potassium with diarrhea	80051
BUN	Elevation shows dehydration	84520
Stool culture	Positive for blood in bacterial or inflammatory process	87046
	Fecal leukocytes may be present when the culture indicates *Campylobacter*	

Differential diagnosis:

- Fecal impaction
- Fecal incontinence
- Colorectal cancers
- Adverse reaction to medications
- Diverticulitis
- Malabsorption
- Pseudomembranous colitis if the patient has been prescribed an antibiotic recently

Treatment: Lost fluids and electrolytes must be replaced. Clear liquids and specially formulated rehydration liquids, such as Gatorade, should be given as tolerated. Clear broths and crackers may be added to the diet when diarrhea has ceased. Patients should avoid caffeine, dairy products, alcohol, fruits, bran, vegetables, and red meats. Solid foods should be added gradually, starting with rice or potatoes. When the patient no longer has loose stools, foods such as applesauce and bananas and skinless chicken can be added. Physical activity should be limited, to avoid unnecessary exertion. Care should be taken to prevent any skin excoriation or pressure sores. Patients with infectious diarrhea should avoid antidiarrheal medications. Antibiotic therapy is specific to the bacterial or parasitic organisms identified from the stool culture:

Campylobacter infection is treated with erythromycin, 250 to 500 mg four times daily for 7 days, or, if sensitivity to erythromycin is present, ciprofloxacin, 500 mg twice daily for 7 days, adjusting the dose for renal function.

G. lamblia infection is treated with metronidazole, 250 mg three times daily for 5 to 7 days.

Severe cases of traveler's diarrhea (enterotoxigenic *E. coli*) can be treated with trimethoprim-sulfamethoxazole, 160/800 mg (double strength) orally twice daily for 5 days, or ciprofloxacin, 500 mg twice daily for 3 days.

Follow-up: Contact outpatients 4 days after the onset of symptoms to determine progress. Request nursing home staff to provide a verbal report of the patient's condition on the third or fourth day; note any further outbreak of gastroenteritis. When contacting the patient at home, question if there have been any additional symptoms, including fever and neurological developments such as paresthesia, motor weakness, and cranial nerve palsies. For older adults with chronic diarrhea or other persistent gastrointestinal symptoms, refer to a gastroenterologist.

Sequelae: Dehydration, anemia, metabolic acidosis, and hypovolemic shock could occur in untreated cases of severe infectious diarrhea.

Prevention/prophylaxis: Older adults with travel plans to foreign destinations should be urged to avoid contaminated water. Avoid ice cubes and brushing teeth with nonbottled water. Discard any foods that contain dairy or egg products that have not been refrigerated for an extended time or have been exposed to warm temperatures. Raw or undercooked meat and seafood should be avoided.

Referral: Refer to a specialist when symptoms persist beyond 4 days, when severe dehydration develops, or when the patient has bloody stools.

Education: Gastroenteritis, although generally self-limiting, can be debilitating. Infections with some microorganisms, such as *G. lamblia,* can become chronic and result in lactose intolerance, which is common in older adults. Any new case of diarrhea not resolved in 3 to 4 days requires health-care provider intervention. Use of OTC antiperistaltic agents, such as loperamide, is contraindicated in infectious diarrhea.

HERNIA

SIGNAL SYMPTOMS a dual dragging sensation with an inguinal hernia; male patients may report pain and swelling in the scrotum; patients with strangulated abdominal hernia usually have a tender mass with associated fever, nausea, and vomiting

Inguinal hernia	ICD-9 CM: 550.90
Femoral hernia	ICD-9 CM: 553.00
Umbilical hernia	ICD-9 CM: 553.1
Incisional hernia	ICD-9 CM: 553.2

Description: A hernia is the protrusion of tissue through a weakened section in the abdominal wall. Abdominal wall hernias usually occur at the groin (inguinal) and umbilicus. Hernias are classified by their severity as reducible, incarcerated, or strangulated. A *reducible hernia* moves easily through the anatomic defect. An *incarcerated hernia* does not return to a normal position automatically or when manipulated externally. A *strangulated hernia* results when an incarcerated hernia develops edema with ischemia to the entrapped bowel.

In addition to these classifications, inguinal hernias may be either direct or indirect. A direct inguinal hernia passes through the posterior inguinal wall, whereas an indirect or congenital inguinal hernia enters in through the internal abdominal inguinal ring along the spermatic cord through the inguinal passage, to exit out the external inguinal ring.

Etiology: Hernia development has been linked to recurrent Valsalva maneuvers and dysfunctional connective tissue resulting from malnutrition or long-term steroid use. In older women, a history of multiple pregnancies and relaxation of the pelvic musculature, combined with loss of extraperitoneal fat, are considered etiologic factors in the development of an obturator hernia.

Occurrence: In the United States, >500,000 herniorrhaphies are performed annually.

Age: The incidence of femoral hernias in women increases with age. The incidence of male indirect (congenital) hernias decreases with age but that of direct inguinal hernias increases.

Ethnicity: No known prevalence exists among ethnic groups.

Gender: Indirect inguinal hernias are 8 to 10 times more common in men than in women, yet the indirect inguinal hernia is the most common type of hernia in women. Older women are three to five times more likely than men to develop a femoral hernia. The obturator hernia is a rare condition that occurs in women only.

Contributing factors: A chronic cough, ascites, abdominal surgery, and symptomatic prostatism can contribute to development of a hernia because of the associated risk factor of increased intra-abdominal or intrathoracic pressure. Chronic straining for bowel movements, straining to urinate, and lifting heavy objects may be precursors to hernia formation. For women, a weakened pelvic floor after childbirth can contribute to the development of femoral herniation. Hernias also may form at the site of a surgical incision or a large scar. Obesity and liver cirrhosis are known contributing factors to the development of hernias.

Signs and symptoms: Patients may report a dual dragging sensation with an inguinal hernia. Male patients may report pain and swelling in the scrotum. Hernias may be asymptomatic, only to be discovered as part of a routine physical examination. A reducible hernia presents as a nontender mass that becomes more pronounced after a Valsalva maneuver. An incarcerated hernia, also a nontender soft mass, is found in the abdominal, femoral, or inguinal area and remains even after gentle manipulation. Patients with strangulated abdominal hernia usually have a tender mass with associated fever, nausea, and vomiting.

Physical examination reveals decreased flatus, high-pitched or tinkling bowel sounds, abdominal distention, and tenderness of the mass. No attempt should be made to reduce a strangulated hernia.

Diagnostic tests: In an uncomplicated asymptomatic hernia, laboratory and diagnostic tests are unwarranted. If there is questionable strangulation from a prolonged incarcerated hernia, laboratory studies for complications may reveal leukocytosis, elevated serum amylase, and guaiac-positive stool. Abdominal series are done postoperatively to look for signs of perforation (free air) or obstruction of the bowel (multiple air-fluid levels).

Test	Results Indicating Disorder	CPT Code
CBC with differential	Leukocytosis	85007, 85009
Serum amylase	Elevated with incarceration	82150
FOBT	Positive with incarceration	82270
Abdominal ultrasound	Diagnostic for inguinal hernia versus pathological lymph node or other palpable mass	76770

Differential diagnosis:
- Femoral lymphadenopathy
- Femoral artery aneurysm
- Psoas abscess
- Undescended testicle
- Muscle strain

Treatment: Surgical repair of strangulated inguinal, umbilical, and femoral hernias is recommended immediately unless the patient is a poor surgical risk. These patients need to be hospitalized, receive intravenous solutions, and remain NPO. Small direct inguinal hernias and painless indirect inguinal hernias do not need immediate attention; however, surgery generally is recommended within 1 week of diagnosis. Patients who are not surgical candidates can be fitted for a truss and monitored for signs of prolonged incarceration. Patients with a small direct, nonpainful hernia should be observed for reduction of the hernia when supine.

Follow-up: For patients with reducible hernias, observation of the hernia during subsequent physical examination is recommended. Patients suspected of having an incarcerated hernia should be followed up within 1 week to determine if they are experiencing any tenderness of the mass and if a general surgeon has seen them. For the postoperative patient who has had a herniorrhaphy, assess for wound healing and recurrence of the hernia.

Sequelae: An untreated inguinal, umbilical, or femoral hernia may become incarcerated and strangulated, with subsequent intestinal gangrene; the likelihood of incarceration is greatest for femoral hernias. Postsurgical complications of a herniorrhaphy include wound hematomas and superficial wound infections. Nerve entrapment is a serious complication of an inguinal herniorraphy. Approximately 50% of hernia recurrence occurs within 5 years, and an additional 20% occur 15 to 20 years after surgical repair of a hernia.

Prevention/prophylaxis: Cessation of cigarette smoking is recommended to reduce intrathoracic pressure from chronic coughing. Encourage the use of fiber, fluids, and stool softeners for patients who strain with defecation. Patients should avoid lifting heavy objects without proper support.

Referral: Refer the patient to a general surgeon when a hernia is detected. A strangulated hernia requires immediate attention.

Education: Inform the patient with a reducible hernia of the potential complications of an untreated hernia. Teach patients to avoid straining to defecate or urinate. Encourage smoking cessation to reduce the probability of a chronic cough. Instruct the patients on proper techniques for lifting heavy objects. Weight reduction should be encouraged for obese patients.

IRRITABLE BOWEL SYNDROME

SIGNAL SYMPTOMS▶ abdominal pain (may be described as colicky, pain relieved by defecation), abdominal distention, mucus in the stool, and the sensation of incomplete evacuation; patients often complain of associated symptoms such as fatigue, flatulence, headache, backache, and dyspepsia

Irritable bowel syndrome	ICD-9 CM: 564.1

Description: IBS is a chronic gastrointestinal disorder characterized by persistent abdominal pain and distressed defecation. The two major classifications of IBS are:

  Spastic colon, in which bowel movements are variable, alternates between periods of diarrhea and constipation.

  Painless diarrhea occurs immediately after a meal or on rising.

Etiology: No anatomic or biochemical cause of IBS is known. This syndrome is a functional disorder of intestinal motility and altered visceral sensation, leading to constipation or diarrhea or both. Stressful and emotional life events often precede or coexist with the presentation of IBS.

Occurrence: A common presentation for patient referral, IBS accounts for almost 50% of all referrals to a gastroenterologist. It is estimated that 23% of adults in the Western world have IBS.

Age: Of cases of IBS, 50% are diagnosed before age 35. Because most cases of IBS present by age 50, this syndrome is often a chronic condition in older adults.

Ethnicity: IBS has a higher prevalence among whites than among other ethnic groups.

Gender: Prevalence of IBS is twice as great in women as in men in the United States.

Contributing factors: Traumatic life events, such as physical or sexual abuse, may trigger the onset of IBS. Stressful psychosocial situations may hasten an exacerbation of IBS. Certain food products, such as fructose, sorbitol, and lactose, have been known to alter bowel motor function.

Signs and symptoms: A thorough dietary history is essential to establish a differential diagnosis of IBS, ruling out the possibility of food intolerance. Explore the patient's psychosocial history to determine the relationships between stressful events and exacerbation of IBS. Determine the onset of symptoms, including the time of day that the pain and gastrointestinal disturbances usually occur. A report of postprandial abdominal pain suggests biliary tract disease, pancreatitis, or PUD. Patients often report loose and frequent stools or alternating constipation and diarrhea. Abdominal pain may be described as colicky. Pain often is relieved by defecation. Abdominal distention, mucus in the stool, and the sensation of incomplete evacuation are other presenting symptoms. Patients often complain of associated symptoms, such as fatigue, flatulence, headache, backache, and dyspepsia.

The physical examination is usually unremarkable. Abdominal tenderness may be elicited, especially in the left lower quadrant, but is not pronounced. Presence of an abdominal mass, lymphadenopathy, hepatosplenomegaly, or ascites in a patient with IBS should prompt further investigation. A routine digital rectal examination generally reveals a tender rectum that is either empty or full of hard firm feces. A pelvic examination in women is recommended to rule out the presence of an ovarian neoplasm.

Diagnostic tests: When ordering diagnostic tests in older adults, determine the length of time since the last evaluation and the nature of the current symptoms. There is no biological indicator for IBS. In general, a CBC and erythrocyte sedimentation rate rule out anemia and inflammation. If diarrhea is the presenting symptom, stool culture and examination for occult blood, ova and parasites, and bacteria are recommended. For older adults with a new onset of IBS, a sigmoidoscopy with air insufflation and a barium enema with contrast administration should exclude other gastrointestinal disorders. Sigmoidoscopy usually reveals normal mucosa except for a mild hyperemic bowel in patients with IBS. Introduction of air in the bowel often triggers abdominal pain and bowel spasms. Patients with documented involuntary weight loss of ≥5% within a 6-month period or with signs of obstruction should have an abdominal CT scan and a small bowel series. Patients with persistent constipation should be evaluated for hypothyroidism. If the presenting symptoms are bloating and abdominal distention with cramping and diarrhea, a 3-week trial of a lactose-free diet is recommended to rule out lactose intolerance.

Test	Results Indicating Disorder	CPT Code
CBC	Anemia, inflammation	85031
Westergren erythrocyte sedimentation rate	May indicate an infectious process	85651 nonautomated 85652 automated
Stool culture	Negative	87045–87046
Sigmoidoscopy with air insufflation	Mild hyperemic bowel	45330
Abdominal CT scan	Rule out other diagnoses	74170–74165, 75635
Thyroid-stimulating hormone	Low (constipation)	80418, 80438– 80440, 84443

Differential diagnosis:

- Food intolerance
- Diverticular disease
- Parasitic diseases
- Biliary tract disease
- Colonic polyps
- Neoplasms
- Pancreatic disease
- Abuse of cathartics
- Latent celiac disease

Treatment: The management of IBS depends on the presentation of the patient's condition. If the patient presents predominately with constipation, psyllium preparations taken with 2 glasses of water and high-fiber food products are recommended. Patients who have been on a low-fiber diet should start gradually with 1 tablespoon of bran daily, building up to at least 3 tablespoons per day. For patients who choose bulk-forming products, a total of 15 to 25 g/day is necessary to achieve results. Caution patients with diabetes about using any products that have a high sugar content. Foods that may exacerbate IBS should be avoided (e.g., caffeinated beverages, alcohol, sorbitol-containing candies or gums, citrus fruits for persons with fructose intolerance, and milk products for persons who have known lactose intolerance). Antispasmodics are not recommended for treatment of IBS in older adults because of the anticholinergic side effects of these medications. Women can be prescribed tegaserod, 6 mg twice daily, for IBS with pain and constipation predominating for 4 to 6 weeks followed by re-evaluation. If diarrhea is severe, loperamide, 2 mg every 4 to 8 hours, can be taken.

Follow-up: With chronic IBS patients, a positive relationship between the health-care provider and the patient is mutually beneficial. Dietary intervention and stress-reduction techniques should be reviewed and evaluated. In patients with newly diagnosed IBS, evaluation of persistent symptoms is necessary because IBS is a diagnosis of exclusion.

Sequelae: Older adults with a chronic history of IBS may have a concomitant illness, such as diverticulosis. Complications may develop because of other pathological processes mistaken for IBS symptoms. Patients with uncontrollable diarrhea are at risk for dehydration because of fluid and electrolyte loss. Fecal impaction may result from chronic constipation, especially in an immobile, cognitively impaired older patient.

Prevention/prophylaxis: The patient should use stress-reduction techniques during emotionally stressful situations. Patients should avoid all food products that are known to irritate their bowels. Patients with known food intolerance must read nutrition labels and be informed of the inactive contents of medications, which may contain irritating substances.

Referral: Refer patients to a gastroenterologist for sigmoidoscopy. Refer again if patients exhibit persistent abdominal pain or uncontrollable diarrhea despite compliance with treatment and if signs of gastrointestinal bleeding are present. Patients may benefit from psychotherapy, biofeedback, or hypnosis.

Education: Inform patients that because the increase of dietary fiber could aggravate their IBS symptoms, they should increase gradually to the recommended dose. It may take 3 to 4 weeks to reach a therapeutic level sufficient to produce results. Inform patients with chronic IBS that although the disease itself does not lead to a more serious illness, any change in symptoms should be reported to the health-care practitioner.

LIVER CANCER

SIGNAL SYMPTOMS ▸ cachexia, jaundice

Liver cancer	ICD-9 CM: 197.7

Description: The liver is the most common organ in the body for metastasis from other cancers. Common sites of primary tumors that metastasize to the liver are the lungs, colon, pancreas, stomach, breast, and gallbladder. Hepatocellular cancer is associated with cirrhosis of the liver.

Etiology: The hepatic filtration of arterial and portal venous blood is a major reason for the high prevalence of metastases from primary cancerous sites in the body to the liver. Metastases also may result from an extension from an abdominal tumor or through the lymphatic system. Malignant tumors of the liver are primarily adenocarcinomas.

Occurrence: Primary liver cancer, rare in the United States, accounts for about 2% of all cancers. A malignant lesion is 20 times more likely to be from a metastatic source than from a primary lesion.

Age: Most common onset of disease is in the 60s to 80s.

Ethnicity: Primary liver cancer is prevalent in people from Africa and

Asia because of the widespread occurrence of hepatitis B virus and hepatitis C virus.

Gender: Liver cancer is more prevalent in men than in women (3 to 4:1).

Contributing factors: The incidence of liver cancer increases for patients who have a history of cirrhosis of the liver, hepatitis B virus, and hepatitis C virus. Exposure to certain chemicals, such as vinyl chloride and arsenic, has been associated with the development of liver cancer.

Signs and symptoms: Complaints of weakness, malaise, weight loss, sweating, and anorexia may be reported. Pain associated with the cancer also may be reported.

Physical examination reveals cachexia. Auscultation may reveal a bruit over the tumor and tenderness of the liver. A mass may be palpable. In more advanced cases, jaundice may appear.

Diagnostic tests: The hematocrit may be normal or elevated owing to the overproduction of erythropoietin by the tumor. Leukocytosis may be present. Serum alkaline phosphatase may be elevated. ALT, AST, and bilirubin usually are elevated. Elevated serum α-fetoprotein, not normally present in adults, is found at levels >500 g/L in patients with primary hepatocellular carcinomas. When the primary site of the malignancy is the gastrointestinal tract, breast, or lungs, elevated levels of CEA may be found. Ultrasound is used to screen for tumors and can detect tumors >3 cm.

Test	Results Indicating Disorder	CPT Code
CBC with differential	Leukocytosis	85007, 85009
Serum alkaline phosphatase	Elevated	84075–84080
ALT	Elevated	84460
AST	Elevated	84450
Bilirubin	Elevated	82247–82248
Abdominal ultrasound	Tumors >3 cm	76700–76705

Differential diagnosis:

- Cirrhosis
- Chronic hepatitis B or C infection
- Metastatic malignancy of the liver

Treatment: Advancements in the surgical treatment of hepatic metastatic cancers include tumor ablation and microscopic glass beads containing a radioactive element. Surgical resection of the liver is beneficial only if the patient has a resectable tumor; even so, the survival rate remains low. Intrahepatic chemotherapeutic agents, such as 5-fluorouracil and floxuridine, may alter the growth of the tumor, but the prognosis remains the same. Older patients with known renal function impairment may require a reduced dosage of these agents compared with younger patients. Often the treatment is palliative at best, however.

Follow-up: Patients and family members should be given the opportunity to explore adjunctive methods of pain relief and relaxation. After diagnosis of liver cancer, the focus should be on holistic palliative care, including the intervention of a hospice and services provided by the American Cancer Society.

Sequelae: The prognosis is poor because the tumor grows rapidly and often metastasizes to the lungs or bones. The survival rate is only 4 to 6 months.

Prevention/prophylaxis: Hepatitis vaccine is recommended for high-risk patients. Avoidance of chemical exposure, as part of occupational safety, is suggested. Annual ultrasound screening for patients with chronic hepatitis B should be considered as a preventive measure for liver cancer.

Referral: Refer the patient to an oncologist when the diagnosis of liver cancer is suspected. Local hospice care services should be contacted for care for the patient and family.

Education: Although no further medical treatment is aimed at reversal of the disease, the patient needs to know that you will collaborate with the hospice nurses to provide for the patient's comfort throughout the disease process. The patient can be referred to www.livertumor.org for basic information about liver cancer.

NEPHROLITHIASIS

SIGNAL SYMPTOMS ▶ vague flank pain, hematuria, renal colic, abdominal pain

Nephrolithiasis	ICD-9 CM: 592.0

Description: In the Western hemisphere, most cases of nephrolithiasis, or kidney stones, are calcium salts, uric acid, cystine, and struvite. Calculi range in size from microscopic to several centimeters in diameter.

Etiology: Kidney stones develop from the supersaturation of urine with stone-forming salts that occurs either by overexcretion of salt or underexcretion of urine. Some preformed nuclei form to create a calculus. Abnormal crystal growth inhibitors are formed as well because of hypocitraturia or magnesium deficiency. Approximately 70% of diagnosed kidney stones contain calcium; 20% to 25% are struvite stones, resulting from urinary tract infections; 5% are uric acid calculi; and 2% contain cystine.

Occurrence: An estimated 500,000 cases of kidney stones are diagnosed in the United States yearly. Approximately 50% of patients who have had previous urinary calculi have a recurrence in 5 to 7 years.

Age: The average age of onset of patients with a kidney stone is in the 30s. The incidence of kidney stones for women peaks again at about age 55.

Ethnicity: The incidence of kidney stones in whites is three to four times greater than in African-Americans.

Gender: Men are more likely than women to form calcium stones; struvite stones are more common in women, however, because of the higher incidence of urinary tract infections. Cystine stone formation occurs equally in men and women.

Contributing factors: A major contributing factor to the development of calculi is decreased fluid intake leading to high concentration of urine. Certain food substances that augment the formation of kidney stones include dairy products, chocolate, and green leafy vegetables (calcium oxalate stones) and eggs, fish, poultry, peanuts, and wheat (cystine stones). Certain medications, such as furosemide, nitrofurantoin, probenecid, silicates, theophylline, triamterene, indinavir, acetazolamide, and vitamins C and D, in a small percentage of cases can contribute to the development of nephrolithiasis. A history of hyperparathyroidism, sarcoidosis, Cushing's syndrome, Paget's disease, and immobilization may contribute to the development of calcium phosphate stones. Chronic urinary tract infections may be precursors to struvite stone formation. Of patients with gout, 50% are predisposed to uric acid stone formation, resulting from prior history or family history of kidney stones or both.

Signs and symptoms: Patients may have abrupt, severe, colicky pain in either flank or pain that originates in the flank and radiates to the groin. The pain sensation can begin as vague flank pain. Pain spreading downward suggests movement of the stone along the ureter. Associated nausea and vomiting may occur. Hematuria may be reported.

Physical examination may reveal local abdominal and costovertebral angle tenderness. Men complaining of groin pain should have a testicular examination to rule out testicular torsion, prostatitis, or epididymitis. Women with pain radiating to the labia should have a pelvic examination to rule out possible ovarian torsion, cysts, or tumors. A cursory physical examination for evidence of systemic diseases, such as sarcoidosis or cancer, should be conducted.

Diagnostic tests: For patients who have yet passed a stone, urine collection for recovery of stones or gravel should be ordered.

Test	Results Indicating Disorder	CPT Code
Urinalysis	Crystalluria	81000–81099
Abnormal pH	Uric acid stones—acidic urine Infection—alkaline urine	83986
Urine for culture and sensitivity	Infection	87086–87088

(continued on the following page)

Test	Results Indicating Disorder	CPT Code
Abdominal x-rays (kidney, ureter, and bladder)	Stones, rule out ileus	74241
IVP	Size, shape, exact location of stone	76770–76778
Ultrasound of kidneys	Hydronephrosis	74400–74415
Noncontrast helical CT scan	Detection of stone	74150

Differential diagnosis:

- Papillary necrosis
- Hydronephrosis
- Ileus
- Diverticulitis
- Appendicitis
- Bowel obstruction
- Mesenteric ischemia
- Ovarian cyst
- Testicular torsion
- Constipation
- Arterial aneurysms

Treatment: Size and location of the stone, coupled with the length of time since the onset of symptoms, directs treatment. Stones ≤4 mm usually pass on their own; stones 4 to 5 mm have a 50% chance of passing without intervention. A stone >5 mm requires *immediate* referral to an urologist for possible extracorporeal shock-wave lithotripsy. Unless contraindicated, intravenous normal saline can be administered, 125 to 150 mL/hr, to help flush out the stone. Instruct patients not in distress and without obstruction to drink 2 L of fluid daily and to strain the urine until a stone has passed. Oral analgesics can be prescribed: 1 tablet of acetaminophen, 300 mg, and codeine phosphate, 30 mg, or 1 or 2 tablets of acetaminophen, 300 mg, and codeine phosphate, 15 mg, every 4 hours, without exceeding 4 g of acetaminophen a day or 2.5 to 5 mg of hydrocodone component with acetaminophen every 4 to 6 hours. An adequate fluid intake should continue throughout the day as part of therapy.

Follow-up: A 24-hour urine collection 6 months after treatment for nephrolithiasis is recommended. At this time, also review with the patient the need for compliance with dietary restrictions and fluid requirements.

Sequelae: Immediate complications of unresolved kidney stones include obstruction and urinary tract infection and sepsis. A high incidence of recurrence of kidney stone formation exists; metabolic causes of kidney stones need to be ruled out when dietary measures are unsuccessful. Additional complications of nephrolithiasis include renal failure, ureteral stricture, perinephric abscess, and pyelonephritis.

Prevention/prophylaxis: An adequate daily fluid intake is essential.

Patients should be encouraged to increase their fluid intake during heavy exercise or when traveling long distances. To prevent recurrent stones, review the patient's dietary habits to discern if there are any excessive food products that may be factors in kidney stone formation (calcium, purine, protein).

Referral: Refer the patient to an urologist when:

Obstruction is detected.

The stone is >5 mm.

The stone has not passed within 24 to 48 hours of the onset of pain.

The patient has complicated diagnostic reports.

The patient has urosepsis, anuria, or renal failure.

Education: Inform all patients with nephrolithiasis that there is a high probability of a second occurrence of a kidney stone. Advise the patient, if possible, to strain urine with the provided strainer when experiencing symptoms of kidney obstruction. A daily fluid intake of 10 large glasses of liquid per day is recommended. Explain to patients that fluid intake needs to be increased when urine appears dark yellow. Provide information about any food restrictions that may be deemed necessary to prevent specific stone formation.

PEPTIC ULCER DISEASE

SIGNAL SYMPTOMS gastric ulcers: history of dyspepsia, epigastric pain, or right upper quadrant pain that radiates to the back after the ingestion of a meal duodenal ulcers: pain 1 to 3 hours after a meal (patients with gastric ulcers have pain immediately on eating nocturnal pain may occur in duodenal ulcers in the older adult, definitive symptoms may be absent vomiting and anorexia may be reported instead of epigastric pain

| Peptic ulcer | ICD-9 CM: 533.90 |
| Duodenal ulcer | ICD-9 CM: 532.90 |

Description: PUD involves ulcerations of the mucus membrane of the esophagus, stomach, or duodenum. The disease is classified according to the nature and anatomic location of the lesion. *Peptic ulcers* usually originate near mucosal transition zones in areas exposed to acid, pepsin, bile, and pancreatic enzymes. *Gastric ulcers* generally are found along the lesser curvature of the stomach between antral and acid-screening mucosa occurring anywhere in the stomach, from the cardia to the pylorus. *Duodenal ulcers* develop in the duodenal bulb or in the immediate postbulbar area.

Etiology: The etiology of PUD is characterized best as an imbalance between the noxious agents to which the gastrointestinal mucosa is exposed (primarily hydrochloric acid and pepsin) and the protective factors (mucus production, bicarbonate secretion) that the mucosa uses to resist destruction from such noxious agents. An increase in destructive influences (e.g., with NSAID use) can destroy the mucosa, leading to the development of an ulcer.

Occurrence: Approximately 25 million Americans have experienced PUD. Annually, >500,000 people are diagnosed with PUD.

Age: The predominant age range for gastric ulcers is 55 to 65, with rare occurrences in people <40 years old. Duodenal ulcers can occur in adults age 25 to 75. Middle-aged men (45 to 64 years old) and women >55 years old have the highest incidence of peptic duodenal disease.

Ethnicity: Prevalence of PUD is higher in African-Americans and Hispanics than in whites.

Gender: Gastric ulcers are more prevalent in older women than in older men because of the increased use of NSAIDs. The occurrence of duodenal ulcers is twice as common in men than in women.

Contributing factors: Use of aspirin and other NSAIDs, because of their ability to inhibit prostaglandin synthesis, and smoking are important risk factors. Drinking alcohol can cause gastritis. The use of caffeine and stressful life situations also contribute to the development of PUD. *H. pylori* infection is a factor in >90% of duodenal ulcers and 80% of gastric ulcers.

Signs and symptoms: Patients with gastric ulcers have a history of dyspepsia, epigastric pain, or right upper quadrant pain that radiates to the back after the ingestion of a meal. Patients with duodenal ulcer have pain 1 to 3 hours after a meal, whereas patients with gastric ulcers have pain immediately on eating. Nocturnal pain may occur. In older adults, definitive symptoms may be absent. Vomiting and anorexia may be reported instead of epigastric pain.

Physical examination of a patient with PUD may be normal. Palpation may reveal upper abdominal tenderness and guarding. Rigidity of the abdomen and absence of bowel sounds may suggest perforation. Patients with chronic duodenal ulcer disease may exhibit signs of dehydration if nausea and vomiting accompany the other symptoms. In patients with suspected gastrointestinal bleeding, signs of shock may be detected. Guaiac stool testing should be done.

Diagnostic tests: In the diagnostic breath test to detect the presence of *H. pylori,* patients are given C-13-labeled or C-14-labeled urea to drink. The marked carbon is absorbed and is measured as carbon dioxide in the patient's expired breath. Hemoglobin and hematocrit values are obtained to detect blood loss. Endoscopic gastroduodenoscopy with a biopsy for the detection of peptic ulcer, malignancy, and *H. pylori* remains the gold standard in diagnostic testing for this disease.

Test	Results Indicating Disorder	CPT Code
CBC	Anemia	85031
C-14 urea breath test for *H. pylori*	Testing for presence of *H. pylori*	78267–78268
C-13 urea breath test for *H. pylori*	Testing for presence of *H. pylori*	83013–83014
Endoscopy with biopsy	PUD, cancer, *H. pylori*	43239

Differential diagnosis:

- Angina
- Gastric carcinoma
- GERD
- Gallbladder disease
- Zollinger-Ellison disease
- Nonulcer dyspepsia
- IBS

Treatment:

The FDA-approved treatment options for *H. pylori*–induced peptic ulcers include[*]:

Lansoprazole, 30 mg twice daily, plus amoxicillin, 1 g twice daily, plus clarithromycin, 500 mg three times daily × 10 (or 14) days; *or*

Omeprazole, 20 mg twice daily, plus clarithromycin, 500 mg twice daily, plus amoxicillin, 1 g twice daily × 10 days (Prevpac); *or*

Omeprazole, 40 mg daily, plus clarithromycin, 500 mg three times daily × 2 weeks, then omeprazole, 20 mg daily × 2 weeks; *or*

Lansoprazole, 30 mg three times daily, plus amoxicillin, 1 g twice daily × 2 weeks (only for persons allergic or intolerant to clarithromycin); *or*

RBC, 400 mg twice daily, plus clarithromycin, 500 mg three times daily × 2 weeks, then RBC, 400 mg twice daily × 2 weeks; *or*

RBC, 400 mg twice daily, plus clarithromycin, 500 mg twice daily × 2 weeks, then RBC, 400 mg twice daily × 2 weeks; *or*

Bismuth subsalicylate, 525 mg four times daily (after meals and at bedtime), plus metronidazole, 250 mg four times daily, plus tetracycline, 500 mg four times daily × 2 weeks (Helidac), plus H_2 receptor antagonist therapy as directed × 4 weeks.

The dosage of the H_2 blockers may be reduced, depending on creatinine clearance, as follows:

If the creatinine clearance is <50 mL/min, the dosage for ranitidine is reduced to 150 mg daily.

[*] Source: www.cdc.gov/ulcer/md.htm.

If the creatinine clearance is 20 to 50 mL/min, the dosage for nizatidine is reduced to 150 mg daily.

If the creatinine clearance is <20 mL/min, the dosage for nizatidine is reduced to 150 mg every other day, or lansoprazole, 30 mg twice daily; amoxicillin, 1 g twice daily; and clarithromycin, 500 mg twice daily, should be given for 14 days.

Encourage patients to complete the therapeutic regimen despite the cessation of pain.

NSAID-induced peptic ulcers can be treated with H_2 blockers.

Follow-up: If a gastric ulcer was detected on endoscopy and the patient continues to have symptoms after 8 weeks of treatment, referral for endoscopic examination with a biopsy is indicated. Periodic stool guaiac testing and blood counts can detect bleeding.

Sequelae: Complications originating from PUD in older adults include gastric bleeding, perforation, and gastric outlet obstruction.

Prevention/prophylaxis: Signs and symptoms of impending recurrence of PUD, including epigastric pain, anorexia, and weight loss, should be identified early. Guaiac stool testing should be performed for all patients taking NSAIDs. Misoprostol, 200 g three times daily, has been approved as prophylaxis against NSAID-induced gastric ulcers.

Referral: Refer the patient to a gastroenterologist for initial endoscopy. Refer again if epigastric pain and dyspepsia persist despite treatment and if signs of gastrointestinal bleeding are present.

Education: Avoidance of aspirin and other NSAIDs and tobacco is essential. Reduction of stressful events, coffee (including decaffeinated forms) and other caffeine products, and alcohol is recommended. Caution patients about taking OTC medication preparations without professional advice. The Centers for Disease Control has established a *H. pylori* information hot line for physicians and patients (888-MYULCER).

REFERENCES

General

American Medical Association: Current Procedural Terminology: CPT 2002, ed 4. AMA Press, Chicago, 2002.

DeGowin, RL, and Brown, D: DeGowin's Diagnostic Examination, ed 7. McGraw-Hill, New York, 2000.

Goroll, A, and Mulley, AG: Primary Care Medicine: Office Evaluation and Management of the Adult Patient, ed 4. Lippincott, Williams & Wilkins, Philadelphia, 2000.

Kennedy-Malone, L, et al: Management Guidelines for Gerontological Nurse Practitioners. FA Davis, Philadelphia, 1999.

Acute Renal Failure

Agrawal, M, and Swartz, R. Acute renal failure. Am Fam Physician 2000. Contact: http://www.aafp.org/afp/20000401/2077.html.

Mehta, RL, et al: Diuretics, mortality, and nonrecovery of renal function in acute renal failure. JAMA 288:2547, 2002.

Bladder Cancer

American Urological Association: Management of Non-Muscle-Invasive Bladder Cancer. American Urological Association, Baltimore, 1999. Contact: http://www.guideline.gov/VIEWS/summary.asp?guideline=001369&summary_type=brief_summary&view=brief_summary&sSearch_string=Non+invasive+bladder+cancer. Retrieved June 18, 2002.

Carlson, K: Urinary bladder cancer. Ostomy Quarterly 39:40, 2002.

Bowel Obstruction

Dang, C, et al: Acute abdominal pain. Geriatrics 57:30, 2002.

Cholecystitis

Agrawal, S, and Jonnalagadda, S: Gallstones, from gallbladder to gut: Management options for diverse complications. Postgrad Med 108:108, 2000.

National Guideline Clearinghouse: Treatment of gallstone and gallbladder disease. J Gastrointest Surg 2:485, 1998.

Society for Surgery of the Alimentary Tract: Treatment of Gallstone and Gallbladder Disease. Manchester, MA, Society for Surgery of the Alimentary Tract, Inc—Medical Specialty Society, 2000.

Chronic Renal Failure

Goolsby, MJ: National Kidney Foundation guidelines for chronic kidney disease: Evaluation, classification, and stratification. Journal of the American Academy of Nurse Practitioners 14:238, 2002.

Lucas, BD: Chronic renal failure: Slowing the onset, changing the course. Patient Care 33:76, 1999.

Manjunath, G, et al: Estimating the glomerular filtration rate: Dos and don'ts for assessing kidney function. Postgrad Med 110:55, 2001.

McCarthy, JT: A practical approach to the management of patients with chronic renal failure. Mayo Clin Proc 74:269, 1999.

National Guideline Clearinghouse: Management of chronic kidney disease and pre-ESRD in the primary care setting. Department of Veterans Affairs (US), Washington, DC, 2001. Contact: http://www.guideline.gov/VIEWS/summary.asp?guideline=002325&summary_type=brief_summary&view=brief_summary&sSearch_string=Management+of+chronic+kidney+disease. Retrieved October 21, 2002.

National Kidney Foundation: K/DOQI clinical practice guidelines for chronic kidney disease: Evaluation, classification, and stratification. 2002. Contact: http://www.kidney.org/professionals/doqi/kdoqi/toc.htm. Retrieved June, 2002.

Parmar, MS: Chronic renal disease. BMJ 325:85, 2002.

Vernarec, E: New anemia drug for use in chronic renal failure. RN 65:90, 2002.

Verove, C, et al: Effect of the correction of metabolic acidosis on nutritional status in elderly patients with chronic renal failure. J Ren Nutr 12:224, 2002.

Cirrhosis of the Liver

Burge, SK, and Schneider, FD: Alcohol-related problems: Recognition and intervention. Am Fam Physician 1999. Contact: http://www.aafp.org/afp/990115ap/361.html. Retrieved May 2002

Riley, T, and Bhatti, AM: Preventive strategies in chronic liver disease: Part I. Alcohol, vaccines, toxic medications and supplements, diet and exercise. Am

Fam Physician 2001. Contact: http://www.aafp.org/afp/20011101/1555.html. Retrieved June 2002

Riley, T, and Bhatti, AM: Preventive strategies in chronic liver disease: Part II. Cirrhosis. Am Fam Physician 2001. Contact: http://www.aafp.org/afp/20011115/1735.html. Retrieved June, 2002.

Colorectal Cancer

Evans, RC, et al: Diet and colorectal cancer: An investigation of the lectin/galactose hypothesis. Gastroenterology 122, 2002.

Pignone, M, and Levin, B: Recent developments in colorectal cancer screening and prevention. Am Fam Physician 66:297, 2002.

Rudy, DR, and Zdon, MJ: Update on colorectal cancer. Am Fam Physician 61:1759, 2000. Contact: http://www.aafp.org/afp/20000315/1759.html. Retrieved December 1, 2002.

Cystitis

Bremnor, JD, and Sadovsky, R: Evaluation of dysuria in adults. Am Fam Physician 2002. Contact: http://www.aafp.org/afp/20020415/1589.html.

Huang, ES, and Stafford, RS: National patterns in treatment of urinary tract infections in women by ambulatory care physicians. Arch Intern Med 162:41, 2002. Contact: WFU School of Medicine database. Retrieved March 22, 2002

O'Donnell, JA, and Hofmann, MT: Urinary tract infections: How to manage nursing home patients with or without chronic catheterization. Geriatrics 57:45, 2002.

Orenstein, R, and Wong, ES: Urinary tract infections in adults. Am Fam Physician 1999. Contact: http://www.aafp.org/afp/990301ap/1225.html.

Rajagopalan, S, and Yoshikawa, T.: Urinary tract infections. In Beers, M, and Berkow, R (eds): Merck Manual of Geriatrics. 2002. Contact: http://www.merck.com/pubs/mm_geriatrics/sec12/ch100.htm. Retrieved October 28, 2002.

Diverticulitis

Buchanan, GN, et al: Diverticulitis. Best Pract Res Clin Gastroenterol 16:635, 2002.

Marcello, P: Understanding diverticular disease. Ostomy Quarterly 39:56, 2002.

Stollman, NH, and Raskin, JB: Diagnosis and management of diverticular disease of the colon in adults. Am J Gastroenterol 94:3110, 1999.

Esophagitis

Ahuja, V, et al: Head and neck manifestations of gastroesophageal reflux disease. 1999. Contact: http://www.aafp.org/afp/990901ap/873.htm. Retrieved December 3, 2002.

Kahrilas, PJ, et al: Esomeprazole improves healing and symptom resolution as compared with omeprazole in reflux oesophagitis patients: a randomized controlled trial. Aliment Pharmacol Ther 14:1249, 2000.

National Guideline Clearinghouse: Procedure guideline for C-14 urea breath test. Society of Nuclear Medicine Procedure Guidelines, version 3.0. 2001. Contact: http://www.guideline.gov/VIEWS/summary.asp?guideline=002173-&summary_type=brief_summary&view=brief_summary&sSearch_string=C%2D14+breath+test. Retrieved June 18, 2002

Pilotto, A, and Malfertheiner, P: An approach to *Helicobacter pylori* infection in the elderly. Aliment Pharmacol Ther 16:683, 2002.

Gastric Cancer

Bowles, MJ, and Benjamin, IS: Cancer of the stomach and pancreas. BMJ 323:1413, 2001.

Kuwada, SK: Gastrointestinal cancers: A three-article symposium. Postgrad Med 107:93, 2000.

Gastritis

ASHP Commission on Therapeutics: ASHP therapeutic position statement on the identification and treatment of *Helicobacter pylori*-associated peptic ulcer disease in adults. Am J Health Syst Pharmacol 58:331, 2001.

Chen, M, et al: Gastritis: Classification, pathology, and radiology. South Med J 94:184, 2001.

Gastroenteritis

National Guideline Clearinghouse: Diagnosis and management of food-borne illnesses: A primer for physicians. MMWR Morb Mortal Wkly Rep 50:1, 2001.

Gastroesophageal Reflux Disease

Ahuja, V, et al: Head and neck manifestations of gastroesophageal reflux disease. Retrieved December 3, 2002 from http://www.aafp.org/afp/990901ap/873.htm.

Fennerty, B, et al: New paradigms for the treatment of acid-related disorders. Patient Care for Nurse Practitioners (special edition), fall 2002.

Hubbard, RA: Update on gastroesopageal reflux disease. Am J Acad Nurse Pract 6:2, 2002.

Hernia

Bax, T, et al: Surgical options in the management of groin hernias. Am Fam Physician 1999. Contact: http://www.aafp.org/afp/990101ap/143.html.

Suleiman, S, and Johnston, D: The abdominal wall: An overlooked source of pain. Am Fam Physician 2001. Contact: http://www.aafp.org/afp/20010801/431.html.

Irritable Bowel Syndrome

Camilleri, M: Management of irritable bowel syndrome. Gastroenterology 120, 2001. Contact: http://www2.gastrojournal.org/scripts/om.dll/serve?article=a0030100652&nav=abs. Retrieved June 18, 2002.

Drossman, DA: Irritable bowel syndrome: How far do you go in the work-up? Gastroenterology 121, 2001. Contact: http://www2.gastrojournal.org/scripts/om.dll/serve?article=a0060101512&nav=full. Retrieved June 18, 2002.

Ringel, Y, et al: Irritable bowel syndrome. Annu Rev Med 52:319, 2001.

Talley, NJ, and Spiller, R: Irritable bowel syndrome: A little understood organic bowel disease? Lancet 360:555, 2002.

Vera, AJ, et al: Management of irritable bowel syndrome. Am Fam Physician 66:1867, 2002.

Liver Cancer

Anonymous. U.S. liver cancer incidence by race/ethnicity. J Natl Cancer Inst 91:1611, 1999.

Fong, Y: A promising technique for liver cancer? Cancer J Sci Am 5:339, 1999.

Nephrolithiasis

Bihl, G: Recurrent renal stones disease—advances in pathogenesis and clinical management. Lancet 358:651, 2001.

Miller, OF, and Kane, CJ: Time to stone passage for observed ureteral calculi: A guide for patient education. J Urol 162:688, 1999.

Portis, AJ, and Sundaram, C: Diagnosis and initial management of kidney stones. Am Fam Physician 63:1329, 2001.

Tawfiek, ER, and Bagley, DH: Management of upper urinary tract calculi with ureteroscopic techniques. Urology 53:25, 1999.

Peptic Ulcer Disease

ASHP Commission on Therapeutics: ASHP therapeutic position statement on the identification and treatment of *Helicobacter pylori*-associated peptic ulcer disease in adults. Am J Health Syst Pharmacol 58:331, 2001.

Graham, DY: Therapy of *Helicobacter pylori*: Current status and issues. Gastroenterology 118:S-2, 2000.

Society of Nuclear Medicine: Procedure Guideline for C-14 Urea Breath Test. Society of Nuclear Medicine Procedure Guidelines, 3rd version. Society of Nuclear Medicine, Reston, Virg., 2001.

Chapter 7

REPRODUCTIVE DISORDERS

ATROPHIC VAGINITIS

SIGNAL SYMPTOMS ▶ dysuria, vulvar and vaginal itching, urinary frequency, blood-tinged vaginal discharge, dyspareunia

Atrophic vaginitis, menopausal	ICD-9-CM: 627.3
Vulvovaginitis	ICD-9-CM: 616.10

Description: Atrophic vaginitis, also called *adhesive vaginitis,* is a non-infectious postmenopausal process in which the female genital tissue thins and becomes fragile.

Etiology: Estrogen deprivation leads to atrophy of the vaginal and vulvar epithelium. Atrophic vaginitis, a common disorder in postmenopausal women, can be surgically induced, created by the natural aging process, or brought on through primary ovarian failure.

Occurrence: This disorder affects all women, to some degree, unless estrogen replacement therapy is provided.

Age: Atrophic vagnitis is predominantly a problem of postmenopausal women. The average age of natural menopause in the United States is 52.5 years.

Ethnicity: Not significant.

Gender: Occurs in women only.

Contributing factors: Estrogen-deficient states accompanying metabolic disorders and changes of normal aging create the risk of atrophic vaginitis. Changes in vaginal epithelium and pH caused by estrogen deficiency provide an environment in which pathogenic bacteria and fungi can flourish. Drugs also may alter vaginal secretions and clinical findings.

Signs and symptoms: Itching, discomfort, burning, dyspareunia, and, at times, a thin blood-tinged vaginal discharge or bleeding after intercourse as the epithelium thins characterize atrophic vaginitis. As vaginal secretions decrease, vaginal dryness can be another bothersome symptom. Complaints of urinary frequency, urgency, and stress incontinence are common. On physical examination, signs include pale, dry, nonrugated vaginal walls with patches of erythema or petechiae or both. A watery white vaginal discharge without foul odor may be found. Estrogen deficiency can lead to loss of uterine support and subsequent uterine descensus.

Diagnostic tests:

Test	Results Indicating Disorder	CPT Code
Pelvic examination with speculum examination and Pap smear (may do wet mount and KOH preparation if infection is suspected)	Pale, dry, nonrugated vaginal mucosa; Pap smear results should be normal	57410 (pelvic exam with speculum) 88141–88167, 88174–88175 (pap smear) 87220 (KOH preparation)
Urinalysis to rule out UTI if symptoms	Variable; if dipstick is positive for white blood cells and nitrites, a culture and sensitivity should be done. If negative, UTI is not cause of symptoms	81000–81099

KOH, potassium hydroxide; Pap, Papanicolaou; UTI, urinary tract infection.

Differential diagnosis:

- Malignancy
- Vulvar dystrophies
- UTI
- Sexually transmitted disease and other infections, such as *Candida albicans* and bacterial vaginosis

Treatment: Vagifem (estradiol vaginal tablets), 25 μg inserted intravaginally daily for 2 weeks, then twice weekly; may take 3 months for full benefits to be realized. Estradiol vaginal cream 0.01% (Premarin vaginal cream) can be used short-term in decreasing dosages. Estring, the vaginal estrogen ring, can be inserted for 3 months at a time. Short-term oral HRT or use of a transdermal patch may be considered. Contraindications to continuous HRT include a history of breast or reproductive organ cancer. Nonpharmaceutical measures, which may or may not be helpful, include taking Sitz baths, wearing cotton underwear, and applying yogurt douches.

Follow-up: Expected response is quick, with resolution of symptoms within 2 to 3 months. If this does not occur, the patient should be re-evaluated and re-examined for other causes of symptoms. Because topical estrogen cream is absorbed and can cause systemic effects, patients should have a follow-up visit 1 to 2 months after beginning oral or vaginal drug therapy. Patients treated with continuous HRT need regular return visits every 3 months to check side effects, blood pressure, and response to therapy. When efficacy is achieved, treatment can be discontinued. If symptoms recur, reinstitute short-term treatment.

Sequelae: With changes in the vaginal pH of postmenopausal women (pH >5.0) and this loss of normal acidity, bacterial species grow in the vagina that are not found there commonly. Infections can become frequent and chronic.

Prevention/prophylaxis: Recognition of early signs and symptoms of atrophic vaginitis can lead to the individual's seeking treatment to prevent atrophy, dryness, infections, urinary and urethral problems, and sexual dysfunction. Intermittent use of topical vaginal estrogen can prevent recurrence of atrophic vaginitis, provide adequate levels of hormone, and give soothing relief. Use of a vaginal lubricant, such as Replens or Astroglide, also may be helpful, especially before coitus.

Referral: Gynecology referral is appropriate for patients who do not respond to treatment or have vaginal bleeding. Patients who present with severe estrogen depletion, evidenced by marked perineal and vaginal changes, along with pelvic floor relaxation, need gynecological referral before initiating topical treatment.

Education: Use water-soluble lubricants for patients with atrophic vaginitis. Counsel the patient regarding benefits of regular sexual activity. Identify each age-related difficulty associated with intravaginal application of creams. Address these needs with sensitivity.

BENIGN PROSTATIC HYPERTROPHY

SIGNAL SYMPTOMS▶ urinary frequency nocturia urgency hesitancy, weak or intermittent urine stream straining to void sensation of incomplete voiding dysuria (with infection)

Benign prostatic hypertrophy (BPH)   ICD-9-CM: 600.0

Description: BPH is the benign growth of the prostate that may lead to obstruction of the bladder outlet.

Etiology: The causes of BPH are unknown. One hypothesis relates BPH to changes in androgen hormones, whereas another alludes to a second growth phase for prostatic tissue. BPH originates in the transitional and periurethral zones.

Occurrence: BPH occurs universally in older men; genetics is thought to play a part in males who develop it at a younger age.

Age: BPH is seen in 50% of men >50 years old and in 80% of men by age 80.

Ethnicity: Not significant.

Gender: BPH occurs in men only.

Contributing factors: Risk factors include male gender, age >40 years, and intact testes.

Signs and symptoms: Symptoms frequently are categorized as irritative or obstructive. *Irritative symptoms* arise from involuntary bladder muscle contractions possibly involving hypersensitivity of the bladder wall. The patient may report frequency, urgency, burning or pain on urination, nocturia, or incontinence. Typical *obstructive symptoms* include straining to urinate, hesitancy, weak or intermittent stream, dribbling, or a sensation of incomplete emptying. These symptoms are related to direct pressure from impingement of prostatic tissue on the urethra or to contraction of muscle fibers in the prostate gland, capsule, and bladder neck from α-adrenergic tone.

The American Urological Association (AUA) has developed a self-administered symptom questionnaire that addresses the occurrence over the past month of the symptoms mentioned here. This questionnaire, contained in the Agency for Health Care Policy and Research guidelines, is helpful in quantifying symptoms, although not specific for BPH.

On physical examination, the prostate may be enlarged or normal-sized. It should feel smooth, with a rubbery consistency. Nodularity or extreme hardness raises suspicions of malignancy. Prostate size does not correlate with degree of obstruction or severity of symptoms. The suggested rationale for this is that rectal examination is limited to palpation of the peripheral zone of the prostate and does not reach the periurethral zone where symptoms originate. In cases of advanced obstruction, the bladder may be palpated on examination. Focal neurological examination assessing the sacral nerve roots is also helpful.

Diagnostic tests:

Test	Results Indicating Disorder	CPT Code
Urinalysis to rule out other conditions (infection, malignancy)	Normal findings if no comorbidities	81000–81099
Serum PSA to rule out coexisting prostate cancer	Variable. Normal is <4 ng/mL. In BPH, 33% have 4–10 ng/mL. Finasteride therapy decreases PSA, so pretreatment PSA should be obtained	84152

PSA, prostate-specific antigen.

Urinalysis is recommended to rule out infection (pyuria or bacteriuria) or malignancy (suggested by hematuria). If the urinalysis is positive for bacteria, culture and sensitivity testing is indicated. Blood urea nitrogen and creatinine should be measured if renal insufficiency or obstructive uropathy is suspected. Most clinicians measure PSA, although expert recommendations differ. PSA may be elevated in BPH, prostatitis, acute urinary retention, prostatic infarction, increased physical activity, ejaculation, and prostatic cancer; the test is used primarily to screen for prostate cancer.

Specialized tests, such as intravenous pyelogram, uroflowmetry, postvoid residual measurement, pressure-flow studies, transrectal ultrasound, and cystourethroscopy, are not indicated routinely. In specific instances, they may be performed as a guide to therapy choices or to rule out other conditions.

Differential diagnosis:

- Prostate cancer (may coexist with BPH)
- Urethral stricture
- Neurogenic bladder
- Medication-induced BPH
- Prostatitis
- Detrusor muscle failure
- Infection
- Bladder neck contracture

Treatment: For patients with minimal symptoms, a program of watchful waiting, with instruction to avoid medications known to worsen symptoms, is prescribed. Medication groups to be avoided include decongestants and other sympathomimetics and anticholinergics, such as antipsychotics, tricyclic antidepressants, antispasmodics, and antihistamines. For mild-to-moderate symptoms, α_1-adrenergic blockers terazosin (Hytrin), prazosin (Minipress), doxazosin (Cardura), and tamsulosin (Flomax) relax smooth muscle of the bladder neck and prostate and can increase peak urinary flow rate. Taking the medication at bedtime minimizes hypotension, the primary side effect. Another medication frequently used is finasteride (Proscar), a 5α-reductase inhibitor that blocks the conversion of testosterone to dihydrotestosterone, the major intraprostatic androgen in men. Side effects include decreased libido, ejaculatory dysfunction, and impotence. Treatment ≥ 6 months is needed for maximal benefit. Finasteride and an α-blocker sometimes are used concurrently. Many patients prefer herbal products because of reduced side effects. South African star grass, saw palmetto berry, African plum tree, stinging nettle, and rye pollen are the most popular products, either singly or in combination. Most of these have shown some efficacy, although product quality and amount of essential ingredients cannot be guaranteed because of lack of regulation. For severe BPH, surgical treatment may be the primary option. In recent years, many treatments have proliferated in this category. Transurethral resection of the prostate (TURP) has been the standard for years, with open prostatectomy for glands of >40 g. Newer treatments include transurethral incision of the prostate (TUIP) for gland enlargement of <30 g, transurethral needle-aspiration ablation of prostate (TUNA), transurethral electrovaporization of the prostate (TVAP), transurethral (TULIP) or visual (VLAP) laser-assisted prostatectomy, insertion of a urethral stent, and transurethral microwave therapy (TUMT). TUIP is associated with fewer complications than TURP; stents usually are reserved for complex cases. Some of the newer laser/microwave procedures may need to be repeated after several years.

Follow-up: Scheduling of follow-up depends on the course of treatment. Advise watchful waiting, and evaluate with the AUA symptoms index every 6 to 12 months. Patients receiving drug therapy should be evaluated for symptoms and side effects every 6 months. Annual digital rectal examination for prostate cancer is indicated, and usually PSA testing and urinalysis are done.

Sequelae: Complications of BPH include urinary retention requiring catheterization, renal insufficiency, urinary tract infections, bladder stones, gross hematuria, prostatitis, treatment complications such as urethral stricture, treatment side effects, and possibly treatment-induced impotence.

Prevention/prophylaxis: No preventive measures are known; BPH occurs with aging.

Referral: Patients may be referred to a urologist if comorbid conditions exist, if the surgical option is feasible or desirable, for initial evaluation for drug therapy, and to rule out acute prostatitis of prostate cancer. Consider collaborative management for drug therapy.

Education: Educate the patient about BPH and its treatment options and side effects. Instruct the patient to avoid spicy foods and any drugs that can increase retention or cause symptoms to flare up, including caffeine, alcohol, sedatives, over-the-counter (OTC) sleeping pills, and OTC cold and allergy remedies. Instruct the patient to report hematuria, UTI symptoms, or increased retention.

BREAST CANCER

SIGNAL SYMPTOMS ▶ none; breast mass

Malignant neoplasm of the breast	ICD-9-CM: 174.9

Description: Breast cancer is the leading cause of death in women age 35 to 54. Each year in the United States, >178,000 women develop breast cancer. Of these, 40,800 die of the disease (American Cancer Society, 2000). The lifetime probability that an American woman will develop breast cancer is 10%. Four out of five women have a relative or acquaintance who has developed breast cancer.

Etiology: Unknown.

Occurrence: Breast cancer incidence and death rate vary by race (Fig. 7–1). The incidence for white women in the United States from 1992 until 1998 was 115 per 100,000.

Age: Between 1973 and 1998, incidence rates of invasive breast cancer increased for women ≥40 years old. Incidence rates did not increase for

Breast Cancer Incidence and Death Rates* by Race and Ethnicity. United States, 1992–1998

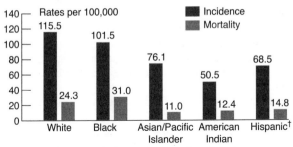

*Rates are age-adjusted to the 1970 US standard population.
†Persons of Hispanic origin may be of any race.
American Cancer Society, Surveillance Research, 2001.
Data source: NCI Surveillance, Epidemiology, and End Results Program.

Female Breast Cancer — United States, 1992–1997

A. 5-Year Survival Rates* by Stage at Diagnosis and Race (%)

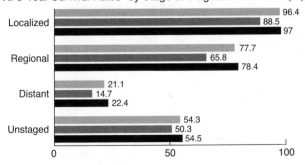

B. Diagnosed by Stage and Race (%)

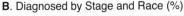

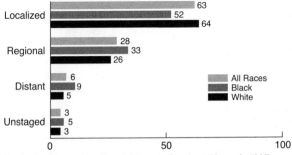

*Survival rates are based on follow-up of patients through 1997.
American Cancer Society, Surveillance Research, 2001.
Data source: NCI Surveillance, Epidemiology, and End Results Program.

Figure 7–1. Female breast cancer incidence.

women <40 years old. The risk of developing breast cancer increases with age. Women <40 years old account for 20% of breast cancer cases. The median age at the time of diagnosis is 54 years, whereas 45% of cases occur in women >65 years old. Half of breast cancer deaths are in women >65 years old.

Ethnicity: Breast cancer is more common in white women than in black women, but the mortality rate for breast cancer is higher in black women. Between 1992 and 1998, incidence rates remained relatively unchanged in women of all racial and ethnic groups.

Contributing factors: Many factors have been associated with increased risk of breast cancer, including:

- Personal or family history of breast cancer; the risk for women who have a first-degree relative with breast cancer is two to three times higher than in the general population
- Biopsy positive for hyperplasia
- Nulliparity and delayed childbearing
- Early menarche
- Late natural menopause

Breast-feeding may decrease the risk for breast cancer.

Other factors that may be associated with breast cancer, but about which the literature is still inconclusive, are diet, exogenous hormones, alcohol consumption, breast trauma, viral infection, higher socioeconomic status, and obesity.

Signs and symptoms: Breast examination is an integral part of a woman's health care. Every woman should be taught to perform breast self-examination. A diagnostic evaluation for breast cancer begins with physical examination and history. Any firm mass suggests malignancy. Fixation to the skin, skin edema, nipple retraction, or deep fixation is further evidence of carcinoma. When a mass is suspected or detected, history should be recorded, with particular emphasis on date of onset, size, and exact location.

Incidence rates of in situ breast cancer have increased considerably. Most of the increase can be explained by the detection of ductal carcinoma with a mammogram. Most cases of ductal carcinoma are detectable only through mammography. Since 1998, although invasive breast cancer rates have remained level, ductal carcinoma incidence has continued to increase. This shift is thought to reflect earlier detection rather than a true increase in occurrence.

Nonpalpable lesions presenting as asymptomatic clusters of microcalcifications require repeat mammography or biopsy. Although most of these lesions are benign, 15% to 20% represent early cancer. Consultation with a radiologist is essential to determine the significance of this finding.

A woman with a *BRCA1* or *BRCA2* altered gene is more likely to develop breast or ovarian cancer than a woman without these alterations. Not every woman who has these genes develops a carcinoma, however. An altered gene alone is not sufficient to cause cancer. Most breast cancer cases do not involve altered genes. At most, 1 in 10 breast cancers involves an altered gene. Finding an altered gene indicates an increased risk for developing cancer, but it does not indicate that it will occur. Knowing that a woman is at risk suggests increased surveillance through mammograms, breast examinations, and ultrasound of the ovaries. Women considering genetic testing should speak to a professional trained in genetics before deciding whether or not to be tested. Information on genetic testing and referral centers can be found through the National Cancer Institute at 1-800-4-CANCER or www.cancer.gov.

Diagnostic tests:

Tests	Results Indicating Disorder	CPT Code
Breast self-examination	Palpable mass present	
Clinical breast examination	Palpable mass present	
Mammogram	Detects >90% of breast cancers	76090–76092
Biopsy	Cytologic examination confirms diagnosis of breast cancer*	19100–19103; 76095 (stereotactic localization)

* Cytologic detection by biopsy is most useful in the diagnosis of breast cancer. A malignant cytologic finding permits immediate planning of treatment and discussion of treatment alternatives. Open biopsy can be performed, as can needle biopsy under radiographic guidance.

Differential diagnosis: Nonmalignant breast mass.

Treatment: Clinical staging determines the therapy for breast cancer. The woman's wishes, the size and histology of the lesion, the size of the breast, and the skill and experience of the oncology team determine the course of surgical treatment. The use of radiation therapy and chemotherapy is determined based on the staging of the disease.

Follow-up: Follow-up depends on the course of therapy. Women may have courses of chemotherapy or radiation therapy before or after surgery. After therapy, women are seen at regular intervals. One regimen involves clinical evaluation every 3 months with annual pelvic examination, mammogram, chest x-ray, and liver function tests. This program continues for 2 years, with an increase to 4-month intervals in the third and fourth years and every 6 months thereafter.

Sequelae: The 10-year survival rate for early-stage lesions ($\leq$2 cm and no node involvement) is 75% to 85%. This rate drops to 40% survival if there is node involvement. Recurrent disease occurs most often in the first 2 years after treatment, but because women continue to die of breast cancer for periods >15 to 20 years after treatment, follow-up must continue indefinitely.

There has been an important reduction in breast cancer deaths in more recent years. Between 1950 and the late 1980s, overall breast cancer mortality was relatively stable. Between 1985 and 1989, the death rate decreased by 1.6%. Between 1995 and 1998, the decrease accelerated to a decline of 3.4% annually. This decline has been attributed to improvements in cancer treatments and to the benefits of mammography screening. During the 1990s, the death rate declines have been most notable in white women. Death rates for women <50 years old declined an average of 3.1% annually between 1990 and 1998. The decline for older women was 2.1% annually.

Prevention/prophylaxis: The combination of breast self-examination, physical examination by a health-care provider, and a mammogram provides the most effective means of screening for breast cancer.

The Breast Cancer Prevention Trial currently is investigating whether tamoxifen can prevent the development of breast cancer in healthy women at risk for the disease. The U.S. Preventive Services reported in 2002 in that tamoxifen and raloxifene reduce the incidence of estrogen receptor–positive breast cancer in women. The absolute risk reduction varies by risk factors for breast cancer and must be balanced against potential harm.

Referral: All palpable masses that do not resolve after menses should be referred for further evaluation. Women with palpable findings should be referred for evaluation regardless of mammogram results. Breast tissue is considerably denser in young women, making a negative mammogram result not always negative for malignancy.

Education: Teach breast self-examination to all women. Menstruating women should perform breast self-examination approximately 7 days after the onset of menses. For women who do not menstruate, a day of the month should be chosen for breast self-examination.

Many women in the United States have breast implants. Examination of the augmented breast should include examination of the natural tissues and evaluation of the implant. During the examination, the implant is displaced with one hand and the breast tissue palpated with the other. Integrity of the implant is evaluated.

DRUG-INDUCED IMPOTENCE

SIGNAL SYMPTOMS▶ none; noncompliance with medication regimen, responses on sexual history query or questionnaire

Sexual, psychogenic	ICD-9-CM: 302.72
Organic origin NEC	ICD-9-CM: 607.84

Description: Impotence, in the strictest sense of the word, is the consistent inability to achieve and maintain erection sufficient for sexual intercourse; it is also referred to as *erectile dysfunction*. In a broader sense, impotence encompasses problems with arousal, libido, orgasm, sensation, and relationships. Drug-induced impotence refers to that which is caused by a drug or drugs.

Etiology: Drug-induced impotence may be caused by many medications or medication interactions (see under Contributing Factors).

Occurrence: An estimated 10 to 15 million American men experience impotence on a chronic basis.

Age: Incidence of erectile dysfunction increases with age. The prevalence is approximately 52% for men between age 40 and 70; in men >70 years old, prevalence is increased further. Men >70 years old with chronic medical problems, such as diabetes, have a prevalence of >90%. Because the condition frequently is underreported, the percentage is probably higher. Approximately 25% of erectile problems are related to drugs.

Ethnicity: Not significant.

Gender: Men.

Contributing factors:

- Stress
- Long-term alcohol use
- Tobacco use
- Recreational drug use
- Antiandrogens
- Anticholinergics
- Anticonvulsants
- Antidepressants (including selective serotonin reuptake inhibitors, monoamine oxidase inhibitors, tricyclic antidepressants)
- Antipsychotics
- Centrally acting depressants (sedatives/hypnotics, tranquilizers, opiates)
- H_2 blockers
- Levodopa
- Lithium
- Stimulants such as amphetamines
- β-Blockers
- Spironolactone
- Methadone
- Chemotherapeutic agents
- Interferon
- Antihypertensives (clonidine, methyldopa, thiazides, calcium channel blockers)
- Urologic drugs (α-blockers)
- Anti-inflammatories (baclofen, naproxen)

Evidence suggests that statins and fibrates may contribute to drug-induced impotence.

Various processes are involved, including effect on libido, neuro-chemical mediation, and drug side effects.

Signs and symptoms: There may be no reported symptoms unless the provider includes a sexual history, is aware of the potential for impotence when prescribing certain medications, and asks about baseline sexual activity at that time, then periodically reassesses this during follow-up visits. The patient should be asked about sexual interest, sexual ability, and sexual activity. Also, if a provider detects noncompliance to a prescribed medication regimen in an otherwise cooperative patient, the provider should inquire whether impotence occurs when the medication is taken. Drug-induced impotence, which has an acute onset, can be associated with starting a new medication.

Medication history including OTC remedies, alcohol use, tobacco use, and use of recreational drugs is also important. The CAGE test for alcoholism, a screening questionnaire for depression, or other psychological screens as needed may be included as part of the history. A history of surgical procedures, especially of procedures involving the prostate, bladder, or colorectal area and including the lymphatic channels, may reveal potential sources of impotence.

Physical examination is performed to rule out other causes of impotence; the cause may be multifactorial, especially in an older patient. Evaluate the patient's overall appearance and mobility, then assess the vital signs, specifically checking for orthostatic hypotension. Palpation of the thyroid may reveal a goiter. Gynecomastia may be related to certain drugs, such as cimetidine. Abdominal or femoral bruits may highlight an abdominal aortic aneurysm or vascular obstruction at the bifurcation of the abdominal aorta.

Diminished peripheral pulses suggest a circulatory problem. Lack of sensation or inability to discriminate between sharp and dull may indicate peripheral neuropathy, especially if the history is positive for diabetes. Abnormal reflexes point to a neurological problem. Decreased mobility may indicate a neurological or musculoskeletal problem contributing to impotence. Examination of the genital area may reveal testicular atrophy or penile plaques, as seen in patients with Peyronie's disease, or an enlarged prostate. Assess for the bulbocavernosus reflex; absence of this reflex indicates penile neuropathy.

Diagnostic tests: Diagnostic testing is not indicated specifically for drug-induced impotence, but it is performed to eliminate other possible causes of impotence, especially vascular and neurological causes, which are the most common. Testing, specific to the etiology suspected, may include a fasting glucose tolerance test, chemistry panel with blood urea nitrogen and creatinine, thyroid-stimulating hormone test, lipid panel, complete blood count, urinalysis, or testing for specific hormonal markers.

Differential diagnosis: Differential diagnosis includes vascular, endocrine, neurological, neurovascular, substance abuse, end-organ disease, psychogenic, and social causes. As stated previously, impotence in elderly persons is frequently multifactorial.

Treatment: Whenever possible, eliminate the medication or substitute another medication from available drugs that do not cause impotence. If this is not possible or if the patient continues to experience the problem after these changes have been made, consider other treatment measures. Counsel the patient regarding alcohol, recreational drug, and tobacco use.

Sildenafil citrate (Viagra) is a selective inhibitor of cyclic guanosine monophosphate (cGMP)–specific phosphodiesterase type 5. During sexual stimulation, nitric acid is released into the corpus cavernosum, resulting in increased cGMP levels, which prevents smooth muscle relaxation and increases blood flow to the penis. Sildenafil enhances this effect by inhibiting an enzyme that degrades cGMP in the corpus cavernosum. It is contraindicated with nitrates and in advanced heart disease; cytochrome influences include increased plasma levels with inhibitors of CYP3A4 or CYP2D9 and decreased plasma levels with inducers of CYP3A4. Side effects include headache, flushing, UTI, abnormal vision (blue-green, blurring, photosensitivity), nasal congestion, diarrhea, dizziness, and rash. It was effective in clinical trials for drug-induced impotence in patients taking antidepressants/antipsychotics and antihypertensives/diuretics. For other types of treatment, such as penile implants or injection, refer the patient to an urologist specializing in this area.

Follow-up: Individualize follow-up according to cause and treatment. Periodic reassessment of treatment for recurrence of the problem is helpful. For medication treatment, monitor for side effects and response.

Sequelae: Disruption of sexual function may result in depression or relationship problems. Complications may arise from treatment.

Prevention/prophylaxis: Whenever possible, avoid prescribing medications with a high risk for causing impotence and include a sexual history in routine history and physical examination whenever prescribing a new medication with impotence as a potential side effect.

Referral: Refer patients to an urologist to evaluate for other causes or multifactorial causes of impotence. Refer to a support group patients who are experiencing the problem. Refer for psychological services when indicated.

Education: Teach the patient about medication side effects. Have the patient report sexual dysfunction. Educate the patient about normal age-related changes in sexual functioning and how to adapt. If sildenafil is prescribed, take as ordered and do not exceed prescribed dosage.

ENDOMETRIAL CANCER

SIGNAL SYMPTOMS postmenopausal bleeding

Endometrial cancer	ICD-9-CM: 182.0

Definition: Cancer of the endometrium is the most common gynecological malignancy in the United States.

Etiology: Adenocarcinoma of the endometrium of the uterus has a histological precursor of atypical endometrial hyperplasia.

Occurrence: Endometrial cancer, which is three times more prevalent than cervical cancer, represents 10% of all cancers in women. Although most women with endometrial cancer present with an early-stage disease and have an excellent chance of cure, approximately 6600 women in the United States died of the disease in 2002. The lifetime probability of developing endometrial cancer for all American women is 3%.

Age: Advancing age is the most important risk factor for endometrial cancer; 5% of tumors occur in women <40 years old. Most tumors occur in women their 60s and 70s.

Ethnicity: Not significant.

Contributing factors: Obesity and glucose intolerance have been correlated with endometrial carcinoma. Strong evidence exists that endogenous or exogenous estrogen has a role in the development of endometrial cancer. There is a high incidence of this cancer in women with polycystic ovarian syndrome. An association exists between menstrual abnormalities and infertility and endometrial cancer. Of women with endometrial cancer, 20% to 30% are nulliparous. The use of estrogen after menopause substantially increases the risk of endometrial cancer. A program of estrogen plus progesterone for postmenopausal therapy has not been associated with endometrial cancer. Low parity, late menopause, and hypertension have been associated with endometrial carcinoma.

Signs and symptoms: Postmenopausal bleeding is the most common symptom associated with endometrial carcinoma.

Diagnostic tests:

Test	Result Indicating Condition	CPT Code
Transvaginal pelvic ultrasound	Endometrial thickness >5mm indicates need for biopsy	76856–76857
Endometrial biopsy	Positive histology	58100–58558
Dilation and curettage hysteroscopy	Verifies diagnosis of endometrial cancer	57800, 57820 58555 (hysteroscopy)

Differential diagnosis:
- Infection
- Atrophy

Treatment: Surgical excision.

Follow-up: Operative and histological findings assign the risk for recurrence. Radiation therapy is used for women with intermediate or high risk. Hormonal therapy and chemotherapy may be used for advanced disease.

Sequelae: Various factors influence the prognosis, including histological differentiation, depth of invasion, and lymph node metastases. Histological type also influences the outcome.

Prevention/prophylaxis: None.

Referral: All cases of suspected endometrial cancer must be referred to a gynecologist for evaluation and treatment. Endometrial sampling should be discussed with a gynecologist for women at risk for endometrial cancer.

Education: Explain the significance of postmenopausal bleeding to every woman at the time of menopause. Estrogen should not be taken without progesterone in the postmenopausal period.

OVARIAN CANCER

SIGNAL SYMPTOMS ▶ none; most women asymptomatic until the disease has metastasized

Ovarian cancer	ICD-9-CM: 183.0

Definition: Cancer of the ovary is the most lethal of pelvic malignancies in women.

Etiology: Unknown.

Occurrence: Each year, >23,000 new cases of ovarian cancer are diagnosed, making ovarian cancer the fifth most common malignancy among U.S. women. For women in the United States, the overall risk for developing ovarian cancer is 1.4% to 1.8%; 12,000 women die of the disease. The lifetime probability of developing the disease is 1 in 70 for American women. Late diagnosis is the primary reason for the poor prognosis. Reliable screening for this disease is not available.

Age: Of ovarian cancers, 80% to 90% occur in women >40 years old. Fewer than 1% of ovarian cancers occur in women <20 years old. The peak incidence of invasive ovarian cancer is age 60. Hereditary ovarian cancers occur approximately 10 years earlier.

Ethnicity: The incidence of ovarian cancer is highest in the United States, Europe, and Israel and lowest in Japan and in the developing countries. Ovarian cancer incidence is higher in white women than in African-American or Asian women.

Contributing factors: Increasing age and family history are the most important risk factors for ovarian cancer. The most significant risk factor for ovarian cancer is family history of the disease. The risk depends on the number of affected first-degree and second-degree relatives and their age at diagnosis with ovarian and breast cancer. This holds true for relatives on the maternal and paternal sides. Families with *BRCA1* and *BRCA2* mutations are at risk for breast and ovarian cancer. Overall lifetime risk for women with this genetic mutation for ovarian cancer is 30%. Some individuals are at risk for ovarian cancer as part of their colorectal cancer genetic risk.

 Clinical Pearl: Only about 5% to 10% of ovarian cancers are familial.

Late menopause may be associated with a slightly higher trend in ovarian cancer. An increase in ovarian cancer risk among nulliparas consistently is reported.

Signs and symptoms: Ovarian cancer may be totally asymptomatic. The woman may experience pelvic pressure, bloating, dull pelvic pain, or bladder pressure. Ovarian cancer may be related to ovarian enlargement.

Diagnostic tests: Annual pelvic examination is recommended in all sexually active women >18 years old. Rectovaginal examination may be necessary to detect ovarian enlargement. Ovarian enlargement cannot always be palpated, making pelvic examination a limited diagnostic test.

Transvaginal ultrasonography with the use of color Doppler images improves the sensitivity for diagnosis of ovarian cancer. Laparoscopy is the gold standard diagnostic tool for ovarian cancer.

There is a great deal of interest in cancer antigen (CA) 125 as a diagnostic tool. Sensitivity of the test currently is 9% to 96%. Specificity is higher in postmenopausal women and lower in women who have not yet experienced menopause. Many women screened for ovarian cancer with this testing method have false-positive results. CA 125 level fluctuates with the menstrual cycle and is elevated in ovarian cysts, fibroid tumors, pregnancy, endometriosis, and pelvic inflammatory disease.

Differential diagnosis:

- Stool-filled sigmoid colon
- Distended bladder
- Pelvic kidney, diverticular abscess
- Cysts (dermoid, functional, cystadenoma)
- Tubo-ovarian abscess

Treatment: Surgical excision.

Follow-up: Chemotherapy and radiation therapy frequently follow surgery. Bone marrow transplants are recommended in selected cases.

Sequelae: On diagnosis, three out of four cases of ovarian carcinoma have spread beyond the ovary. Ovarian cancer is less common than breast cancer but has the highest case-fatality rate. Ovarian cancer is the fifth leading cause of cancer mortality in women with 14,000 deaths annually.

More women die from ovarian cancer than from all the other gynecological malignancies combined.

Prevention/prophylaxis: Use of the oral contraceptive pill reduces the risk of ovarian cancer by 35% to 50%. Women reduce their risk of ovarian cancer by 40% to 60% by taking oral contraceptives for 4 to 8 years. Pregnancy reduces the risk by 50%; increasing the number of pregnancies further reduces the risk. Tubal ligation and possibly hysterectomy seem to reduce the risk of ovarian cancer.

Referral: Women with a significant family history of ovarian cancer or breast cancer should be referred for genetic counseling. Women with a significant family history should be referred to a gynecological oncologist for discussion of prophylaxis.

Education: Routine screening for women without family history of ovarian cancer is not currently recommended. Stress the importance of an annual pelvic examination for all women.

PROSTATE CANCER

SIGNAL SYMPTOMS▶   none initially; nocturia, frequent urination, difficulty starting urination, dysuria, inability to urinate, weak or interrupted urine flow

Prostate, neoplasm	ICD-9-CM: 222.2

Description: Prostate cancer is a malignant neoplasm of the prostate. Of prostate cancers, 95% are adenocarcinoma occurring in the peripheral areas of the prostate.

Etiology: Genetic and environmental factors are believed to influence the development of prostate cancer. Although testosterone is a tumor promoter, its role in the development of prostate cancer is poorly understood.

Occurrence: Carcinoma of the prostate is the most frequently diagnosed cancer in the United States, and it accounts for 13% of all cancer deaths. In men ≥55 years old, this cancer is the second leading cause of cancer deaths. The American Cancer Society estimated that 189,000 men would be diagnosed in 2002, and 30,200 of these men would die. Asymptomatic, previously undiagnosed prostate cancer is seen during autopsy in approximately 30% of American men.

Ethnicity: In the United States, African-American men have a 30% higher incidence of prostate cancer than white men. Prostate cancer tends to be more advanced and poorly differentiated at the time of diagnosis in African-American and Hispanic men than in their white counterparts.

Gender: Prostate cancer occurs only in men.

Age: The mean age at diagnosis is 71; 83% of cases are found in men >64 years old.

Contributing factors: Increasing age contributes to the development of prostate cancer. A family history of the disease increases the risk for prostate cancer twofold to threefold. African-American race is a risk factor. Some studies suggest that a diet high in animal fats is a risk factor. Currently, studies are looking at use of supplements and increasing fruits and vegetables as negative risk factors. Although some studies have suggested vasectomy as a risk factor, most studies do not support this.

Signs and symptoms: Prostate cancer is often asymptomatic in early stages. Nonspecific complaints that may suggest prostate cancer include dysuria, difficulty voiding, urinary frequency, urinary obstruction, back or hip pain, hematuria, hemospermia, and impotence. Occasionally, deep vein thrombosis, pulmonary embolus, lower extremity lymphedema, or spinal cord compression may be due to advanced metastatic prostate cancer.

Diagnostic tests: The following tests are screening tests and can indicate the presence of abnormalities. Only a biopsy is definitive for prostate cancer at this time.

Test	Results Indicating Disorder	CPT Code
Digital rectal examination: annually age 50; African-Americans or family history, start at age 40	Early stage cannot be felt; later stages felt as hard, irregular nodules	
PSA: annually age 50; African-Americans or family history, start at age 40. If total PSA is 4–10 ng/mL, the following tests are advised:	4–10 ng/mL is indeterminate; >10 ng/mL suggests prostate cancer	84153
Free-to-total PSA	<25% in men with total PSA 4–10 ng/mL strongly suggests prostate cancer	84154
Complexed PSA	Increased in prostate cancer compared with BPH	84152
Transrectal ultrasonography with biopsy (if screening abnormal)	Positive histological confirmation of prostate cancer	76872, 76873 (prostate ultrasound)

Differential diagnosis:

- BPH
- Prostatitis
- Prostatic inflammation and urethral obstruction

Treatment: Treatment options should be determined by careful consideration of patient age, general health, and stage of cancer. Watchful waiting may be the treatment of choice in men who have a life expectancy of

<10 years and a low-grade tumor. Treatment options include surgery (radical prostatectomy), radiation treatment, hormonal therapy, and chemotherapy. Experimental therapies with gene therapy, immunotherapy, and tumor suppressors show promise for the future.

Follow-up: Serial PSA testing, every 3 to 4 months for 3 years, then every 6 months for 2 years, then annually, is recommended after surgical resection or radiation treatment. At the same intervals, patients should be evaluated for recurrent or new symptoms and for any complications of treatment, including a focused physical examination. Reduction in PSA by 50% to 75% is a positive sign.

Sequelae: Complications of treatment include impotence, incontinence, and radiation cystitis. Metastasis by direct extension may cause obstruction or damage to the seminal vesicles, rectum, bladder, and bowel. Lymphatic metastasis may result in lymphadema and thrombosis. Vascular metastasis to the bones of the axial skeleton is the most common metastasis, but the lungs, colon, or bladder also may become involved.

Prevention/prophylaxis: Screening should focus on high-risk groups, including African-American men and all men ≥40 years old with a family history of prostate cancer. Other men >50 years old should be screened annually. Screening for prostate cancer includes a symptom review and digital rectal examination annually. Studies are under way to evaluate dietary strategies and supplementation with vitamin D or E or both in the prevention of prostate cancer. Currently, green tea and lycopene contained in tomato products are considered helpful.

Referral: Refer patients to an urologist, oncologist, and radiologist.

Education: Review risk factors with patients and encourage yearly screening. Teach dietary guidelines covering the increased risk for cancer associated with a high-fat diet.

PROSTATITIS

SIGNAL SYMPTOMS ▶ nonbacterial: perineal pain, sacral or suprapubic pain, penile pain, painful ejaculation, dysuria chronic: recurrent UTI, irritative voiding pattern, possible obstructive symptoms, pain;
acute: fever, chills, dysuria, arthralgia, perineal pain, systemic symptoms

| Prostatitis, acute | ICD-9-CM: 601.0 |
| Prostatitis, chronic | ICD-9-CM: 601.1 |

Description: Prostatitis, the inflammation or infection of the prostate gland, may occur in four common forms:

- Acute bacterial
- Chronic bacterial

- Chronic nonbacterial inflammatory and chronic nonbacterial noninflammatory (formerly prostatodynia)
- Asymptomatic

Etiology: The most common causes of acute bacterial and chronic bacterial prostatitis are gram-negative organisms, such as *Escherichia coli, Pseudomonas aeruginosa, Serratia, Klebsiella, Proteus*; less frequently, gram-positive enterococci, *Chlamydia, Mycoplasma, Ureaplasma,* and viruses have been linked to the development of nonbacterial prostatitis. A small percentage of men are infected with two or more pathogens at one time.

Occurrence: It is estimated that 25% to 50% of all men are diagnosed with prostatitis at least once in their lifetime.

Age: Prostatitis is common in sexually active men; chronic prostatitis is more common in men >50 years old. Prostatitis is the third most common urological diagnosis in men >50 years old.

Ethnicity: Not significant.

Gender: Prostatitis occurs only in men.

Contributing factors: Patients with a history of UTIs are at risk for developing bacterial prostatitis. Other factors that have been linked to the development of prostatitis include noncircumcision, anal intercourse, urological procedures, chronic bladder catheterization, sexually transmitted diseases, bladder neck dysfunction, and pelvic floor spasm with intraprostatic urinary reflux. Patients with neuromuscular dysfunction that includes ejaculatory dysfunction, abnormalities of urinary flow (especially a pulsating flow), and urinary hesitancy are at risk for developing prostatitis. Interstitial cystitis, fibromyalgia, and back pain frequently coexist with chronic nonbacterial, noninflammatory prostatitis.

Signs and symptoms: In older men, frequency, dribbling, hesitancy, and urgency may be the presenting symptoms, although dysuria also can occur. Question patients about the quality of their urinary flow; a pulsating flow is common in patients with chronic noninflammatory prostatitis. Inquire if the patient has had penile discharge, painful ejaculations, or hematuria. Irritative voiding is common in chronic prostatitis. It is important to discern if the patient has a history of UTIs; in patients with nonbacterial and noninflammatory prostatitis, a history of UTIs is rare. In acute prostatitis, fever and severe pain also may occur. Patients may complain of myalgia or arthralgia, especially in the lower back, perineum, groin, scrotum, or suprapubic area. Physical examination of patients presenting with symptoms of prostatitis may reveal suprapubic tenderness. Percuss the bladder to note if there is distention. A digital rectal examination should be avoided in men presenting with acute symptoms to minimize pain. In examination for chronic prostatitis, the prostate may feel tender or boggy.

Diagnostic tests:

Test	Results Indicating Disorder	CPT Code
Complete blood count if acute prostatitis is suspected	Leukocytosis with shift to left	85022-85025
Urinalysis	Acute: pyuria, bacteriuria, hematuria; chronic bacterial, nonbacterial: normal urinalysis	81000-81099
Urine culture and sensitivity (in acute prostatitis to identify organism for treatment)	Culture shows pathogen and antimicrobials that it will respond to	87086
Culture of expressed prostatic secretions (*note:* prostatic massage is contraindicated in acute prostatitis owing to risk of sepsis)	Chronic bacterial: culture shows pathogen Nonbacterial: increased numbers of leukocytes but negative culture Nonbacterial, noninflammatory: normal numbers of leukocytes, negative culture	87070

Differential diagnosis:

- Urethritis
- Bladder infection
- Interstitial cystitis
- Diverticulitis
- Pyelonephritis
- Prostatic abscess
- BPH
- Urethral stricture
- Neurogenic bladder
- Proctitis
- Epididymitis
- Bladder or prostatic carcinoma

Treatment: Patients presenting with high fever, leukocytosis, or delirium should be hospitalized for hydration and empirical broad-spectrum intravenous antibiotics; aminoglycosides should be used with caution in older adults but are the treatment of choice. When the patient is stabilized, oral antibiotic therapy with quinolones should be continued for 4 to 6 weeks (adjust dosage for creatinine clearance and renal function). Evaluate the need for stool softeners and analgesics. Primary management for this population is by urology. Follow-up urine culture and prostatic secretions evaluation should be done to confirm elimination of infection.

Treat patients with chronic prostatitis with trimethoprim-sulfamethoxazole or a quinolone for 1 to 3 months (adjusting the dosage as needed for renal function). Nonsteroidal anti-inflammatory drugs (NSAIDs) are prescribed for symptom relief; patients also can be instructed to use Sitz baths two to three times a day as needed. In some cases, long-term suppressive antibiotic therapy may be indicated. Patients with chronic, nonbacterial prostatitis may benefit from a trial of erythromycin, tetracycline, or doxycycline for 2 to 4 weeks; some sources advocate use of quinolones in lieu of the other antibiotics. For patients in any of the three nonacute categories who experience pelvic pain, use of NSAIDs and α-blockers such as terazosin (Hytrin), doxazosin (Cardura), or tamsulosin (Flomax) is helpful. In men who experience significant irritative voiding and suprapubic pain, consider pentosan polysulfate (Elmiron), an anti-inflammatory glycosaminoglycan that has been used for the treatment of interstitial cystitis, for 6 months. Finasteride, a 5α-reductase inhibitor used in BPH, reduces symptoms in some patients with category chronic nonbacterial inflammatory prostatitis, particularly men who are >40 years old and have a large boggy prostate. Finasteride must be used for a minimum of 6 months to be effective. Skeletal muscle relaxants such as diazepam (Valium) and baclofen (Apo-Baclofen) combined with physical and medical therapies are helpful. For refractory cases, pelvic floor, perineal, or prostate massage; myofascial trigger point therapy; biofeedback; or microwave hyperthermia should be considered.

Follow-up: For patients with acute prostatitis, a repeat culture and prostate examination are recommended after completion of the antibiotic regimen. Patients with chronic prostatitis who have a relapse should continue receiving long-term therapy. Consider suppression therapy of low-dose antibiotics if the infection is not eradicated and repeating the prostatic localization cultures in 6 months to 1 year.

Sequelae: Quality of life is severely compromised because of pain in all types of prostatitis. Unresolved acute prostatitis can lead to bacteremia or pyelonephritis. Patients with chronic infection may develop small prostatic stones.

Referral: Refer patients who also have symptoms of BPH or an intractable infection to an urologist. Initial management of acute prostatitis should be by a specialist in an inpatient setting. Complex or recurrent cases of nonacute prostatitis may need referral for further evaluation and management.

Education: Inform patients of the importance of increasing fluid intake during symptomatic periods. Emphasize the need to complete the antibiotic regimen to eradicate the organism. Symptomatic patients should avoid bladder irritants, such as alcohol and caffeine. The use of certain medications, such as anticholinergics, should be restricted while the patient is symptomatic. Patients should be advised that prostatitis can recur and to report symptoms when detected.

REFERENCES

Atrophic Vaginitis

Bernier, F, and Jenkins, P: The role of vaginal estrogen in the treatment of urogenital dysfunction in postmenopausal women. Urol Nurs 17:92, 1997.

Bremnor, JD: Evaluation of dysuria in adults. Am Fam Physician 65:1589, 2002.

Curtis, LA: Acute urinary retention and urinary incontinence. Emerg Med Clin N Am 19:591, 2001.

Cutson, TM: Managing menopause. Am Fam Physician 61:1391, 2000.

Egan, ME: Diagnosis of vaginitis. Am Fam Physician 62:1095, 2000.

Eriksen, B: A randomized, open, parallel-group study on the preventive effect of an estradiol-releasing vaginal ring (Estring) on recurrent urinary tract infections in postmenopausal women. Am J Obstet Gynecol 180:1072, 1999.

Flisser, A: Evaluation of incontinence in women. Urol Clin N Am 29:515, 2002.

Heim, LJ: Evaluation and differential diagnosis of dyspareunia. Am Fam Physician 63:1535, 2001.

Kaunitz, A: Gynecologic problems of the perimenopause: Evaluation and treatment. Obstet Gynecol Clin N Am 29:455, 2002.

Keenan, NL: Vaginal estrogen creams: Use patterns among a cohort of women. J Am Geriatr Soc 47:65, 1999.

Leclair, DM: Effects of estrogen deprivation: Vasomotor symptoms, urogenital atrophy, and psychobiologic effects. Clin Fam Pract 4:27, 2002.

Mounsey, AL: Postmenopausal bleeding: Evaluation and management. Clin Fam Pract 4:173, 2002.

Notelovitz, M: Estradiol absorption from vaginal tablets in postmenopausal women. Obstet Gynecol 99:556, 2002.

Ouslander, JG: Estrogen treatment for incontinence in frail older women. J Am Geriatr Soc 47:1383, 1999.

Pandit, L: Postmenopausal vaginal atrophy and atrophic vaginitis. Am J Med Sci 314:228, 1997.

Quan, M: Vaginitis: Meeting the clinical challenge. Clin Cornerstone 3:36, 2000.

Rioux, JE: 17β-estradiol vaginal tablet versus conjugated equine estrogen vaginal cream to relieve menopausal atrophic vaginitis. Menopause 7:156, 2000.

Szumigala, JA: Vulvovaginitis, estrogen deficient. In Ferri FF (ed): Ferri's Clinical Advisor: Instant Diagnosis and Treatment, 2003 ed. Mosby, St. Louis, 2003, p 875.

Benign Prostatic Hypertrophy

Bremnor, JD: Evaluation of dysuria in adults. Am Fam Physician 65:1589, 2002.

Dull, P: Managing benign prostatic hyperplasia. Am Fam Physician 66:77, 2002.

Epperly, TD: Health issues in men: Part I. Common genitourinary disorders. Am Fam Physician 61:3657, 2000.

Fagelman, E: Herbal medications in the treatment of benign prostatic hyperplasia (BPH). Urol Clin North Am 29:23, 2002.

Ferri, FF: Ferri's Clinical Advisor: Instant Diagnosis and Treatment, 2003 ed. Mosby, St. Louis, 2003, p 671.

Grossfeld, GD: Benign prostatic hyperplasia: Clinical overview and value of diagnostic imaging. Radiol Clin North Am 38:31, 2000.

Khosravi, J: Insulin-like growth factor I (IGF-I) and IGF-binding protein-3 in benign prostatic hyperplasia and prostate cancer. J Clin Endocrinol Metab 86:694, 2001.

Medina, JJ: Benign prostatic hyperplasia (the aging prostate). Med Clin North Am 83:1213, 1999.

Roberts, RG: Evaluation of dysuria in men. Am Fam Physician 60:865, 1999.

Santucci, R: Urethral reconstruction of strictures resulting from treatment of benign prostatic hypertrophy and prostate cancer. Urol Clin North Am 29:417, 2002.

Walsh P, et al (eds): Campbell's Urology, ed 8. WB Saunders, Philadelphia, 2002.

Breast Cancer

McKeon, VA: The breast cancer prevention trial, advanced evidence-based practice. Women's Health Suppl JOGNN 28:1, 2000.

Shapiro, TJ, and Clark, P: Breast cancer: What the primary care provider needs to know. Nurse Practitioner 20:36, 1995.

Sheps, C: Chemoprevention of breast cancer. Ann Intern Med 137:59, 2002.

Drug-Induced Impotence

Gutierrez, MA: Management of and counseling for psychotropic drug-induced sexual dysfunction. Pharmacotherapy 19:823, 1999.

Hale, TM: Antihypertensive drugs induce structural remodeling of the penile vasculature. J Urol 166:739, 2001.

Jensen, J: The prevalence and etiology of impotence in 101 male hypertensive outpatients. Am J Hypertens 12:271, 1999.

Lue, TF: Physiology of penile erection and pathophysiology of erectile dysfunction and priapism. In Walsh P, et al (eds): Campbell's Urology, ed 8. WB Saunders, Philadelphia, 2002, p 1609.

Master, VA: Ejaculatory physiology and dysfunction. Urol Clin North Am 28:363, 2001.

Nehra, A: Neurologic erectile dysfunction. Urol Clin North Am 28:289, 2001.

Pautler, SE: Priapism: From priapus to the present time. Urol Clin North Am 28:391, 2001.

Piccirillo, G, et al: Effects of sildenafil citrate (viagra) on cardiac repolarization and on autonomic control in subjects with chronic heart failure. Am Heart J 143:703, 2002.

Rizvi, K: Do lipid-lowering drugs cause erectile dysfunction? A systematic review. Fam Pract 19:95, 2002.

Saper, CB: Autonomic disorders and their management. In Goldman (ed): Cecil Textbook of Medicine, ed 21. WB Saunders, Philadelphia, 2000.

Seagraves, RT: New treatment for erectile dysfunction. Curr Psychiatry Rep 2:206, 2000.

Swerdloff, RS, and Wang, C: The testis and male sexual dysfunction. In Goldman (ed): Cecil Textbook of Medicine, ed 21. WB Saunders, Philadelphia, 2000.

Endometrial Cancer

Gupta, JK, et al: Ultrasonographic endometrial thickness for diagnosing endometrial pathology in women with postmenopausal bleeding. Acta Obstet Gynecol Scand 81:799, 2002.

Plaxe, S, and Saltzstein, S: Impact of ethnicity on the incidence of high risk endometrial carcinoma. Gynecol Oncol 65:8, 1997.

Porter, S: Endometrial cancer. Semin Oncol Nurs 18:200, 2002.

Ovarian Cancer

Collins, W, et al: Screening strategies for ovarian cancer. Curr Opin Obstet Gynecol 10:33, 1998.

Holschneider, C, and Berek, J: Ovarian cancer: Epidemiology, biology and prognostic factors. Semin Surg Oncol 19:3, 2000.

Lea, J, and Miller, D: Optimum screening interventions for gynecologic malignancies. Tex Med 97:49, 2001.

Paley, P: Ovarian cancer screening: Are we making any progress? Curr Opin Oncol 13:399, 2001.

Prostate Cancer

Bostwick, DG: Treatment changes in prostatic hyperplasia and cancer, including androgen deprivation therapy and radiotherapy. Urol Clin North Am 26:465, 1999.

Burack, RC: Screening for prostate cancer: The challenge of promoting informed decision making in the absence of definitive evidence of effectiveness. Med Clin North Am 83:1423, 1999.

Carducci, MA: Prostate specific antigen and other markers of therapeutic response. Urol Clin North Am 26:291, 1999.

DePrimo, S E: Prevention of prostate cancer. Hematol Oncol Clin N Am 15:445, 2001.

Fleshner, NE: Vitamin E and prostate cancer. Urol Clin North Am 29:107, 2002.

Gupta, S: Green tea and prostate cancer. Urol Clin North Am 29:49, 2002.

Hahnfeld, LE: Prostate cancer. Med Clin North Am 83:1231, 1999.

Isaacs, JT: The biology of hormone refractory prostate cancer: Why does it develop? Urol Clin North Am 26:263, 1999.

Konety, BR: Vitamin D and prostate cancer. Urol Clin North Am 29:95, 2002.

Middleton, RG: Prostate Cancer Clinical Guidelines Panel: Summary report on the management of clinically localized prostate cancer. The American Urological Association. J Urol 154:2144, 1995.

Miller, EC: Tomato products, lycopene, and prostate cancer risk. Urol Clin North Am 29:83, 2002.

Morton, RA, and Lepor, H: Prostate disorders: Benign and malignant. In Noble (ed): Textbook of Primary Care Medicine, ed 3. St. Louis: Mosby, St Louis, 2001, p 1418.

Nudell, DM: Imaging for recurrent prostate cancer. Radiol Clin North Am 38:213, 2000.

Screening for prostate cancer. U.S. Preventive Services Task Force Guideline, Guide to Clinical Preventive Services, 2/e. 1996.

Seidenfeld, J: Relative effectiveness and cost-effectiveness of methods of androgen suppression in the treatment of advanced prostate cancer. Evidence Report/Technology Assessment (Summary) 4:1, 1999.

Shekarriz, B: Salvage radical prostatectomy. Urol Clin North Am 28:545, 2001.

Slovin, SF: Vaccines as treatment strategies for relapsed prostate cancer: Approaches for induction of immunity. Hematol Oncol Clin N Am 15:477. 2001.

Small, EJ: New treatment strategies in advanced prostate cancer. Radiol Clin North Am 38:203, 2000.

Taplin, ME: Clinical review 134: The endocrinology of prostate cancer. J Clin Endocrinol Metab 86:3467, 2001.

Walsh, P: Epidemiology, etiology, and prevention of prostate cancer. Walsh P, et al (eds): Campbell's Urology, ed 8. WB Saunders, Philadelphia, 2002.

Yip, I: Nutrition and prostate cancer. Urol Clin North Am 26:403, 1999.

Yu, KK: The prostate: Diagnostic evaluation of metastatic disease. Radiol Clin North Am 38:139, 2000.

Zoorob, R: Cancer screening guidelines. Am Fam Physician 63:1101, 2001.

Prostatitis

Anderson, RU: Management of lower urinary tract infections and cystitis. Urol Clin North Am 26:729, 1999.

Anderson, RU: Management of chronic prostatitis—chronic pelvic pain syndrome. Urol Clin North Am 29:235, 2002.

Bremnor, JD: Evaluation of dysuria in adults. Am Fam Physician 65:1589, 2002.

Curtis, LA: Acute urinary retention and urinary incontinence. Emerg Med Clin N Am 19:591, 2001.

Epperly, TD: Health issues in men: Part I. Common genitourinary disorders. Am Fam Physician 61:3657, 2000.

Ferri, FF: Practical Guide to the Care of the Medical Patient, ed 5. Mosby, St. Louis, 2001.

Klein, NC: New uses of older antibiotics. Med Clin North Am 85:125, 2001.

Lefort, A: Antienterococcal antibiotics. Med Clin North Am 84:1471, 2000.

Litwin, MS, et al: The National Institutes of Health chronic prostatitis symptom index: Development and validation of a new outcome measure. Chronic Prostatitis Collaborative Research Network. J Urol 162:369, 1999.

Lummus, WE: Prostatitis. Emerg Med Clin N Am 19:691, 2001.

Nickel, JC: Prostatitis: Evolving management strategies. Urol Clin North Am 26:737, 1999.

Nickel, JC: Prostatitis and related conditions. Walsh P, et al (eds): Campbell's Urology, ed 8. WB Saunders, Philadelphia, 2002, p 603.

Oliphant, CM: Quinolones: A comprehensive review. Am Fam Physician 65:455, 2002.

Stoller, ML, et al: Prostatitis. In Tierney, LM, et al (eds): Current Medical Diagnosis and Treatment 2001. Lange Medical Books/McGraw-Hill, New York, 2001, p 936.

Rajagopalan, S: Antimicrobial therapy in the elderly. Med Clin North Am 85:133, 2001.

Stevermer, JJ: Treatment of prostatitis. Am Fam Physician 61:3015, 2000.

Chapter 8

MUSCULOSKELETAL DISORDERS

FRACTURES

SIGNAL SYMPTOMS soft tissue swelling, ecchymosis, local tenderness, pain with any motion

Cervical vertebra	ICD-9-CM: 805.0–805.1
Carpal	ICD-9-CM: 814
Clavicle	ICD-9-CM: 810
Humerus	ICD-9-CM: 812
Tibia, fibula	ICD-9-CM: 823.0–823.1
Radius	ICD-9-CM: 813.0

Description: Fractures or breakage of bone or cartilage are a common cause of disability in older adults. A compound fracture or open fracture occurs when fragments of the bone pierce the skin or mucosa; an impacted fracture occurs when bone fragment is forced into another bone. In older adults, common sites for fractures include proximal humerus, distal radius, pelvic ramus, proximal femur, proximal tibia, and thoracic and lumbar vertebral bodies.

Etiology: Most fractures can be traced to an injury. Vertebral fractures may result from an activity such as lifting or bending that puts great stress on the spine. A relationship exists between the severity of bone mineral loss and the chance of sustaining a fall. In a pathological fracture caused by multiple myeloma, bone marrow is replaced by malignant plasma cells, and bone is destroyed.

Occurrence: Estimates show 30% of people ≥65 years old fall each year; of that group, 5% of the falls result in fractures. Specifically, 1 million fractures in the United States have been associated with a diagnosis of osteoporosis.

Age: Women >50 years old have a 15% chance of experiencing a hip fracture; by age 90, one out of three women and one out of six men experience a hip fracture.

Ethnicity: White and Asian-American women have a higher prevalence of fractures than African-American women because of the risk of osteoporosis in these two groups.

Gender: The prevalence for fracture is higher in women because of the higher incidence of osteoporosis in women.

Contributing factors: Factors that can contribute to the incidence of fractures in older adults include advanced age, female gender, osteoporosis, family history of osteoporosis, osteopenia, confusion, Parkinson's disease, prolonged bed rest, motor vehicle trauma, cerebrovascular accident, urinary retention, peripheral neuropathy, peripheral edema, and bone metastases. Additional factors that are known contributors to falls in older adults include environmental hazards, reduced visual acuity, change in depth perception, vestibular dysfunction, postural hypotension, and certain medications that include alcohol.

Signs and symptoms: Patients present with a history of recent injury to the affected area. For vertebral compression fractures, however, trauma may not be necessary for the insult to occur. Generally, for any type of fracture, an older adult may report pain, pressure, spasms, and swelling in the injured area. A patient with a femoral neck fracture may report groin pain. Physical examination reveals soft tissue swelling, ecchymosis, local tenderness, and pain with any motion.

 Clinical Pearl: In a hip fracture, the affected leg appears shorter than the other leg and externally rotated.

Diagnostic tests:

Test	Results Indicating Disorder	CPT Code
Radiograph of affected area	Standard procedure in diagnosing a fracture	73100 (wrist two views) 73060 (humerus, minimum of two views) 73510 (hip complete, minimum of two views) 73560 (knee, two views)
CBC	Determine if there has been any internal blood loss when there has been major trauma	85031
Westergren ESR	Elevated ESR may indicate an infectious process	85651 (nonautomated) 85652 (automated)

CBC, complete blood count; ESR, erythrocyte sedimentation rate.

Differential diagnosis:

- Fracture associated with an infectious process/osteomyelitis
- Fracture that can be attributed to a neoplastic process/multiple myeloma
- Fracture caused by osteoporosis

Treatment: For the pain related to the fracture, analgesics and nonsteroidal anti-inflammatory drugs (NSAIDs), if not prohibited, are helpful. Depending on the site of the fracture, casting, elastic wrapping, splints, immobilization, traction, or surgical intervention may be used. The most common surgical intervention for a fractured hip is open reduction internal rotation, especially for fractures of the intertrochanteric or subtrochanteric region.

Follow-up: The long-term management of a patient with a fracture depends not only on the location of the fracture, but also on the etiology of the fracture, whether osteoporosis, an infectious process, or neoplasia. Patients may have return appointments with an orthopedist, physical therapist, or both. Patients should be questioned about any muscle weakness or paresthesia after the incident. The function of the affected area should be evaluated. Determine what impact the injury had on the patient's activities of daily living (ADLs) and instrumental ADLs.

Sequelae: The complications resulting from a fracture depend on many factors, including comorbidities, health status of the patient before the injury, and the location of the fracture. Patients are susceptible to hypovolemic shock, infection, incontinence, decubiti, subdural hematoma, dehydration, electrolyte imbalance, hypothermia, and phlebitis after sustaining the injury and throughout the recovery period. For hip fractures, approximately 10% to 17% of patients are readmitted to the hospital during the first 6 months. There is also a high mortality rate associated with hip fractures. Loss of physical and social function also may follow an injury.

Prevention/prophylaxis: Related to osteoporosis, estrogen replacement therapy reduces the incidence of hip fractures 50% to 75%. Exercise programs and cataract surgery in patients whose vision is impaired reduce the number of fractures. The modification of the patient's environment, including removal of hazards such as throw rugs and small pieces of furniture; improvements in lighting; and installation of grab bars, raised toilet seats, and ramps, helps prevent injuries.

Referral: Depending on the radiographic findings and location of the fracture, patients may need to be referred immediately to orthopedist. A physical therapy consultation is often necessary to teach patients exercises to improve or maintain function. The patient should be referred to an occupational therapist for recommendations for the need for adaptive equipment, such as grabbers, reachers, and elevated toilet seats, when the patient has suffered loss of function.

Education: After an injury, older adults are often hesitant or afraid to repeat the activity that led to the incident. Patients with osteoporosis need to be instructed on safe practices for lifting, bending, and reaching for objects. If the injury occurred after a fall, assessment of the home environment and consideration of adaptive equipment are suggested.

GOUT

SIGNAL SYMPTOMS ▶ polyarticular in older adults, soft tissue tenderness, tophi, podagra (metatarsophalangeal [MTP])

| Gout | ICD-9 CM: 274.9 |

Description: Gout, an inflammatory disease associated with malfunctioning metabolism of purine, leading to overproduction or underexcretion of uric acid, results in deposits of sodium urate crystals in the joints, periarticular tissues, subcutaneous tissues, and kidneys. Primary gout is the clinical disease caused by hyperuricemia; secondary gout usually occurs as a result of extended use of agents that decrease uric acid excretion.

Etiology: Clinically, hyperuricemia is defined when the serum urate level is >7 mg/dL. With levels >10 mg/dL, the chance of an acute attack of gout is >90%. In 70% to 90% of patients with diagnosed gout, underexcretion of urate rather than a metabolic overproduction causes elevation of the plasma urate level.

Occurrence: For every 100,000 people in the United States, 100 cases of gout occur.

Age: Primary gout usually begins in the 40s to 60s, whereas a new presentation of gout in the older adult occurs in the 60s to 70s.

Ethnicity: There is a high prevalence in Pacific Islanders, people from Samoa and the Philippines.

Gender: Primary gout is 20 times more prevalent in men than in women; however, among the elderly, gout occurs predominantly in women.

Contributing factors: Factors associated with primary gout in men include positive family history, obesity, trauma, hypertension, hyperlipidemia, hypertriglyceridemia, alcohol consumption, fasting, binge-eating, analgesic nephropathy, nephrolithiasis, and polycystic kidney disease.

Clinical Pearl: In women or men >60 years old, with a first-time presentation of gout, a relationship between long-term use of thiazide diuretics, salicylate use, hypertension, and renal insufficiency is observed.

Gout usually occurs after menopause in women. Patients taking nicotinic acid, cyclosporine, and ethambutol are at risk for gout. Acute gout attacks have been linked to stressors such as surgery or illness. Certain malignancies, such as hemolytic anemia, lymphoreticular cancers, and leukemias, can lead to secondary gout because of the accelerated turnover of cells that occurs with these conditions, leading to increased purine biosynthesis. Lead intoxication and consumption of illegal or moonshine whiskey has been found to be a contributor to saturnine gout. **Signs and symptoms:** Review the patient's history for evidence of excessive alcohol consumption, dietary habits, medical diagnosis of gout, family history of gout, exposure to lead, consumption of illicit whiskey, trauma, and all medication use. The following questions are helpful to ask the patient, to understand the presentation of symptoms:

Did the pain occur suddenly or become noticeable gradually?

Has the pain ever occurred before?

If so, how long did it last, and was the swelling in the same joint?

In middle-aged men, the classic presentation of an acute gout attack is a hot, swollen MTP joint of the great toe. Usually, in the first presentation of gout in middle-aged men, joint involvement is monarticular. In elderly women, joint involvement with gout is usually polyarticular. The proximal interphalangeal (PIP) joints and the distal interphalangeal (DIP) joints should be examined and the instep, heel, ankle, knee, wrist, and olecranon bursa palpated for signs of swelling and tenderness. Tophi, subcutaneous deposits of sodium urate, are common in chronic gout. Examine the helix of the ear, olecranon bursa, prepatellar bursa, Achilles tendon, over Heberden's nodes, and finger pads for signs of tophi. Fever may be present. Although rare, gout may be found in the spine (Fig. 8–1).

Diagnostic tests:

Test	Results Indicating Disorder	CPT Code
Synovial aspirate	Aspiration of monosodium urate crystals is the gold standard to diagnose gout and rule out sepsis	20600 (small joint, bursa, ganglion, or cyst) 20605 (intermediate joint, bursa, ganglion, or cyst) 20610 (major joint, bursa, ganglion, or cyst)
24-hour urine collection	Urate overproducers when urate is 600 mg/dL on a purine-free diet or 800 mg/dL on a regular diet	81050 (volume measurement for timed collection)
Plain radiography	Rule out other disorders; initially show soft tissue swelling Chronic gout shows oval punched-out erosions	76006 (stress views any joint)
Serum uric acid	>7.5 mg Serum uric acid may be normal in patients taking uricosuric drugs	84550
White blood count	Mild leukocytosis	85048
BUN	Renal insufficiency	84520
Serum creatinine	Renal insufficiency Serum creatinine level needed to calculate creatinine clearance level	82565

BUN, blood urea nitrogen.

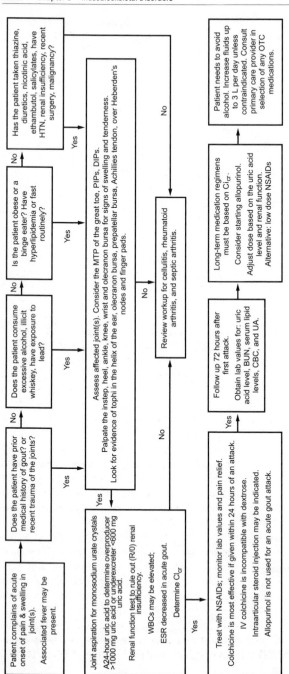

Figure 8–1. Gout.

Differential diagnosis:

- Pseudogout (calcium pyrophosphate rhomboidal crystals are present)
- Traumatic joint injury (radiographs)
- Septic arthritis
- Cellulitis
- Hemarthrosis
- Rheumatoid arthritis (RA) (when subcutaneous tophi are present)
- Osteoarthritis (OA)
- Seronegative spondyloarthropathies

Treatment: Management of the older adult with gout requires careful monitoring. Older adults are susceptible to renal insufficiency, may have other concomitant diseases, and experience hypersensitivity to some of the medications used to treat younger patients with gout. NSAIDs are the drugs of choice for older adults with gout. Indomethacin is effective in the treatment of acute gout; the usual dose is 25 to 50 mg orally two to three times daily until the symptoms cease, then begin to taper the dose for 5 to 7 days. Other NSAIDs, such as naproxen, ibuprofen, fenoprofen, and sulindac, can be tried. As with any NSAID, renal function must be monitored. NSAIDs can endanger existing renal function, especially when the creatinine clearance is ≤30 mL/min. Colchicine can be given for acute gout attacks either intravenously or orally. It is most effective if given within 24 hours of an attack. Intravenous dosage is 1 to 2 mg in 10 to 20 mL of normal saline, followed by 1 mg once or twice more at 4-hour intervals. *Note: Colchicine is incompatible with dextrose because precipitation occurs. I.V. cholchicine is contraindicated in patients who have had recent oral colchicine.* The oral colchicine dose is 0.5 mg every 2 hours until relief is felt; maximum total dose is 8 mg/24 hour period. Gastrointestinal toxicity commonly precedes a therapeutic response. Because oral colchicine is associated with more side effects than intravenous colchicine, it should not be administered to patients with impaired renal or hepatic function or gastrointestinal disease or to postoperative patients because of the potential for vomiting. Patients for whom colchicine and NSAIDs are contraindicated may be given intra-articular steroid injections. Allopurinol and uricosuric agents should not be prescribed for an acute gout attack.

Follow-up: Patients having a first acute attack of gout should be followed up 72 hours after initiating treatment to determine effectiveness and presence of any side effects. Patients who have more than three attacks of gout in a year are considered to have chronic disease. Before initiating a long-term medication regimen, uric acid level, BUN, serum lipid level, CBC, and urinalysis should be ordered.

Patients with chronic gout may require a uric acid–lowering agent, such as allopurinol. The starting dose for allopurinol is 100 mg/day, to be increased until the desired uric acid level is achieved (<6.5 mg/dL).

A dose of 200 mg/dL is probably the maximum dose that should be prescribed if the creatinine clearance is 50 to 60 mL/min; the dosage is lower if the creatinine clearance is 30 mL/min. The usefulness of probenecid in the older adult is limited because it is effective only when the creatinine clearance is <50 mL/min and is contraindicated in patients with renal insufficiency and on diuretics. Alternative treatment for chronic gout includes indomethacin, 25 mg twice daily, or another low-dose NSAID, reducing the dose in patients with documented hepatic or renal disease.

Sequelae: Older adults who have preexisting hypertension or primary renal disease or who use NSAIDs and diuretics are at risk for developing renal insufficiency, urate nephropathy, and acute hyperuricemia nephropathy. Uric acid nephrolithiasis is also a complication of gout. Untreated chronic gout may lead to multilobular, tender subcutaneous tophaceous gout, which can be deforming and impair ADLs.

Prevention/prophylaxis: Thiazide diuretics and salicylates should be avoided in patients with gout.

Referral: Patients may need a referral to a rheumatologist if they require intra-articular injections of steroids or joint aspiration, have complications from treatment, or have unusual presentation of the disease. A patient also may benefit from a referral to a dietitian for information on how to follow a low-purine diet.

Education: Patients need to be informed that during an acute attack they should rest the affected area and limit weight bearing if the first MTP joint is involved. Intake of 3 L/day of fluids is recommended unless contraindicated. The use of alcohol should be discouraged. Patients should consult their primary-care provider regarding selection of any over-the-counter medications.

OSTEOARTHRITIS

SIGNAL SYMPTOMS morning stiffness lasting <30 minutes, stiffness that improves with activity, Bouchard's nodes (PIP joints), Heberden's nodes (DIP joints), crepitus

Osteoarthrosis and allied disorders   CD-9 CM: 715.0

Description: OA, still also referred to as *degenerative joint disease,* is a degenerative disease of the joint cartilage. It is the second leading cause of disability in older adults in the United States. OA most commonly affects the hips, knees, and cervical and lumbar spine. Joint deformity with minimal pain is found in the DIP and PIP joints of the hand and the first carpometacarpal joint.

Etiology: The etiology of OA is unknown; however, it is known that OA is not age dependent. Conditions that change joint mechanics, such as untreated hip dislocation, may predispose an individual to OA.

Occurrence: Approximately 21 million people in the United States have OA.

Age: OA is common in older adults. An estimated 33% to 90% of the population >65 years old are thought to have OA.

Ethnicity: OA of the knee is more common in African-American women than in white women. Also, the prevalence of OA in male and female Alaskan natives is considerably lower than in whites.

Gender: Among people ≥55 years old, women are affected more often than men.

Contributing factors: Increasing age, obesity, previous joint injury, occupation, hobby, and prolonged sport activity involving the weight-bearing joints contribute to the development of OA. Other factors include calcium pyrophosphate or uric acid crystal deposits in the joints, Wilson's disease, acromegaly, hyperparathyroidism, and diabetes mellitus.

Signs and symptoms:

 Clinical Pearl: Complaints of morning stiffness lasting <30 minutes or stiffness that improves with activity and accompanying muscle spasms may indicate OA.

Persistent pain and limitation of motion in the affected joint may be reported. Bouchard's nodes (nontender nodules of the PIP joints), Heberden's nodes (nontender nodules of the DIP joints of the hands and feet), or both may be found. In women, inflammatory OA often occurs in the PIP joints and DIP joints, manifesting red, tender joints. MTP joints also may be involved.

On examination, patients with OA of the hip and knee may present with an antalgic gait. Crepitus of the affected joint is common. Internal and external hip rotation may be reduced. Some patients may complain of knee locking and unsteadiness. Patients with OA of the cervical spine often complain of paresthesias and numbness in the arms waking them from their sleep; this sensation generally improves when the limb is lightly shaken. Examination of the cervical spine may show some restricted joint movement and muscle tenderness.

When OA affects the lumbosacral spine, patients may report pain across the lower back with radiation to the buttocks and posterior thigh; if nerve root compression has occurred, patients may complain of pain in the lower leg. It is important to assess the patient's current functional status and pain level initially and at every subsequent visit.

Diagnostic tests:

Test	Results Indicating Disorder	CPT Code
Radiographs of affected area	Joint space narrowing Subchondral cyst formation Subchondral bony sclerosis Proliferative spurs	72010 (entire spine)
CT scan	Rule out spinal disorders or nerve entrapment	72131 (CT lumbar spine without contrast material) 72132 (CT lumbar spine with contrast material) 72133 (CT lumbar spine without contrast material, followed by contrast material and further sections) 72125 (CT cervical spine without contrast material) 72127 (CT cervical spine without contrast material followed by contrast material and further sections) 72128 (CT scan thoracic spine without contrast material) 72129 (CT scan thoracic spine with contrast material) 72129 (CT thoracic spine without contrast material, followed by contrast material and further sections)
Arthrocentesis (joint effusions)	Confirm noninflammatory process and rule out crystalline disease or infection	20600 (small joint, bursa, ganglion, or cyst) 20605 (intermediate joint, bursa, ganglion, or cyst) 20610 (major joint, bursa, ganglion, or cyst)
CBC (monitoring drug therapy)	Evaluate for anemia and elevated prothrombin time	85031
LFTs (monitoring drug therapy)	Evaluate to determine baseline and increases in LFT after initiation of drug therapy	80076
Renal function (monitoring drug therapy)	Evaluate for baseline and to look for increases in BUN and serum creatinine in response to drug therapy	82565 (creatinine) 84520 (BUN)

CT, computed tomography; LFT, liver function test.

Differential diagnosis:

- Osteoporosis (radiographs)
- Metastatic disease (radiographs)

- Multiple myeloma (bone marrow is infiltrated; lytic lesions are common in the axial skeleton)
- Anserine bursitis (knee involvement)

Treatment: Nonpharmacological therapies such as walking can be beneficial. Water therapy has been shown improve the function of patients with OA with no evidence of inflammation. In patients with no evidence of inflammation, acetaminophen is the medication of choice in doses of 2.6 to 4 g/day. For patients not getting relief from acetaminophen and exercise, the cyclooxygenase type 2 selective agents should be tried, especially in patients with a history of gastrointestinal bleeding and who are anticoagulated. Starting doses are celecoxib, 50 to 100 mg twice daily; rofecoxib, 12.5 to 25 mg daily; and valdecoxib, 10 mg once a day. The lowest starting does should be used in the elderly, especially in elderly patients weighing <50 kg. Selection of an NSAID should be based on dosing frequency, toxicity potential, and cost to the patient. Older adults should be started on a low dose of an NSAID, increasing the dose gradually. The use of NSAIDs should be avoided in older adults with a calculated creatinine clearance <35 mL/min. Tramadol can be given, 50 mg every 4 to 6 hours; maximum dose in patients ≥75 years old should not exceed 300 mg/day. Reports have shown that glucosamine and chondroitin sulfate (1500mg/1200mg per day) may relieve the pain of OA. Selection of capsaicin cream 25%, applied twice daily to the affected joint, also has been shown to reduce pain. When only one or a few joints are inflamed, intra-articular corticosteroid injections may be beneficial; however, use of these injections should be limited to only a couple of times each year. Viscosupplementation is another nonpharmacological option for patients with OA; an intra-articular injection of the highly viscous joint lubrication has been shown to be effective for 6 months. Patients with severe pain and restricted mobility may benefit from surgical intervention or reconstructive joint surgery.

Follow-up: Patients should be re-evaluated in about 2 to 3 weeks initially, to determine the effectiveness of the treatment. At this time, the patient should be weighed if obesity is a contributing factor; diet and exercise should be reviewed. The patient should be asked about benefits received from heat, cold, and massage. Response to pharmacological measures can be re-evaluated in patients who have been prescribed NSAIDs. A CBC and creatinine clearance and LFTs should be ordered at this time, then every 3 months. Question the patient about any new onset of dyspepsia, abdominal pain, or bleeding.

Sequelae: Because OA is a slowly progressive disease, joint deformity and functional disability may occur in individuals who have difficulty responding to the therapeutic regimen.

Prevention/prophylaxis: Weight reduction and avoidance of joint trauma may prevent further joint deformity in patients with OA. Studies have suggested that estrogen replacement therapy may reduce the risk of OA of the hip and knee in women. Similarly, work has indicated that the occurrence and progression of the disease might be slowed by maintaining normal levels of vitamin D.

Referral: Patients may need a referral to a rheumatologist if they have complications from treatment or an unusual presentation of the disease. Patients with involved joint deformities should be referred to an orthopedic surgeon for possible joint replacement.

Education: Patients should be given a treatment plan that includes information about the importance of exercise, such as water exercise and aerobic and resistance exercises as tolerated. Other nonpharmacological therapies shown to be beneficial to patients with OA are scheduled rest periods; weight reduction; and the safe use of heat, cold, and medication to control or alleviate pain. Information should be provided about acquiring necessary assistive devices, such as walkers, canes, elevated toilet seats, and any orthotics needed. Patients may require instruction on how to use these devices safely and should be measured properly for walker and cane size. It is essential to review all medications, especially over-the-counter drugs, to avoid duplication of NSAIDs.

OSTEOPOROSIS

SIGNAL SYMPTOMS▶ gibbous, decreased height, vertebral fractures, severe back pain

Osteoporosis:	ICD-9-CM: 733.0

Description: Osteoporosis is a systemic skeletal disease resulting in a reduction in bone mass and microarchitectural deterioration of bone tissue, which increases susceptibility to fractures. Fractures are common in the vertebrae, proximal femur, and distal forearm.

Etiology: Osteoporosis results from an imbalance between bone resorption and bone formation, causing a reduction in bone tissue. Two types of primary osteoporosis are type I, which occurs mainly in postmenopausal women and is characterized by increased bone resorption, reduced production of parathyroid hormone, and a decreased activation of vitamin D; and type II, or senile osteoporosis, which develops in persons ≥70 years old. In type I osteoporosis, trabecular bone loss is accelerated. Women who have estrogen deficiency as a result of early natural or surgical menopause are at risk for developing this type of osteoporosis. In type II osteoporosis, trabecular and cortical bone loss occurs. Type I and type II osteoporosis may overlap. Secondary osteoporosis may result from hormone excess, malignancy, genetic disorders, chronic disease, and certain medications.

Occurrence: Of Americans, > 25 million have osteoporosis; 80% are women.

Age: Type I osteoporosis is found in persons age 55 to 75; type II is found in persons age 70 to 85.

Ethnicity: The risk for osteoporosis is twice as great in white women compared with African-American women. Asian-American women are also at a high risk. About 15% of Mexican-American women have osteoporosis. White men are at greater risk for developing osteoporosis than African-American men.

Gender: The ratio of women to men for developing type I osteoporosis is 6:1; the ratio decreases to 2:1 for type II osteoporosis.

Contributing factors: Many risk factors predispose individuals to osteoporosis, including female gender, white or Asian race, small body structure, light hair and complexion, and family history of the disease. A history of tobacco abuse and excessive alcohol and caffeine intake increases the risk of developing osteoporosis. A diet that limits calcium and vitamin D but contains large quantities of protein and phosphorus may put persons at greater risk. Patients taking certain medications, such as corticosteroids, thyroid hormones, anticonvulsants (e.g., phenytoin), anticoagulants, lithium, certain chemotherapeutic agents, aluminum antacids, and tetracyclines, are at increased risk. Patients diagnosed with hyperthyroidism, type 1 diabetes mellitus, RA, chronic renal failure, past or present history of Cushing's syndrome, previous gastric surgery, and major organ transplantation, liver disease, epilepsy, alcoholism, malabsorption states, anorexia nervosa, and hyperparathyroidism; women having menopause before age 40 without hormonal replacement; and persons who are immobile also are susceptible to osteoporosis. A history of fracture or of a tendency to fall puts a person at risk for sustaining an osteoporotic fracture. Anyone with a history of a sedentary lifestyle and limited exercise also is at risk for developing osteoporosis.

Signs and symptoms: Patients with osteoporosis may be asymptomatic. Patients need to be questioned about all of the risk factors for osteoporosis. Inquire about family history of fractures and obtain a thorough menstrual history in women; questions about libido and potency in men are important.

The patient's height should be measured at the initial visit and yearly. The mouth should be examined to assess dentition and any evidence of oral bone loss, and the thyroid gland should be palpated. The spine should be examined in detail, including configuration. Any tenderness to palpation over the spinous processes and evidence of swelling, tenderness, and ecchymosis present at the sight of the injury should be noted. Range of motion should be determined, noting limitations or painful movement. An abdominal examination reveals whether the abdomen is protuberant from spinal changes; the distance between the rib cage and the anterior iliac crest should be recorded. Physical examination may reveal loss of height with associated kyphosis of the spine. The most common site for vertebral fractures in patients with osteoporosis is the lower thoracic (T12) or upper lumbar (L1) region. The patient may appear humpbacked; the sharp angle in the flexion of the spine is called a *gibbous*. Gait should be assessed objectively, and the patient's body mechanics should be observed at this time.

Diagnostic tests:

Test	Results Indicating Disorder	CPT Code
CBC	Evaluate nutritional status and rule out myeloma	85031
TSH	Rule out presence of hyperthyroidism	84443
Blood chemistries, including calcium, phosphorus, creatinine, and electrolyte levels	Serum calcium and phosphate is normal in osteoporosis Alkaline phosphatase may be elevated if there is a fracture	80048 (basic metabolic panel) 84075 (alkaline phosphatase)
Dual-energy x-ray absorptiometry	Normal: BMD <1 SD of the young adult reference mean Osteopenia: BMD <1–2.5 SD below the young adult reference mean Osteoporosis: BMD >2.5 SD below the young adult reference mean	76075
Radiographs of affected area	Fractures	72010 (entire spine)

TSH, thyroid-stimulating hormone; BMD, bone mineral density.

Differential diagnosis:

- Multiple myeloma (bone marrow infiltrated; lytic lesions common in the axial skeleton)
- Hyperparathyroidism (serum calcium >10.5 mg/dL)
- Osteomalacia (abnormal serum calcium, alkaline phosphatase, and phosphate levels)
- Hyperthyroidism (decreased TSH levels)
- Cushing's syndrome (serum cortisol levels >7.5 g/dL)
- Paget's disease (serum alkaline phosphate is distinctly elevated)

Treatment: The management of osteoporosis is comprehensive. Patients should be educated on the importance of preventing injury and altering changeable risk factors. Dietary adjustments should include supplementation with 1500 mg of elemental calcium for patients not receiving hormone replacement therapy or 1000 mg of calcium for patients who are receiving hormone replacement therapy, unless the patient has hypercalciuria. Calcium carbonate is 40% elemental calcium by weight but may cause constipation; calcium citrate, which is 22% elemental calcium by weight, is absorbed better and has fewer gastrointestinal side effects. Recommend elimination of tobacco, elimination of excessive alcohol and caffeine, and a reduction in the amount of high-phosphorus foods. Patients should engage in regular weight-bearing exercises. Measures to enhance safety in the home and surrounding environment should be emphasized. Options for pharmacological measures to treat osteoporosis in postmenopausal women include vitamin D, bisphosphonates, calcitonin, and fluoride. Treatment plans must be individualized. An intake of 250 to 400 U/day of vitamin D in the form of a multivitamin or fortified dairy products is recommended. Salmon calcitonin is available as an injection or a nasal spray for patients who cannot tolerate estrogen; the dosage is 50 IU three times weekly to 100 IU daily subcutaneously or intramuscularly. The dosage for the nasal spray is 1 puff daily (0.09 mL, 200 IU) in alternating nostrils. Another option for postmenopausal women is alendronate, 10 mg once daily in the morning swallowed whole with 8 oz. of plain water; the patient must remain fully upright for 30 minutes and when at least that amount of time has elapsed consume the first meal of the day. Alternatively, alendronate, 70 mg once weekly, can be prescribed for treatment of postmenopausal osteoporosis and for men. Alendronate is not recommended for patients with creatinine clearance >35 mL/min. Risedronate, 5 mg/day on awakening with 8 oz. of water on empty stomach with no oral intake for at least 30 minutes, is another one of the bisphosphonates. Risedronate at 35 mg once weekly for the treatment of osteoporosis is also available. The dose for raloxifene is 60 mg daily; raloxifene is a selective estrogen receptor modulator; it may be taken with or without meals. Teriparatide, a form of parathyroid hormone, has been approved for the treatment of osteoporosis in postmenopausal women and men who are at high risk for fracture.

Follow-up: For persons at risk for osteoporosis, monitor their height, exercise patterns, habits, and diet; review the safety measures for the home and proper body mechanics; and evaluate the need for adaptive equipment. Repeat bone densitometry may be indicated. For patients receiving pharmacological therapy, review the medication regimen, assess for side effects, and repeat laboratory tests as indicated. The patient should also be assessed for fractures and for the need for analgesics. Patients with osteoporosis should be enrolled in fall prevention programs.

Sequelae: Osteoporosis-related fractures are major complications. Of the 250,000 people who sustain a hip fracture yearly, 12% to 20% die within the first year after the injury, and >50% of patients require long-term care. Because patients often have a fear of falling and injury, a loss of social and physical function may occur.

Prevention/prophylaxis: As part of the routine examination, patients should be screened to determine their level of risk for the development of osteoporosis. Dietary history, exercise patterns, and habits should be reviewed with patients. A measurement of height should be recorded at least yearly for all adults. The benefits of changing lifestyle patterns should be emphasized to patients even in advanced age. For patients with identifiable risk factors for osteoporosis, bone mass measurement should be considered. Dual-photon and dual-energy x-ray absorptiometry and quantitative CT scans can determine whether a patient has lost enough bone mass to be at risk for fracture. Both Alendronate and Risedronate have been approved to be prescribed for prevention of osteoporosis for patients at risk.

Referral: Women who will be beginning hormone replacement therapy may be referred to a gynecologist. For patients who have sustained a fracture, depending on its location, an immediate referral to an orthopedist is recommended. Patients may require referral for physical therapy to be evaluated for weight-bearing exercises and for demonstration of safe transferring, lifting, and bending. Patients with functional limitations need instruction on the use of adaptive equipment (e.g., walkers, grabbers).

Education: Patients can contact the National Osteoporosis Foundation at 1232 22nd Street NW, Washington, DC 20037 (202-223-2226), for educational materials. The web site for the foundation is www.nof.org. Patients also should be given information about local support groups for persons with osteoporosis, senior exercise classes, and dietary counseling.

POLYMYALGIA RHEUMATICA

SIGNAL SYMPTOMS ► stiffness in neck, shoulders, pelvic girdle, unable to get out of bed in the morning without extreme difficulty, difficulty in lifting arms over one's head

Polymyalgia rheumatica (PMR)   ICD-9 CM: 725.0

Description: PMR is a clinical syndrome characterized by fatigue, pain, and stiffness primarily in the neck, shoulders, hips, and pelvic girdle, occurring primarily in older adults. Round cell infiltration and synovial proliferation are found in patients with PMR. An elevated Westergren ESR is essential in the diagnosis of PMR.

Etiology: The etiology of PMR is unknown. A relationship between the presence of the HLA-DR4 haplotype and presentation of PMR has been suggested.

Occurrence: PMR affects 1 in 1000 individuals ≥50 years old in the United States.

Age: This disease occurs predominantly in adults >50 years old. PMR and giant cell arteritis occur 10 times more frequently in adults >80 years old than in adults <60 years old.

Ethnicity: PMR is six times more common in whites than in African-

Americans. A genetic factor, the HLA-DR4 haplotype, is found in patients with PMR.

Gender: PMR occurs twice as often in women as in men.

Contributing factors: Advanced age and a possible genetic predisposition are thought to contribute to the development of PMR.

Signs and symptoms: Patients often complain of fatigue and generalized malaise. Fever is common; patients may report night sweating. Additionally, patients usually have bilateral, proximal aching and stiffness in the neck, shoulders, upper arms, hips, thighs, and lower back. Stiffness occurs in the morning and may last >30 minutes. Anorexia, weight loss, apathy, fear, and depression are also constitutional symptoms of PMR. Musculoskeletal pain and related symptoms last about 1 month.

Muscle weakness usually is not elicited on physical examination. Tenderness may be elicited on palpation to the muscle groups mentioned earlier. Check for signs of carpal tunnel syndrome, such as paresthesia of the thumb and index and middle fingers. Patients may complain of numbness and tingling in the fingers and a decreased ability to grasp small objects. Diagnostic studies may reveal anemia; checking for signs of pallor is important. Because giant cell arteritis is associated with PMR, the workup should include questions to evaluate for giant cell arteritis, such as complaints of occipital or temporal headaches, transient visual disturbances, jaw or ear pain, sore throat, hoarseness, and cough and painful scalp. Assess for tender temporal arteries and visual acuity. Funduscopic examination may reveal retinal hemorrhages, cotton-wool patches, and edema of the optic disc (Fig. 8–2).

Diagnostic tests:

Test	Results Indicating Disorder	CPT Code
Westergren ESR	50 mm/hr May be >100 mm/hr	85651
CBC	May show normocytic, normochromic anemia	85031

 Clinical Pearl: Patients with PMR initially may have normal ESRs but be symptomatic with a milder form of the disease.

Differential diagnosis:

- RA (by the absence of synovitis)
- Polymyositis (normal muscle enzymes and muscle biopsy)
- Fibromyalgia
- Hypothyroidism (TSH would be normal in absence of previous thyroid disease)
- Osteoarthritis
- Carcinomatosis

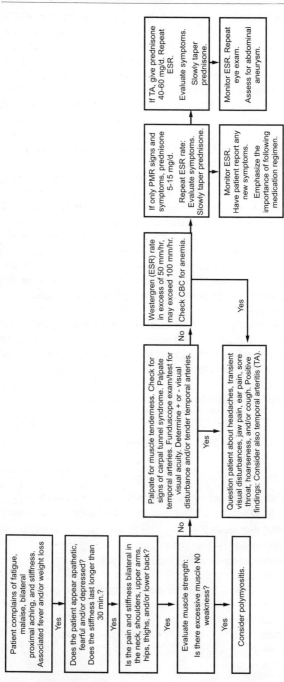

Figure 8–2. Polymyalgia rheumatica.

Treatment: If the patient presents with signs and symptoms only of PMR, start low-dose prednisone (5–20 mg/day). Symptoms should begin to resolve after 24 hours, and the ESR should normalize in 7 to 10 days. Prednisone is tapered off slowly, continuing over months, when the symptoms have resolved and the ESR rate is normal. NSAIDs such as ibuprofen may be used instead of steroids when the patient is stable. Patients presenting with visual disturbances or other symptoms of giant cell arteritis need a higher dose of oral corticosteroids; prednisone, 40 to 80 mg in divided daily doses, is the suggested starting dose, again with a gradual tapering depending on symptoms and laboratory values. Treatment may last 6 months to 1 year.

Follow-up: For patients with PMR, the ESR is monitored until it decreases and previously reported symptoms resolve. Given the risk of developing osteoporosis from long-term steroid use, patients with PMR and giant cell arteritis should be scheduled to have a baseline dual-energy x-ray absorptiometry scan. Consider prophylactic therapy to prevent osteoporosis. Patients also presenting with giant cell arteritis need to be monitored in the same way, with repeated eye examinations as warranted. Because patients with giant cell arteritis are at risk for developing aortic aneurysm, follow-up abdominal examination for aortic aneurysm is needed.

Sequelae: The diagnosis of PMR is confirmed when a response to the corticosteroid is noted. Usually the patient begins to exhibit a reduction in symptoms within 24 hours after starting treatment. Patients should be alerted to the signs of giant cell arteritis. Patients with untreated giant cell arteritis are at risk for blindness. Patients should be informed they must complete all of the prescribed medication to avoid a relapse.

Prevention/prophylaxis: No preventive measures exist for PMR, but because the disease can recur, patients should be advised to contact their health-care providers when any of the prevailing signs and symptoms reappear.

Referral: For patients with signs of visual disturbance, funduscopic changes, or both, referral to an ophthalmologist is warranted if the patient can be evaluated immediately. If not, these patients should be referred to an emergency department for immediate evaluation. Consultation with a rheumatologist is beneficial for patients who have giant cell arteritis or who do not respond to treatment for PMR.

Education: Patients should be taught the precautions needed when steroids are being taken; in addition to being at risk for osteoporosis, the likelihood for developing infections, fractures, diabetes, peptic ulcers, cataracts, depression, and weight gain increases with steroids. Patients should be instructed to include an adequate amount of calcium in their diets. Patients who do not have temporal arteritis should be alerted to potential symptoms, such as visual disturbance, headache, temporal tenderness, and jaw pain.

RHEUMATOID ARTHRITIS

Rheumatoid arthritis	ICD-9 CM: 714.0

Description: RA is a chronic systemic inflammatory process evidenced by symmetrical polyarthritis; it is the most common inflammatory arthropathy. Patients generally experience episodes of remission and acute exacerbations of the disease. Extra-articular presentations of RA include vasculitis, rheumatoid nodules, scleritis, pericarditis, neuropathy, interstitial fibrosis, Sjögren's syndrome, and Felty's syndrome.

Etiology: The cause of RA is unknown. Susceptibility to the disease is genetic; a relationship between presence of class II human leukocyte antigen (HLA) and RA has been identified.

Occurrence: RA occurs in 0.3% to 1.5% of the U.S. population. Estimates have shown that 2.1 million people have RA.

Age: The usual age of onset is 20 to 60 years, and initial presentation of the disease peaks between ages 35 and 45. Elderly-onset RA begins after age 60.

Ethnicity: Native Americans have a prevalence of 3.5% to 5.3%. A familial tendency also exists.

Gender: RA affects women two to three times more frequently than men.

Contributing factors: Factors associated with the development of RA include family history of RA, female gender, Native American ethnic background, and presence of the HLA haplotype.

Signs and symptoms: The clinical presentation for patients with long-standing RA before age 60 reflects the duration of the individual's disease and concomitant conditions. For patients with elderly-onset RA, the initial presentation may be a gradual onset of morning stiffness, swelling, and pain in multiple joints. In others, the first attack may be more acute. In older adults, constitutional symptoms with RA may include low-grade fever, anorexia, weight loss, malaise, and depression. In elderly-onset RA, larger joints, such as the shoulders, often are involved more frequently than in patients with earlier onset RA, in whom smaller joints usually are affected. Joint deformities prevalent in patients with a history of RA include hyperflexion of the PIP joints and flexion of the DIP joints (called *swan-neck deformity*), flexion of the PIP joints and extension of the DIP joints (called *boutonnière deformity*), ulnar deviation of the metacarpophalangeal joint, and knee and ankle effusions.

The metacarpophalangeal, wrist, PIP, MTP, shoulder, ankle, and elbow joints should be examined for range of motion, tenderness, erythema, warmth, and swelling. The skin should be checked for subcutaneous nodules, which are generally <1 to 3 cm in diameter and feel firm and fixed on palpation; these often are found proximal to the elbow. Systemic evaluation also includes an eye examination to check for keratoconjunctivitis, scleritis, and corneal ulcers. The lungs are evaluated to determine if pleuritis or pneumonitis is present. Pericarditis, a possible manifestation of RA, warrants a cardiac examination. The clinician also should examine the patient for evidence of nerve entrapment and sensory neuropathy. All patients should be questioned about the impact of RA on their lifestyle and current ability to carry out ADLs.

Diagnostic tests:

Test	Results Indicating Disorder	CPT Code
CBC	May show normochromic, normocytic anemia, mild leukocytosis, thrombocytosis	85031
Rheumatoid factor	Positive in 50% of all cases, although rheumatoid factor can be elevated in older adults	86430 (qualitative) 86431 (quantitative)
Radiographs	Soft tissue swelling initially Symmetrical joint space narrowing Subluxations, erosions	76006 (stress views any joint)
Westergren ESR	ESR may be normally elevated in older adults	85651
C-reactive protein	Elevations indicate an active inflammatory process and are known to correlate with bone destruction	86140–86141

Differential diagnosis:

- Erosive OA (radiographs)
- PMR (rapid response to corticosteroid therapy)
- Polyarticular gout (monosodium urate crystal determination is the gold standard to diagnose gout and rule out sepsis)
- Pseudogout (calcium pyrophosphate rhomboidal crystals are present)
- Chronic infection
- Occult malignancy
- Systemic lupus erythematosus or drug-induced lupus
- Scleroderma
- Polymyositis (normal muscle enzymes and muscle biopsy)

Treatment: The three classes of drugs used to treat RA are the NSAIDs, corticosteroids, and disease-modifying antirheumatic drugs (DMARDs). For patients who have been treated for years for RA, modifications in the drug regimen may be necessary to protect against renal toxicity, NSAID-induced gastritis, and central nervous system toxicity. Early referral to a rheumatologist is essential for the newly diagnosed RA patient because new clinical guidelines indicate that treatment early in the course of the disease using DMARDs within 3 months of diagnosis may alter the progression of the disease (American College of Rheumatology

Subcommittee on Rheumatoid Arthritis, 2002). Combination therapy is often necessary in treating RA patients. When using NSAIDs to treat older adults with RA, the NSAID selection should be based on the medications' half-lives, giving favor to those with short half-lives, using the lowest effective dose. Low-dose oral corticosteroids may provide relief, starting with doses of <10 mg, then tapering off to determine the lowest effective dose. The DMARDs used for treating RA include injectable gold salts, oral gold, hydroxychloroquine, sulfasalazine, methotrexate, penicillamine, leflunomide, etanercept, azathioprine, and cyclosporine. Often more than one DMARD is prescribed at a time to improve efficacy. Patients require extensive monitoring for potential toxic effects. RA patients with comorbidities on combination therapy along with other medication regimens for other conditions are at high risk for drug interaction.

Follow-up: Initially, it is important to determine if the disease is in an active or inactive state. Routine evaluations for patients with RA should include the patient's response to pharmacological and nonpharmacological therapy for pain management and functional ability. Medications should be adjusted if the patient does not obtain symptomatic relief from the current therapy. Assess for duration of morning stiffness and fatigue. Progression of articular and extra-articular disease should be monitored through a focused physical examination. Any change in the patient's ability to carry out ADLs and his or her psychosocial status as well as the impact the disease process is having on quality of life should be evaluated at each visit using standardized instruments, such as the Arthritis Impact Measurement Scale or the Health Assessment Questionnaire.

Sequelae: Older adults who have had RA for years eventually experience more severe disease with increased joint deformities. Comorbidities, such as septic arthritis, Sjögren's syndrome, Felty's syndrome, and pericarditis, may exist in patients with a history of RA. Patients with elderly-onset RA may tend to have a milder course of the disease, with periods of remission; however, patients experiencing a more rapid decline also have been reported. Complications from the medication regimen need to be considered.

Prevention/prophylaxis: Although RA cannot be prevented, a program of gentle range-of-motion exercises can help maintain function and muscle strength.

Referral: Newly diagnosed RA patients should be referred to a rheumatologist for initial evaluation and selection of therapeutic agents and for the monitoring of RA activity and drug toxicity, unless specific arrangements have been made for the primary-care provider to monitor the patient's RA therapeutic regimen. Patients also can benefit from referral to a physical therapist and an occupational therapist, to assist them in their exercise programs, splinting needs, and adaptive equipment requirements, all aimed at maintaining function and independence for as long as possible. Patients with high levels of pain with limited range of motion and loss of function should be referred to a surgeon for consideration of surgical procedure.

Education: Patients should be taught the importance of incorporating periods of rest and exercise into their daily lives. Information on devices to protect joints, ways to conserve physical energy while maintaining optimal functioning, and prescribed exercise program should be reinforced with patients at each visit. Medication education is important in RA because of the potential for side effects associated with a complicated drug regimen. Because there is no cure for RA, patients must be skeptical about antidotes promised for RA and check with their health-care providers if they have any concerns about treatments. Patients can contact the Arthritis Foundation (800-282-7800) for information; a booklet, "Overcoming Rheumatoid Arthritis," is available.

REFERENCES

General

American Medical Association: Current Procedural Terminology: CPT 2002, ed 4. AMA, Chicago, 2002.

Callahan, LF, and Jonas, BL: Arthritis. In Ham RJ, et al (eds): Primary Care Geriatrics: A Case-Based Approach, ed 4. Mosby, St Louis, 2002.

DeGowin, RL, and Brown, D: DeGowin's Diagnostic Examination, ed 7. McGraw-Hill, New York, 2000.

Goroll, A, and Mulley, AG: Primary Care Medicine: Office Evaluation and Management of the Adult Patient, ed 4. Lippincott Williams & Wilkins, Philadelphia, 2000.

Kennedy-Malone, L, et al: Management Guidelines for Gerontological Nurse Practitioners. FA Davis, Philadelphia, 1999.

Lawrence, RC: Estimates of the prevalence of arthritis and selected musculoskeletal disorders in the United States. Arthritis Rheum 41:778, 1998.

Fractures

Brown, JS, et al: Urinary incontinence: Does it increase the risk of fall and fractures? J Am Geriatr Soc 48:721, 2000.

Kannus, P: Preventing osteoporosis, falls, and fractures among elderly people: Promotion of lifelong physical activity is essential. BMJ 318:205, 1999.

Wallace, RB: Bone health in nursing home residents. JAMA 284:1018, 2000.

Gout

Harris, MD, et al: Gout and hyperuricemia. Am Fam Physician 60:925, 1999.

Kase, E, and Ostrov, B: Intricacies in the diagnosis and treatment of gout. Patient Care 35:33, 2001.

Meiner, SE: Gouty arthritis: Not just a big toe problem. Geriatr Nurs 22:132, 2001.

Mekelburg, K, and Rahimi: Gouty arthritis of the spine: Clinical presentation and effective treatment. Geriatrics 55:71, 2000.

Pittman, JR, and Bross, MH: Diagnosis and management of gout. Am Fam Physician 59:1799, 1999.

Osteoarthritis

American College of Rheumatology Subcommittee on Osteoarthritis Guidelines: Recommendations for the medical management of osteoarthritis of the hip and knee. Arthritis Rheum 43:1905, 2000.

American Geriatrics Society Panel on Exercise and Osteoarthritis: Exercise prescription for older adults with osteoarthritis pain: Consensus practice recommendations. J Am Geriatr Soc 49:803, 2001.

Birchfield, PC: Osteoarthritis overview. Geriatr Nurs 22:124, 2001.

Felson, DT: An update on the epidemiology of knee and hip osteoarthritis with a view to prevention. Arthritis Rheum 41:1343, 1998.

Hinton, R, et al: Osteoarthritis: Diagnosis and therapeutic considerations. Am Fam Physician 2002. Contact: http://www.aafp.org/afp/20020301/841.html.

McCarberg, BH, and Herr, KA: Osteoarthritis: How to manage pain and to improve function. Geriatrics 56:14, 2001.

Miller, CA: Newer and safer options for osteoarthritis. Geriatr Nurs 22:165, 2001.

Reginster, JY: Long-term effects of glucosamine sulphate on osteoarthritis progression: A randomized, placebo-controlled clinical trial. Lancet 357:251, 2001.

Osteoporosis

Brunader, R, and Shelton, DK: Radiologic bone assessment in the evaluation of osteoporosis. Am Fam Physician 2002. Contact: http://www.aafp.org/20020401/1357.html.

National Osteoporosis Foundation: Update on medications: US FDA-approved pharmacologic options for prevention and treatment of osteoporosis. 2002. Contact: http://www.nof.org/physguide/pharmacologic_NOFupdate.htm.

Osteoporosis prevention, diagnosis and therapy. NIH Consensus Statement Online 2000 March 27–29. 17:1, 2000.

Wishnia, G: Challenges in the care of adults with osteoporosis. Geriatr Nurs 22:160, 2001.

Polymyalgia Rheumatica

Apgar, B: Corticosteroids in patients with polymyalgia rheumatica. Am Fam Physician 60:954, 1999.

Brigden, ML: Clinical utility of the erythrocyte sedimentation rate. Am Fam Physician 60:1443, 1999.

Epperly, TD, et al: Polymyalgia rheumatica and giant cell arteritis. Am Fam Physician 64:778, 2000.

Kennedy-Malone, L, and Enevold, G: Assessment and management of polymyalgia rheumatica and temporal arteritis in older adult. Geriatr Nurs 22:152, 2001.

Leslie, M: When the ache is not arthritis. RN 63:38, 2000.

Mikanowicz, C, and Leslie, M: Polymyalgia rheumatica and temporal arteritis. Nurs Clin North Am 35:245, 2000.

Rheumatoid Arthritis

American College of Rheumatology Subcommittee on Rheumatoid Arthritis Guidelines 2002 update. Arthritis Rheumatism 46:328, 2002.

Ignatavicius, DD: Rheumatoid arthritis and the older adult. Geriatr Nurs 22:139, 2001.

Browning, MA: Rheumatoid arthritis: A primary care approach. J Am Acad Nurse Practitioners 13:399, 2001.

Martyn, R, and Zurier, RB: Rheumatoid arthritis: Update on therapeutic agents. Clin Geriatr 2001. Contact: http://www.mmhc.com/cg/articles/CG9901/martyn.html.

Ollivier, JE: Advances in the management of osteoarthritis and rheumatoid arthritis. J Am Acad Physicians Assistants 14:22, 2001.

Pisetsky, DS, and Williams St. Clair: Progress in the treatment of rheumatoid arthritis. JAMA 286:2787, 2001.

Chapter 9

PERIPHERAL VASCULAR DISORDERS

ABDOMINAL AORTIC ANEURYSM

SIGNAL SYMPTOMS persistent or intermittent pain in the middle or lower abdomen often radiating to the lower back; most are asymptomatic

Abdominal aortic aneurysm (AAA)	ICD-9-CM: 441.4
Dissecting AAA	ICD-9-CM: 441.02
Ruptured AAA	ICD-9-CM: 441.3

Description: The abdominal aorta is the large artery that provides blood to the abdominal organs and the lower extremities. It extends from the descending aorta to the iliac arteries. An AAA is a dilation of the abdominal aorta that is 1.5 to 2 times greater than the size of the aorta and involves all layers of the artery.

Etiology: Most AAAs are atherosclerotic in nature; other causes include trauma, infection, and inflammation. Most AAAs are infrarenal (65%), occurring below the renal arteries.

Occurrence: AAAs are the 13th leading cause of death in the United States. Operative mortality rates for ruptured aneurysms are 70% to 90% compared with 5% operative mortality for elective repair.

Age: More frequent in adults >50 years old; prevalence rate is 2% to 4%.

Gender: Onset occurs around age 50 for men and 60 for women. Incidence steadily increases with age and peaks at age 80. AAA is five times more likely in men than women.

Ethnicity: There is no dominant ethnic group that develops AAA, but there is a familial history associated with AAA development.

Contributing factors: Risk factors for developing AAA include arteriosclerotic heart disease and arteriosclerotic changes of other vessels, smoking history, hypertension, chronic obstructive pulmonary disease, obesity, family history of AAA and diabetes mellitus, cystic medial necrosis, Marfan syndrome, and previous spinal cord injury.

Signs and symptoms: Most patients with AAAs are asymptomatic (66–75%) except in the presence of dissection, rupture, or impending rupture. A pulsatile abdominal mass at or slightly above the umbilicus in the epigastrium revealed by palpation of the abdomen may be an AAA. These are easier to palpate in thin individuals; however, if noted in an obese individual, they are usually large. AAA should be suspected in individuals with a femoral or popliteal aneurysm because one third of individuals with a peripheral aneurysm also have an AAA. In patients with symptomatic AAAs, the complaints are of mild-to-severe abdominal, flank, or lower back pain. Other symptoms include nausea and vomiting, gastrointestinal bleeding, and lower extremity ischemia. Rupture is the most lethal clinical presentation. Symptoms include sudden onset of severe abdominal and back pain, hypotension, and the presence of a pulsatile mass. There is a high mortality rate associated with ruptured AAAs; its diagnosis should be considered in any elderly patient with abdominal or flank pain.

Diagnostic tests:

Test	Result Indicating Disorder	CPT Code
Abdominal ultrasound	Determines size, shape, and location of aneurysm	76700
Contrast-enhanced computed tomography	Preoperative assessment of the AAA. Provides accurate measures of aneurysm and surrounding anatomy	74160
MRI and MRA	Accurate but expensive method of measuring aneurysm. Exclude patients with metallic devices or claustrophobia	74181 (MRI) 74185 (MRA)

MRI, magnetic resonance imaging; MRA, magnetic resonance angiography

Differential diagnosis: Because various agents can produce aortic aneurysms, it is important to search for hypertension and heart disease because AAA management includes blood pressure control and recognition of heart function. An ectatic abdominal aorta without aneurysm may be palpated and confused with AAA. Other acute causes of abdominal and back pain may mimic a ruptured AAA and must be ruled out.

Treatment: The rate of AAA growth for an individual is unpredictable. Some aneurysms may remain stable for long periods, whereas others may enlarge quickly. Medical management of an asymptomatic, small AAA should include blood pressure control and smoking cessation. β-Blockers have been shown to slow the long-term growth of aortic aneurysms.

There are two options for excising an AAA when it becomes symptomatic or becomes >5 cm in diameter: open surgical repair and endovascular repair. Elective operative repair has a mortality rate of 2% to 5%. Urgent repair of an intact symptomatic AAA has a mortality rate of 18%. In emergent repair in which the AAA has ruptured, there is a 50% mortality rate in patients who reach the hospital. Average postoperative length of stay for an uncomplicated recovery is 4 to 5 days. The major cause of death after AAA repair is myocardial infarction. Other complications include renal failure, limb ischemia, ischemic colitis, hemorrhage, and paraplegia (which occurs rarely).

Endovascular grafts are a more recent addition to the treatment modalities for elective AAA repair. The graft is deployed through the femoral artery. Not all AAAs are anatomically appropriate for stenting. Experimental AAA stent trials began in 1993 in the United States. Current success rates are >90% with a mortality rate of <2%. Most patients are discharged from the hospital in 1 to 2 days. Complications after endovascular treatment include arterial injury at site of access, arterial embolization, endoleak (blood flow outside the lumen of the graft but within the aneurysmal sac), postimplant syndrome (back pain and fever without elevated white blood cell count or other signs of infection), and graft limb thrombosis.

Follow-up: Initial management of patients with small aneurysms (<4 cm) should include serial evaluation with ultrasound every 3 to 6 months. Any symptomatic AAA or an asymptomatic AAA >5 cm should be repaired using either open surgical or endovascular technique.

Sequelae: The most common complication of AAA is rupture. Infrequent complications are thrombi to the lower extremities and infection of the aneurysm, with *Salmonella* and *Staphylococcus aureus* being the most commonly identified organisms.

Prevention/prophylaxis: Because most AAAs are atherosclerotic in nature, the same preventive measures for reducing coronary artery disease should be applied. These include lifestyle modification, controlling hypertension and diabetes mellitus, and early screening for individuals in high-risk categories, including first-degree relatives of individuals who already have been diagnosed. The prevalence of AAA in affected families is reported to be 15% to 33%.

Referral: Referral to a vascular surgeon or specialist is essential for all patients with symptomatic AAAs.

Education: Patients and their families should be taught the importance of follow-up; how to manage hypertension, smoking, and other risk factors; and to recognize symptoms that should be reported to the physician immediately (sudden onset of abdominal or back pain, dizziness). The risks of operative versus nonoperative treatment should be explained thoroughly to the patient and family.

PERIPHERAL VASCULAR DISEASE

SIGNAL SYMPTOMS ▶ pain, intermittent claudication of the feet

Claudication	ICD-9-CM: 440.21
Gangrene	ICD-9-CM: 440.24
Rest pain	ICD-9-CM: 440.22
Bypass graft	ICD-9-CM: 440.30
Ulceration	ICD-9-CM: 440.23

Description: Peripheral vascular disease (PVD) refers to a disease or process that limits blood flow to the extremities and vital organs other than the heart. These processes may involve the arterial, venous, or lymphatic systems but most often are due to enlarging atherosclerotic plaques in the distal aorta or in major bifurcations or areas of angulation in the iliac, femoral, and popliteal arteries.

Etiology: Atherosclerotic plaques may be fatty streaks, fibrous plaques, or complicated lesions. Fatty streaks are early lesions that occur in the intima of arteries. Fibrous plaques, areas of intimal thickening, are the most frequently occurring type of lesion. Complicated plaques, calcified fibrous plaques with potential for necrosis and thrombosis, are associated most often with symptoms.

Occurrence: PVD is referred to as an age-related disease. More diabetics than nondiabetics are diagnosed with PVD. Nearly 30% of older adults in the general population have PVD. This percentage is expected to increase as the number of elderly individuals in the population increases.

Age: Nearly 20% of individuals >70 years old have PVD compared with <8% of individuals <70 years old.

Gender: Symptomatic disease is two to five times more prevalent in men than women.

Ethnicity: There are few available data to support an ethnic predisposition for the development of PVD.

Contributing factors: Smoking remains the most important risk factor; 80% of cases of intermittent claudication are associated with tobacco use. Diabetes mellitus is another important risk factor; >80% of diabetics surviving 20 years from the time of diagnosis have some type of arterial disease. Of patients with a gangrenous lesion of the feet requiring amputation, >50% are diabetic. Other associated risk factors include hypertension, high serum cholesterol, obesity, sedentary lifestyle, and strong family history.

Signs and symptoms: Intermittent claudication is the early sign of PVD. It is described as a painful cramping of the muscles of the leg during walking. It goes away when the patient stops walking and resumes after the patient starts walking again. It also may be described as a sensation of tiredness or fatigue. One third of patients with proven arterial stenosis report symptoms of claudication. Ischemic rest pain occurs constantly and is differentiated easily from claudication. It is described as a burning sensation and localizes to the metatarsal heads or to an ischemic ulcer. Pain is often worse at night when the leg is elevated. Relief is often dependency of the foot. Ischemic rest pain requires immediate attention. Ulceration or gangrene develops at an area of external pressure or at the sight of a minor injury. Gangrene is the end stage of PVD. Acute arterial ischemia results from arterial thrombosis, embolism, or trauma. Its symptoms are sudden in onset. It often causes the five *P*s: pain, pallor, pulselessness, paresthesia, and paralysis. Other signs include decreased sensation and mottling of the extremity. A thorough patient history and physical examination are essential to determining the stage of vascular disease.

Diagnostic tests:

Test	Results Indicating Disorder	CPT Code
ABI	Compares ankle blood pressure with arm pressure. In claudication, the ABI range is 0.50–0.75; ABI is 0.30–0.50 with rest pain and <0.30 in patients with gangrene	93922
Pulse volume recording	Pressure volumes are recorded waveforms examined for changes between various levels of the leg and between both legs	93922
Angiography	Accurate determination of occlusion but invasive and risky	75710–75790

ABI, ankle brachial index.

Differential diagnosis: Buerger's disease and Raynaud's phenomenon should be considered when diagnosing PVD. Buerger's disease often is found in men <35 years old who are smokers; it affects the upper and the lower extremities. Raynaud's phenomenon affects the fingertips, the tips of the ears and nose, and the feet. Patients with Raynaud's phenomenon tend to have cool hands and feet. Other diagnoses that mimic the symptoms of PVD include gout, arthritis, diabetic neuropathy, and venous insufficiency.

Treatment: The main goal of treatment is slowing the progression of the disease. Treatment may be conservative, pharmacological, operative, or endovascular.

Conservative Treatment

Conservative treatment involves modification of risk factors, including smoking. Smoking is the number one modifiable risk factor; numerous methods are available to help individuals stop smoking. In addition, managing diabetes, hypertension, and hyperlipidemia is key. Exercise is key to managing PVD. Collateral vessels are strengthened with the onset of an exercise program, mainly walking. Formalized vascular rehabilitation programs exist; however, they are not currently recognized by insurers and rarely are reimbursed. Home exercise programs should focus on exercising three or more times per week for 30 minutes per day. Patients should be instructed to walk until pain develops, then rest until pain goes away, then resume walking. Over time, the patient should be able to walk further with fewer rest breaks. Meticulous foot care is important to prevent complications of ulceration and gangrene. Patients should be instructed about wearing properly fitting footwear, daily inspection of feet and legs, walking barefoot, proper hygiene for feet and legs, and cutting toenails straight across.

Pharmacological Treatment

Pharmacological treatment is provided with conservative treatment. Currently, aspirin (81–325 mg daily) is frequently used. Aspirin has been shown to prevent progression of disease in patients with claudication. Pentoxifylline (Trental) is available for treatment of claudication; however, studies have not shown significant improvement in claudication symptoms. Vasodilators and anticoagulants have not proved effective in relieving pain symptoms. Clopidogrel (Plavix) (75 mg daily) is a new antiplatelet medication that helps to reduce the risk of stroke, heart attack, and other atherosclerotic problems. Medications for the management of hypertension, diabetes, and hyperlipidemia also may need to be considered.

Surgical Treatment

Surgical treatment of PVD involves revascularization of the affected extremity. Surgical options should be considered when pain limits the patient's lifestyle or there is ulceration or gangrene present. Surgical options involve using vein graft or synthetic graft material.

Endovascular Treatment

Endovascular options for the treatment of PVD include balloon angioplasty and endoluminal stents, which are minimally invasive for the patient. Angioplasty involves inflating a balloon across a stenotic lesion. Stents are devices that are deployed in a stenotic lesion to keep the vessel open.

Follow-up: Follow-up should include patient response to pharmacological intervention and progression of risk factor modification.

Sequelae: A history of intermittent claudication approximately doubles the risk of mortality resulting from ischemic heart disease. In patients with claudication, 1 out of 4 develop worsening symptoms, and 1 out of 20 require an amputation.

Prevention/prophylaxis: Prevention of PVD focuses on slowing the progression of disease in patients with symptoms. This can be accomplished through risk factor modification as discussed earlier. Good foot care can prevent the development of tissue loss or gangrene.

Referral: Referral for surgical or endovascular treatment should occur when claudication becomes disabling to the patient, when ischemic rest pain or gangrene is present, or when nonhealing ulceration is present.

Education: Education needs to focus on proper follow-up and the modification of risk factors as discussed earlier; patients need to be taught to report any new onset of symptoms, including nonhealing ulcers.

REFERENCES

General

Ernst, CB, and Stanley, JC: Current Therapy in Vascular Surgery, ed 4. Mosby, St. Louis, 2001.

Fahey, V: Vascular Nursing, ed 2. WB Saunders, Philadelphia, 1994.

Assessment

Jarvis, C: Physical Examination and Health Assessment. WB Saunders, Philadelphia, 1992. Woods, B: Clinical evaluation of the peripheral vasculature. Cardiol Clin 9:413, 1991.

Abdominal Aortic Aneurysm

Ahronheim, J: Handbook of Prescribing Medications for Geriatric Patients. Little, Brown, Toronto, 1992.

Anderson, LA: Abdominal aortic aneurysm. J Cardiovasc Nurs 15:1, 2001.

Carpenito, L: Nursing Diagnosis: An Application to Clinical Practice, ed 3. JB Lippincott, Philadelphia, 1989.

Friedman, S: Peripheral vascular diseases. In Abrams, W, and Berkow, R (eds): The Merck Manual of Geriatrics. Merck Sharp & Dohme Research Laboratories, Rahway, NJ, 1990.

Gadowski, G, et al: Abdominal aortic aneurysm expansion rate: Effect of size and beta adrenergic blockade. J Vasc Surg 19:727, 1994.

Ham, R, and Sloane, P: Primary Care Geriatrics: A Case-Based Approach. Mosby Year Book, St Louis, 1992.

Jones, C: Peripheral vascular disease and arterial aneurysms. In Barker, L, et al (eds): Principles of Ambulatory Medicine, ed 4. Williams & Wilkins, Baltimore, 1995, p 1298.

Kalinowski, H: Aortic stent grafting: A new approach to a deadly diagnosis: One hospital's findings in defining new care processes. Lippincott's Case Management 6:79, 2001.

MacSweeney, S, et al: Smoking and the growth of small abdominal aortic aneurysms. Lancet 344:651, 1994.

Meadors, F: Outpatient surveillance of abdominal aortic aneurysms. J Ark Med Soc 91:85, 1994.

Palec, D: Endovascular repair of abdominal aortic aneurysm: New technology is helping to save lives. Am J Nurs 101:24AA, 2001.

Sung, J, et al: Racial differences in mortality from cardiovascular disease in Atlanta, 1979–1985. J Natl Med Assoc 84:259, 1992.

Upton, C, and Graham, M: Clinical Guidelines in Adult Health. Barmarrae Books, Gainesville, Fla., 1993.

Woods, B: Clinical evaluation of the peripheral vasculature. Cardiol Clin 9:413, 1991.

Yoshikawa, T, et al: Ambulatory Geriatric Care. CV Mosby, St Louis, 1993.

Peripheral Vascular Disease

Ahronheim, J: Handbook of Prescribing Medications for Geriatric Patients. Little, Brown, Toronto, 1992.

Allen, SL: Perioperative nursing interventions for intravascular stent placements. AORN J 61:689, 1995.

CAPRIE Steering Committee: A randomised, blinded trial of clopidogrel versus aspirin in patients at risk of ischaemic events (CAPRIE). Lancet 348:1329, 1996.

Carpenito, L: Nursing Diagnosis: An Application to Clinical Practice, ed 3. JB Lippincott, Philadelphia, 1989.

Christman, SK, et al: Exercise training and smoking cessation as the cornerstones of managing claudication. J Cardiovasc Nurs 15:64, 2001.

Friedman, S: Peripheral vascular diseases. In Abrams, W, and Berkow, R (eds): The Merck Manual of Geriatrics. Merck Sharp & Dohme Research Laboratories, Rahway, NJ, 1990.

Ham, R, and Sloane, P: Primary Care Geriatrics: A Case-Based Approach. Mosby Year Book, St Louis, 1992.

Hiatt, WR: Drug therapy: Medical treatment of peripheral arterial disease and claudication. N Engl J Med 344:1608, 2001.

Jones, C: Peripheral vascular disease and arterial aneurysms. In Barker, L, et al (eds): Principles of Ambulatory Medicine, ed 4. Williams & Wilkins, Baltimore, 1995, p 1298.

Lewis, CD: Peripheral arterial disease of the lower extremity. J Cardiovasc Nurs 15:45, 2001.

Sung, J, et al: Racial differences in mortality from cardiovascular disease in Atlanta, 1979–1985. J Natl Med Assoc 84:259, 1992.

Uphold, C, and Graham, M: Clinical Guidelines in Adult Health. Barmarrae Books, Gainesville, Fla., 1993.

Woods, B: Clinical evaluation of the peripheral vasculature. Cardiol Clin 9:413, 1991.

Yoshikawa, T, et al: Ambulatory Geriatric Care. CV Mosby, St Louis, 1993.

Chapter 10

CENTRAL AND PERIPHERAL NERVOUS SYSTEM DISORDERS

ALZHEIMER'S DISEASE AND RELATED DISORDERS

SIGNAL SYMPTOMS ▶ amnesia, anomia, agnosia, apraxia

Alzheimer's disease (AD) AD	ICD-9 CM: 331.0 with behavioral disturbance (294.11) ICD-9 CM: 331.0 without behavioral disturbance (294.01)
Multi-infarct (cerebro- vascular) dementia	ICD-9 CM: 290.40 uncomplicated
Arteriosclerotic dementia	ICD-9 CM: 290.40 dementia with delirium
Cerebral atherosclerosis	ICD-9 CM: 437.0 (additional code is required)

Description: AD, a progressive neurodegenerative disease of the brain, ultimately results in significant dementia and dependence. The most common type of dementia, AD is defined by diminished cognitive function accompanied by affective and behavioral disturbances, manifested by memory loss and an inability to calculate and determine visuospatial orientation. AD is one of the leading contributing causes of death and premature institutionalization among older adults. Vascular dementia, including multi-infarct dementia, lacunar dementia, and Binswanger's disease, is the second most common type of dementia. Vascular dementias tend to have a more abrupt onset after multiple infarcts than AD. AD and vascular dementia may coexist.

Etiology: The cause of AD is unknown, and disease progression varies. AD is characterized by the presence of neurofibrillary tangles and neuritic plaques. The process of the neuron destruction is unknown. The degeneration of the neurons is believed to occur first in the hippocampus, spreading from there to other parts of the brain.

Occurrence: An estimated 10% of adults $\geq$65 years old have AD, increasing to 47% for adults >85 years old. An estimated 4 million Americans have from AD.

Age: The prevalence of AD increases with age. Onset can occur as early as the 40s. Binswanger's disease begins around age 50. The onset of multi-infarct dementia generally occurs between age 60 and 75.

Ethnicity: Not significant for AD. Vascular or multi-infarct dementia is responsible for 60% of dementia in the Asian population.

Gender: AD is twice as common in women as in men. Vascular dementia is more common in men.

Contributing factors: Family history of a first-degree relative with AD, genetic predisposition, and Down syndrome have been shown to increase the risk of developing AD. The presence of apolipoprotein E-e4, infrequent use of nonsteroidal anti-inflammatory drugs, little or no use of postmenopausal estrogen replacement, deficiency of antioxidant nutrients, history of head injury with loss of consciousness, and family history of Down syndrome also may increase the risk.

Risk factors for vascular dementia include history of hypertension, cardiovascular disease, smoking, diabetes mellitus, alcoholism, advancing age, hyperlipidemia, and history of transient ischemic attacks (TIAs) or cerebrovascular accidents (CVAs) or both. An inherited form of multi-infarct dementia is found in patients known to have cerebral autosomal dominant arteriopathy with subcortical infarcts and leukoencephalopathy.

Signs and symptoms: Patients or family members report difficulty with errors of judgment and subtle memory loss. The ability to comprehend, assimilate, and interpret new information is impaired, and attention to usual social amenities is decreased. In addition to the amnesia that occurs with AD, cognitive deficits noted early in AD include anomia (inability to name common objects), agnosia (an inability to recognize objects), and apraxia (inability to perform voluntary activities despite no objective weakness). Ask the patient and family if there has been a change in performance, difficulty with language, difficulty with orientation to time or place, or any personality or mood changes, including depression. Determine whether these occurrences have been gradual or sudden. Review all medications with the patient and family. A nutritional history is important to determine presence of nutritional deficiencies and malnutrition.

The *7-minute screen,* which consists of four tests that evaluate orientation, memory, clock drawing, and verbal fluency, can be used as an initial screening tool. One also can administer the Mini Mental Status Examination (MMSE) or other objective test of cognition to obtain baseline information. It is important to determine the patient's baseline functional status. The Functional Activities Questionnaire can be used to evaluate the patient's performance of 10 complex activities. The Hachinski Ischemic Scale can be used to differentiate between multi-infarct dementia and AD. A score of ≥ 7 on the scale suggests multi-infarct dementia; a score < 7 indicates AD.

Direct the physical examination toward looking for primary causes of dementia and determining if any coexisting conditions may be contributing to the patient's decline in mental or functional status. In the absence of concomitant disease processes, findings on the overall physical examination are usually normal. Pay particular attention to the vascular and neurological parts of the examination. In general, the cranial nerves, sensation, and motor function are intact. Special neurological examination techniques may elicit primitive reflexes, such as the palmar grasp reflex; the glabellar reflex, in which a patient with dementia continues to blink after the examiner has stopped tapping on the patient's forehead; and the plantar reflex. Patients with AD can lose the sense of taste and smell, so these senses should be evaluated. In the early stages of AD, the patient may have difficulty initiating ambulation. There may be some muscle rigidity as a result of increased muscle tone. For patients with suspected vascular dementia, it is important to evaluate for hypertension and diabetes.

Diagnostic tests: Selection of tests is not inclusive and is based on clinical judgment.

Test	Results Indicating Disorder	CPT Code
CBC	Rule out anemias, infection, and hemoglobinopathies	85031
Creatinine	Evaluate for kidney impairment	82565
Westergren (ESR)	Elevation indicates inflammatory process Elevation of ESR in older adults	85651
Blood urea nitrogen	Evaluate for kidney impairment	84520, 84525
Vitamin B_{12} (depending on CBC results)	Evaluate for vitamin B_{12} deficiency, which can contribute to neurological deficits	82607–82608
Folate (depending on CBC results)	Evaluate for folate deficiency, which can contribute to neurological deficits	82746
TSH	Assess for hypothyroidism or hyperthyroidism, which may cause changes in mental status	80418
HIV-1	AIDS dementia complex	87390
Urinalysis	Urinary tract infection	81000, 81001
Comprehensive metabolic profile	Assess for electrolyte and chemical abnormalities	80053
Toxicity screen for heavy metals	Chemical poisoning	83015
ECG	Arrhythmias	93000

Test	Results Indicating Disorder	CPT Code
Chest x-ray	Pneumonia	71010–71035
CT scan	Helpful in diagnosing masses or other space-occupying lesions	70450 (without contrast enhancement) 70470 (with and without contrast enhancement)
MRI	Preferred test for diagnosis of suspected brain tumor or bleeding in the brain	70551
EEG	Creutzfeldt-Jakob disease	95816
Lumbar puncture	Neurosyphilis or neoplastic meningitis	62270
VDRL	Test for syphilis if neurosyphilis is suspected	86592

CBC, complete blood count; ESR, erythrocyte sedimentation rate; TSH, thyroid-stimulating hormone; HIV-1, human immunodeficiency virus type 1; AIDS, acquired immunodeficiency syndrome; ECG, electrocardiogram; CT, computed tomography; MRI, magnetic resonance imaging; EEG, electroencephalography; VDRL, Venereal Disease Research Laboratory.

Differential diagnosis:

- Multi-infarct or vascular dementia: Neuroimaging reveals single or multiple strokes.
- Binswanger's disease: Neuroimaging shows increased prominent white matter ischemia.
- Lewy body dementia: The presence of the protein ubiquitin in the hippocampus differentiates Lewy body dementia from AD.
- Frontotemporal dementia: This generally occurs in patients <65 years old. Memory may remain intact, but the patient may exhibit the following behaviors: loses sexual inhibition, develops compulsive rituals, lacks spontaneous conversation.
- Dementia associated with Parkinson's disease: Graphic visual hallucinations are common. Generally the ability to perform high-level executive functions is more impaired than in AD.
- Pick's disease: Disinhibition and inappropriate sexual behavior are characteristic features early in the disease.
- Progressive supranuclear palsy: This presents with supranuclear gaze abnormality, facial spasticity, and axial rigidity.
- Metabolic, endocrine, and nutritional dementia.
- Dementia associated with long-term alcoholism.
- Early-stage depression: A screening instrument, such as the Geriatric Depression Scale, should be administered.
- Creutzfeldt-Jakob disease: This presents as a rapid progressive syndrome of mental deterioration, lead pipe rigidity, myoclonus, aphasia, apraxia, and hallucinations. EEG is diagnostic of Creutzfeldt-Jakob disease.

- Cerebral tumors: Tumors can be ruled out by CT or MRI.
- Subdural hematoma: Persistent headache after trauma with poorly defined intellectual impairment may be ruled out by CT or MRI.
- Head injuries.
- Encephalitis: This may be ruled out with a lumbar puncture.
- Syphilis and neurosyphilis: Neurosyphilis may occur at any time during an infection, up to 35 years later. Diagnosis is based on cerebrospinal fluid abnormalities and a reactive serological test for syphilis.
- AIDS: AIDS dementia is characterized by excessive preoccupation with certain topics, slow thought process, and progressive cognitive decline. Laboratory studies confirm diagnosis of AIDS.
- Normal pressure hydrocephalus: This condition often presents with dementia, gain disturbances, and incontinence of bladder or bowel. Neuroimaging is diagnostic for normal pressure hydrocephalus.
- Heavy metal exposure, pollutants, drugs, alcohol, and carbon monoxide: Toxicology reports indicate chemical exposure.

Treatment:

Behavioral

Treatment of AD consists of first optimizing the patient's environment by maintaining safety and consistency, fostering or preserving independence with activities of daily living (ADLs), and minimizing restraint for behaviors that do not represent a danger to the patient or others. Any behavioral change requires medical evaluation to address the intervening illness.

Pharmacological

Pharmacological treatment for patients with AD is not curative. The cholinesterase inhibitor donepezil has been shown to delay cognitive decline. Initial starting dosage is 5 mg daily before bedtime. Patients can be re-evaluated 4 to 6 weeks after starting initial dosage to determine efficacy, presence of side effects, and whether an increase to 10 mg/day is warranted; dosage should not be increased before the initial trial period. Rivastigmine is another cholinesterase inhibitor. This drug should be taken with food. Initial dosage is 1.5 mg twice daily. Dosage may be increased at 2-week intervals to 3 mg, then 4.5 mg, to a maximum dose of 6 mg twice daily. A liquid solution of rivastigmine is also available. Galantamine, another reversible cholinesterase inhibitor, is used to treat mild-to-moderate AD. Dosage should begin at 4 mg twice daily with morning and evening meals. The dose may increase gradually at 4-week intervals to 8 mg twice daily, then to a maximum of 12 mg twice daily. It is important to start low and increase the dosage gradually as needed to avoid adverse effects. Some clinicians support the benefit of patients with

AD taking vitamin E. The use of ginkgo biloba has been refuted as beneficial in the treatment of dementia.

Preliminary findings (Erkinjuntti, et al, 2002) indicate that patients with vascular dementia benefited from taking galantamine. Treatment for vascular dementia traditionally has focused on controlling the contributing conditions, such as diabetes, hypertension, and hyperlipidemia. Smoking cessation and reduction of alcohol consumption should be discussed with the patient and caregivers of patients with vascular dementia.

Management of the behavioral symptoms of dementia, such as aggression, delusions, hallucinations, depression, and verbal outbreaks, need additional pharmacological and nonpharmacological interventions depending on the individual and any concomitant conditions. Options for treating dementia patients with behavioral symptoms include atypical antipsychotics, trazodone, selective serotonin reuptake inhibitors, and buspirone. Memantine, an antiglutamatergic, has been shown to reduce clinical deterioration in patients with moderate to severe Alzheimer's disease.

Follow-up: Patients should be seen every 3 to 6 months from the time of diagnosis of AD, depending partly on the patient's physical, mental, and emotional status. At follow-up appointments, the patient's competence to drive (if applicable) and to manage household responsibilities and finances should be assessed. Determine efficacy of pharmacological interventions; evaluate for evidence or decline in overall level of functioning and if any side effects are present from the medications. Periodic re-evaluation of mental status, ADLs, and instrumental ADLs is recommended. An annual decrease of four points in the MMSE is expected in a patient with AD. Determine whether patient is having episodes of aggression, sleep disturbances, wandering, communication difficulties, depression, or failure to recognize familiar surroundings or family members.

At each follow-up visit, review the patient's diet, monitor the patient for weight loss, and obtain a history of change in continence of bowel and bladder. A rectal examination is performed to determine the competency of the internal and external sphincters and to test for occult blood. All concurrent medical illnesses should be managed to avoid further compromising the patient's cognitive function. Dehydration; infection; anemia; and respiratory, cardiovascular, and endocrine disorders should be treated to maintain the patient's quality of life. Determine the current ability of family members to provide care for the patient with dementia if he or she is residing at home. Family members should be informed of the prognosis of the disease to make plans for the environment, estate, and caregiving needs.

Sequelae: Survival for patients with AD has been estimated to be 2 to 20 years from time of diagnosis. The numerous complications that can arise in the patient with AD have been categorized as behavioral, psychiatric, and metabolic. Patients can exhibit behavioral and psychiatric changes throughout the course of the disease. Depression and anxiety may develop early in the disease. Hostility, wandering, and agitation may occur at a later stage. The sudden onset of a behavioral or psychiatric change may indicate an underlying infection or metabolic disturbance. Some patients experience evening confusion or sundowning. Ambulatory patients with AD are at risk for sustaining injuries such as falls, burns, or accidental poisoning. In the final stages of AD, patients are unable to communicate verbally or ambulate. Bowel and bladder incontinence occurs, and patients may be unable to swallow and eat. These patients are at risk for malnutrition, aspiration pneumonia, and decubitus ulcers. Death occurs usually from an unresolved infection. Patients with vascular dementias tend to decline more rapidly than patients with AD; often the cause of death is related to myocardial infarction or CVA.

Prevention/prophylaxis: No primary prevention measures are known for AD; prevention measures for patients who already have AD include providing a safe environment with a consistent structure and routine. Regular intake of antioxidant nutrients as a means of reducing cognitive decline in age is currently being examined. The risk factors for vascular dementias for the most part are controllable; careful management of cardiac disease, diabetes, hypertension, and hyperlipidemia is crucial for the prevention of further strokes. A healthy diet, exercise, and reduction of alcohol and smoking are highly recommended.

Referral: After reversible causes of dementia have been excluded, patients with abnormal mental status examination findings but without functional changes or vice versa should have further neuropsychological testing. Patients who are not responding to medications, who are experiencing symptoms of paranoia or psychosis, who have complex comorbidity, and who have severe impairment also may be referred for specialist management. The National Alzheimer's Association can be contacted at 1-800-272-3900 and www.alz.org. Families can ask for information about programs closest to their area; every state has at least one local chapter. The national office is located at 919 North Michigan Avenue, Chicago, IL 60611.

Education: In the early stages of AD and related disorders, the patient and the family need to be provided with information on how to create a safe, nonthreatening environment for the patient. Reminder aids and reinforcing cues, such as large signs and calendars, can help patients maintain orientation.

When AD is diagnosed early, patients and family members have time to plan household responsibility management, retirement from the work force, and resolution of transportation issues. As the disease progresses, the family should consider acquiring special identification cards and bracelet for the patient, especially if wandering has become problematic. For additional information, encourage the family to contact The

Alzheimer's Disease Education and Referral Center, PO Box 8250, Silver Spring, MD 20907; the telephone number is 1-800-438-4380 and the web site is www.alzheimers.org/adear.

BRAIN TUMOR

SIGNAL SYMPTOMS▶ severe morning headaches, headache with vomiting not associated with nausea, focal seizures

Brain tumor (benign)	ICD-9 CM: 225
Brain tumor (unspecified)	ICD-9 CM: 239.2

Description: A brain tumor is a malignant or benign neoplasm of the brain or its supportive structures, which may arise from glial cells, blood vessels, connective tissue, meninges, pituitary, or pineal glands. The most common primary brain tumor in adults is glial neoplasm, which arises from the astrocytes. Other types of primary brain tumors include oligodendroglioma, arising from the oligodendrocytes; central nervous system (CNS) lymphoma, from lymphocytes; meningioma, from the meninges; ganglioma, from the neurons; and ependymoma from the ependyma.

Etiology: The etiology of brain tumor is largely unknown. Some hereditary syndromes exist.

Occurrence: Since 1984, there has been a 50% increase in the incidence of primary brain tumors. Approximately 17,000 new cases of brain and other nervous system cancers were diagnosed in the United States in 2002. The incidence among elders 65 to 79 years old is 18 cases per 100,000. Brain tumors occur most commonly in children <15 years old and in adults in their 50s and 60s. Gliomas account for 65% of brain tumors seen in adults; pituitary adenoma, acoustic neuroma, and meningiomas also occur in adults but almost never in children. The incidence of CNS lymphoma among adults is increasing.

Ethnicity: Not significant.

Gender: Brain tumors occur equally among males and females.

Contributing factors: There is no proven association between environmental factors and primary brain tumors except that of vinyl chloride exposure and gliomas. Some association does exist between Epstein-Barr virus and CNS lymphoma. The increase in CNS lymphoma also is associated with AIDS. Prior radiation and chemotherapy are associated with brain tumors.

Signs and symptoms: Constant or paroxysmal headaches may be due to tumor infiltration of nervous tissue, displacement of brain structures by tumor mass, or increased intracranial pressure. These headaches tend to be more severe in the morning, when upright, and with position changes. They may be relieved by analgesics and rarely interfere with sleep.

Clinical Pearl: Headaches related to brain tumors are *usually holocephalic* and may be accompanied by vomiting, which is often *not preceded* by nausea.

Brain tumor should be part of the differential diagnosis for any headaches of recent onset, headaches differing from the patient's usual pattern of headaches, or headaches accompanied by a migraine-like aura that persists after the pain is gone. Nausea, appetite changes, and hiccups occur less frequently.

Partial motor, sensory, or grand mal seizures occur in 20% to 30% of patients with brain tumors. New-onset focal seizures in individuals >40 years old are suspicious for brain tumor until proved otherwise. Psychomotor function may slow down in patients with primary brain tumors. Personality changes may be marked or subtle, including changes in mood, concentration, and intellectual functions.

Focal neurological changes are related to the area of the brain invaded by tumor. Frontal and parietal lobe tumors may cause changes in memory, behavior, and cognitive function. Memory, hearing, vision, and emotions are affected most often by temporal lobe tumors. Symptoms of temporal lobe tumors may mimic symptoms of affective or psychotic thought disorders. Visual changes can occur with occipital lobe tumors, in addition to speech, motor, and sensory changes for left-sided occipital masses and an inability to grasp abstract concepts for right-sided occipital masses. Lesions in the cerebellum affect balance and coordination. Pituitary tumors may present with the symptoms of hypothyroidism, hypercortisolism, diabetes insipidus, or visual changes (Fig. 10–1).

Diagnostic tests:

Test	Results Indicating Disorder	CPT Code
CBC	Assesses for anemia or infection	85031
Westergren ESR	Elevation indicates an inflammatory process. Elevations of ESR in older adults can occur in the absence of inflammation	85651
TSH	Assesses for hypothyroidism or hyperthyroidism, which may cause changes in mental status	84443
VDRL	Test for syphilis if neurosyphilis is suspected	86592
Comprehensive metabolic profile	Assess for electrolyte and chemical abnormalities	80053
CT scan	Helpful in diagnosing masses in the brain or space-occupying lesions	70470 (with or without contrast enhancement) 70450 (without contrast for patients with a history of allergy to contrast dye)
MRI	Preferred test for diagnosis of suspected brain tumor or bleeding	70551

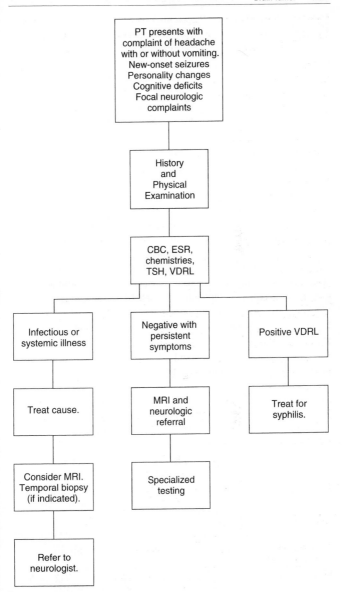

Figure 10–1. Brain tumor.

A careful history of symptoms is invaluable. Complete physical examination should include skin survey for stigmata of neurocutaneous syndromes or melanoma, lymph node examination, abdominal examination for hepatomegaly or splenomegaly, and rectal examination with guaiac stool testing. Breast and pelvic examination in women and cardiopulmonary examination are recommended. The neurological evaluation should include a mental status evaluation, testing for cognitive deficits or memory loss, and assessment for personality changes. Family members may be able to provide clues about subtle personality changes. Ophthalmic examination is essential to assess for papilledema, although this may not be present in patients 55 years old and older. Test also for asymmetry of strength, sensation, visual fields, reflex activity, cranial nerve function, and radicular signs.

Laboratory studies should include CBC, ESR, blood chemistry analyses, TSH levels, and VDRL to rule out infectious, inflammatory, or systemic illnesses. MRI of the brain, with or without contrast enhancement, is the recommended diagnostic examination for suspected brain tumor. CT scan with contrast enhancement is acceptable in special circumstances, such as when a patient is uncooperative or when MRI is unavailable. Positron emission tomography is not used to diagnose tumors of the CNS but may have an ancillary role after treatment. Specialized testing that may be ordered by a neurologist/neurosurgeon. EEG is useful for evaluating possible seizure activity. Lumbar puncture should not be performed before MRI or CT scan because of the potential for fatal brain herniation to result. Lumbar puncture can yield pressure readings and fluid for cytology, protein, glucose, and tumor markers. Also testing blood for tumor markers, α-fetoprotein, or β-human chorionic gonadotropin is useful for the diagnosis of some brain tumors. Histological examination of a biopsy specimen of brain tissue may be required.

Differential diagnosis:

- CVA: There is acute onset of headache with persistent focal neurological deficits for >24 hours. CT or MRI is diagnostic.
- Aneurysm: In acute rupture, there is a sudden intense headache, often with signs of meningeal irritation. MRI is preferred for diagnosis.
- Arteriovenous malformation: There is chronic unilateral throbbing headache with no prodromal or associated symptoms. CT or MRI may be diagnostic.
- Meningitis: Headache usually is associated with fever and nuchal rigidity. Cerebrospinal fluid is obtained through a lumbar puncture for diagnosis.
- Abscess: This often is associated with fever or other signs of infection.

- Syphilis: Neurosyphilis may occur at any time during infection, up to 35 years later. Symptoms vary according to the area infected. Diagnosis is based on cerebrospinal fluid abnormalities and a reactive serological test for syphilis.
- HIV: Various neurological manifestations can be caused by the virus or opportunistic infections; the incidence of CNS lymphoma is increasing in these patients.
- Subdural hematoma: Persistent headache occurs after trauma, with poorly defined intellectual impairment. This may be ruled out by CT or MRI.
- Postconcussion syndrome: A dull, constant headache occurs within 24 hours of trauma. The patient may complain of loss of concentration, giddiness, irritability, and anxiety.
- Trauma: History of injury to the head or neck is present.
- Temporal arteritis: This usually is characterized by a slow-onset headache that is worse at night, temporal in more than half of patients, often with jaw claudication and temporal artery tenderness, and elevated ESR.
- Normal pressure hydrocephalus: This condition often presents with dementia, gait disturbances, and incontinence of bladder or bowel.
- Multi-infarct dementia: This may present with impaired cognition and symptoms of upper motor neuron disease in patients with a history of hypertension, atrial fibrillation, diabetes, carotid artery disease, or history of smoking.
- AD: This presents with progressive dementia, memory disturbances, and behavior changes.
- Chemical poisoning: History of exposure to chemicals, such as carbon monoxide, pesticides, or industrial materials, is present.
- Migraine: Migraine is characterized by an often-unilateral headache with a pulsating quality, associated with nausea and vomiting, photophobia, or phonophobia; prodromal or aura symptoms may be present.

Treatment: Treatment of brain tumor includes surgery, radiation, chemotherapy, glucocorticoids, anticonvulsants, immunotherapy, and gene therapy.

Follow-up: Prognosis depends on the tumor type, age, functional neurological status, extent of resection, tumor location, and extent of metastasis at diagnosis. During the first year after treatment, the patient should have a focused history and physical examination, including a neurological and funduscopic examination every 3 months. MRI of the head is recommended at the same intervals during the first year. The patient should be seen every 6 months during years 2 through 5, with yearly MRI. Patients receiving palliative care should be seen as necessary for pain and symptom control; hospice care is recommended for these patients.

Sequelae: Various neurological deficits, personality changes, seizure disorders, and chronic head pain can result from brain tumor. Paraplegia, hemiplegia, and quadriplegia are also consequences of brain tumor. Bradycardia, hypertension, and respiratory arrest can occur with increased intracranial pressure. Brain herniation is a life-threatening emergent complication.

Prevention/prophylaxis: Instruct patients to avoid radiation exposure.

Referral: Refer patients to a neurosurgeon, oncologist, radiation oncologist, and hospice, as appropriate.

Education: Genetic counseling is warranted in hereditary syndromes of brain tumor.

CEREBROVASCULAR ACCIDENT (STROKE)

SIGNAL SYMPTOMS▶ weakness, paralysis, aphasia

Cerebrovascular accident	ICD-9 CM: 436

Description: A CVA, or stroke, occurs when a disruption in blood flow to the brain leads to brain tissue ischemia and infarction. The consequent impairment depends on the location and extent of the infarction.

Etiology: There are two major types of strokes: ischemic, indicating blockage of an artery, and hemorrhagic, usually resulting from a tear in an artery wall. *Ischemic* events account for approximately 80% of all strokes and generally are classified as one of three types: thrombotic, embolic, or lacunar. Thrombotic strokes occur when an artery in the brain is blocked by a blood clot that forms as a result of an inflammatory response to an unstable atherosclerotic plaque. Embolic strokes occur when a blood clot forms elsewhere and becomes lodged in a brain artery. Embolic strokes are associated with atrial fibrillation, valvular disorders, and heart failure. Lacunar infarcts are a subtype of thrombotic strokes that occur in the smaller arteries that branch from main cerebral arteries.

Hemorrhagic strokes result from trauma or a hypertensive episode when a weakened area of an artery in or around the brain ruptures. Arteriovenous malformations also may cause hemorrhagic strokes.

Occurrence: CVA (or stroke) is the leading neurological cause of death and disability in the United States, affecting an estimated 500,000 to 750,000 people each year.

Age: Stroke occurs mostly in persons >65 years old; the incidence increases exponentially with advancing age. Approximately 28% of strokes occur in persons <65 years old.

Ethnicity: Native Americans, Hispanics, and African-Americans are at higher risk for stroke and stroke mortality than whites. Among middle-aged adults, African-Americans are two to three more times likely to have a stroke than their white peers.

Gender: CVA incidence seems to be more prevalent in men than women, but women have a higher likelihood of stroke mortality.

Geography: People in the southeastern United States have been reported to have a higher risk of stroke over the past several years, but the stroke risk may be shifting westward. Socioeconomic differences do not fully explain these higher risk areas.

Contributing factors: Risk factors for stroke include advanced age, family history of stroke, prior history of TIA, hypertension, diabetes, carotid stenosis, atrial fibrillation, hyperlipidemia, heart disease, sedentary lifestyle, smoking, alcohol abuse, obesity, and some infections (respiratory tract, periodontal disease). Additional risk factors include sleep apnea, antiphospholipid antibody, hyperhomocystinemia, drug abuse, hypercoagulability disorders, hormone replacement therapy or oral contraceptive use, sickle cell anemia, and other inflammatory processes.

Signs and symptoms: History may indicate a prior TIA. Patients having an ischemic stroke may report any of the following symptoms, usually with a sudden onset: weakness, numbness, or paralysis in the face, arm, or leg (usually unilateral); difficulty speaking or understanding verbal communication; blurred or decreased monocular or binocular vision; loss of balance or coordination; and severe headache. Patients with a hemorrhagic stroke may report any of the aforementioned symptoms and nausea and vomiting, altered mental status, sensitivity to light, and neck stiffness.

Physical signs may include one or more of the following: decreased visual acuity or field cut; diplopia; slurred speech; and hemiparesis or sensory changes of the face, arm, or leg. A decrease in coordination or balance can occur. Acute confusional state and elevated blood pressure are also common. Any other focal signs on neurological examination should be assessed carefully. Physical examination should include repeated measures of vital signs and examination of the head and neck for signs of trauma and infection, checks of the peripheral and carotid pulses, auscultation of the neck for bruits, and a complete neurological examination for focal abnormalities (Fig. 10–2).

Diagnostic tests: Selection of tests is not inclusive and is based on clinical judgment.

Test	Results Indicating Disorder	CPT Code
CBC	Anemias, hemoglobinopathies	85031
PT PTT	Coagulopathies	85610–85611 (PT) 85730–85732 (PTT)

(Continued on page 365)

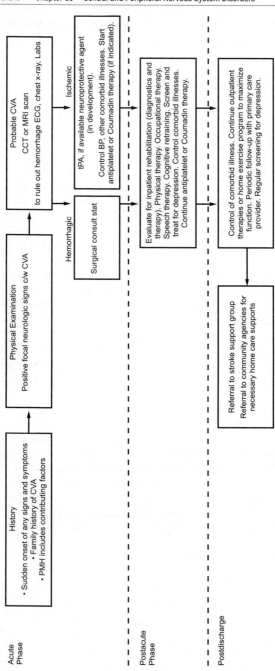

Figure 10–2. Cerebrovascular accident.

Test	Results Indicating Disorder	CPT Code
Blood chemistries, including calcium, phosphorus, creatinine, and electrolyte levels	Serum calcium and phosphate is normal in osteoporosis Alkaline phosphatase may be elevated if there is a fracture	80048 (basic metabolic panel) 84075 (alkaline phosphatase)
Glutamate	Indicates neuronal cell damage	82965
Serum blood glucose	Hypoglycemia or hyperglycemia	82847
ECG	Arrhythmias	93000
Holter monitor	Arrhythmias	93224, 93235
Carotid duplex studies	Reveal extracranial carotid disease	93880, 93882
Magnetic resonance angiography	Stenosis in extracranial or intracranial cerebral arteries	70544, 70546
MRI	Early infarction, hemorrhage	70551–70553
CT scan	Infarction (after 48 hours), hemorrhage	70450 (without contrast enhancement)
Arteriography	Gold standard to evaluate the condition of cerebral arteries	75600–75630

PT, prothrombin time; PTT, partial thromboplastin time.

Laboratory tests should include an ECG with cardiac monitoring for arrhythmia, echocardiogram, pulse oximetry, chest x-ray, CBC, platelet count, PT, PTT, serum electrolytes, glutamate level, and blood glucose level. Inflammatory markers also may indicate stroke (C-reactive protein, troponins, and ESR).

A head CT scan reveals 95% of hemorrhagic strokes immediately. Ischemic events may not be visible on CT scan for 24 to 48 hours and may be noted anywhere in the cerebral cortex, cerebellum, or brainstem. MRI is helpful in early diagnosis of ischemic or hemorrhagic strokes but may not be available in rural areas. Magnetic resonance angiography is a non-invasive method of showing vascular occlusion in the head or neck. If a hemorrhagic stroke is confirmed, the patient should be referred to a neurosurgeon immediately. Several alternative types of imaging techniques can identify more precisely the location and volume of infarct, but many are not yet widely available.

Differential diagnosis:

- Temporal arteritis: This condition is ruled out based on history, physical examination, ultrasound of temporal arteries, and laboratory tests (elevated ESR, alkaline phosphatase) if indicated.
- Vertebral disc disease: This condition is ruled out based on history, physical examination, and x-rays as indicated.
- Migraine: This is ruled out based on history and physical examination.

- Head trauma: Trauma is ruled out based on history, physical examination, and brain imaging studies as indicated.
- Brain tumor: Tumor is ruled out based on history, physical examination, and brain imaging studies as indicated.
- Meningeal infection: This is ruled out based on history, physical examination, and lumbar puncture if indicated.

Treatment: Emergency transport should be initiated for patients with suspected stroke.

Patients should be made NPO (given nothing by mouth), and intravenous fluids should be started to maintain euvolemic status in most patients. Patient with fever may be treated with antipyretics, and an aggressive search for the source of fever should be initiated. Careful use of analgesics for headache is appropriate. Hypertension associated with stroke usually resolves spontaneously over the first 24 hours; aggressive use of antihypertensives may reduce cerebral perfusion further. If the stroke is hemorrhagic, elevated blood pressures >200 mm Hg systolic and >100 mm Hg diastolic should be treated. In the presence of ischemic stroke, blood pressure should be reduced if systolic blood pressure is >220 mm Hg or diastolic blood pressure is >110 mm Hg on repeated measurements made over 30 to 60 minutes; if cardiac ischemia, heart failure, and aortic dissection have been identified; or if thrombolytic therapy is used.

If the patient presents within 3 hours of the onset of symptoms and a hemorrhagic event is ruled out, intravenous tissue plasminogen activator (tPA), a thrombolytic agent, may minimize the size of the infarct. Patients taking aspirin are eligible for tPA treatment; patients taking warfarin or heparin should not be considered for tPA. After 3 hours, anticoagulants (heparin) may be used for patients with a suspected cardioembolic source or documented large vessel stenosis. If selected, heparin should be given without a bolus and titrated to a PTT 1.5 to 2.0 times control. If tPA and heparin are contraindicated, antiplatelet agents (aspirin 50–325 mg) have been shown to improve functional outcome if started within 48 hours after symptom onset. Hemorrhagic events should be referred for neurosurgical consultation. Control of any other comorbid disease also is indicated. Patients should be monitored for signs of cerebral edema.

Follow-up: Indications for follow-up depend on the type and extent of the infarct. Referral to inpatient rehabilitation usually is indicated for individualized therapy: physical, occupational, speech, or cognitive retraining with the focus on restoring optimal levels of function. After a stroke, patients should be followed regularly by a primary care provider to assess periodically changes in level of function and to control for comorbid illnesses.

Sequelae: Stroke survivors are most commonly at high risk for complications related to immobility, such as skin breakdown, loss of muscle strength, and pulmonary compromise. Speech and swallowing difficulties also may persist after a stroke. Depression and anxiety are also common consequences of stroke. Patients are at highest risk for these problems during the first 2 years after stroke; however, because they may occur at any time, screen patients for depression regularly and treat as indicated. Monitor the physical and emotional well-being of patients and families. Finally, all stroke survivors are at risk for recurrent stroke and other cardiovascular events. Appropriate strategies should be implemented for prevention/prophylaxis.

Prevention/prophylaxis: Strategies to prevent stroke are similar to strategies used to prevent other cardiovascular diseases. Control hypertension, diabetes, hyperlipidemia, and cardiac disease through lifestyle and pharmacotherapeutic agents. Encourage patients to increase physical activity levels, lose weight, and stop smoking. Prophylactic treatment with antiplatelet agents is recommended for patients with prior TIA or stroke and/or identified carotid disease unless otherwise contraindicated. Many clinicians now utilize combinations of antiplatelet agents to inhibit platelet aggregation at multiple points on the clotting cascade. Prophylactic warfarin therapy is recommended in patients with known arrhythmias or hypercoagulation states, but the international normalized ratio (INR) must be monitored regularly and kept within the range of 2.0 to 3.0. Carotid endarterectomy may be considered for stenosis >50%.

Referral: Referrals depend on the type and severity of impairment from the stroke and the influence of any comorbid illnesses. Referrals to physiatry (rehabilitation medicine), neurology, psychiatry, and cardiology for consultation are common.

Education: Education for patients after a stroke should emphasize cause of the stroke, limitation of risk factors to prevent future events, and early identification and treatment of recurrent stroke. A home exercise program or other therapies to maintain or improve functional levels should be introduced. Exercise has been shown to improve functionality many years after the index stroke. Access to support groups for patients and caregivers should be provided. Patients should be taught the importance of periodic follow-up with the primary care provider. The National Stroke Association can be contacted at www.stroke.org and 1-800-STROKES (1-800-787-6537).

PARKINSON'S DISEASE

SIGNAL SYMPTOMS▶ resting tremor, rigidity, bradykinesia

Parkinson's disease: idiopathic primary	ICD-9 CM: 332.0
Parkinson's disease: secondary	ICD-9 CM: 332.1

Description: Parkinson's disease, a gradually degenerative condition, results in a loss of melanin-containing dopaminergic nerve cells in the substantia nigra and a progressive loss of the inhibitory neurotransmitter dopamine. The imbalance between dopamine and acetylcholine is primarily responsible for an overall worsening of symptoms leading to immobility and debilitation. The cardinal features of Parkinson's disease include resting tremor, rigidity, bradykinesia, and gait disturbances. Before clinical features become evident, 60% to 80% of the substantia nigra neurons and striatal dopamine must be lost. Subtle motor impairment may precede by many years the development of overt clinical signs and symptoms.

Etiology: The cause of idiopathic primary Parkinson's disease is unknown. Secondary Parkinson's disease (Parkinson's syndrome) may be caused by toxins; drugs; and other conditions, such as head trauma, encephalitis, Shy-Drager syndrome, progressive supranuclear palsy, hypoparathyroidism, and Wilson's disease.

Occurrence: Approximately 1% of the population (100 to 150 cases in 100,000) are diagnosed with Parkinson's disease.

Age: Parkinson's disease is found predominantly in older adults beginning at age 55 to 69; however, 15% of newly diagnosed cases occur in persons <49 years old.

Ethnicity: Parkinson's disease can be found in all cultures; however, it is less prevalent in African-Americans in the United States and in the Japanese than in the general population.

Gender: The ratio of Parkinson's disease in men and women is 1.4:1, indicating an almost-equal prevalence in gender.

Contributing factors: Some evidence exists linking environmental toxins, viral infections, and a possible genetic tendency to the development of Parkinson's disease.

Signs and symptoms: An initial clinical symptom of Parkinson's disease is a resting tremor, often initially unilateral, that disappears with movement. Tremor also is noted in the lips, chin, and tongue. Patients may make a motion of the thumb and forefinger known as pill rolling. Although common, tremor is not present in every patient with Parkinson's disease. Rigidity, as shown by increased resistance to passive range of motion, is a classic sign. Cogwheel rigidity can be noted in the wrists and elbows. Patients experience a slowing of movements called *bradykinesia*. Patients also report having difficulty initiating movement. Autonomic movements, such as the normal pattern of arm swinging during ambulation, are decreased.

Other associated manifestations include masked facial expression, decreased blinking, and delayed ability to show facial expressions. Patients also experience an associated softening of the voice, hypophonia, and drooling. The size of the patient's handwriting often changes (micrographia). Flexed posture is common, with a bowed head, kyphotic back, and a trunk that leans forward. The gait may become faster, with the body propelled forward (festination). Ask the patient about associated presentations, such as constipation, seborrhea, myalgia, impotence, and urinary incontinence. Depression is common in Parkinson's disease (>50% of patients may experience depression). Dementia may occur with or without associated AD involvement in 20% to 30% of people with Parkinson's disease. Patients and family members may report mood swings, hallucinations, and insomnia.

Clinical examination should begin with observation of the patient's stature to note any kyphosis and bending of the head forward. Have the patient ambulate and observe the gait, including arm swing. Test the patient for postural instability while the patient is standing, by gently pushing the patient forward and then backward and noting whether the postural reflexes are absent. Check the patient's ocular movements; impairment of upward or downward gaze is common in progressive supranuclear palsy and not in Parkinson's disease. Examine the patient's upper and lower extremities. Test for range of motion and strength, noting any cogwheel rigidity. Strength generally does not deteriorate despite the rigidity. Tendon reflexes are almost always normal. To test for tremor, have the patient rest the arms on the legs while seated. Note the frequency and amplitude of the tremor. The patient's blood pressure should be checked on every visit because hypotension is common in patients with Parkinson's disease. An orthostatic blood pressure check with the patient lying and standing is recommended at each examination. The presence of two cardinal signs—bradykinesia and resting tremor, rigidity, or postural instability—is crucial to establishing the diagnosis of Parkinson's disease.

Diagnostic tests:

Test	Results Indicating Disorder	CPT Code
MRI	Rule out suspected brain lesions or abnormalities such as normal pressure hydrocephalus	70551–70553
Positron emission tomography	Generally ordered before surgery	78608

No histologic markers can establish the diagnosis of Parkinson's disease. MRI may be ordered by a neurologist to rule out suspected brain lesions or abnormalities such as normal pressure hydrocephalus.

Differential diagnosis:

- Drug-induced parkinsonism: This is confirmed by withdrawal of suspected medication, such as neuroleptics and metoclopramide.
- Cortical basal ganglionic degeneration: This is distinguished by unilateral coarse tremor, ideomotor ataxia limb dystonia, and lack of response to levodopa.

- Essential (benign familial) tremor: Tremor is an action tremo 6 to 8 Hz compared with Parkinson's disease tremor, which is 3 to 6 Hz.
- Huntington's disease: This disorder is genetic in origin and characterized by chorea, clumsiness, and cognitive decline.
- Shy-Drager syndrome: This syndrome is distinguished by early and prominent autonomic nervous system dysfunction and poor response to dopamine.
- Progressive supranuclear palsy: Supranuclear gaze abnormality, facial spasticity, and axial rigidity are present; tremor is usually absent.
- Creutzfeldt-Jakob disease: This is a rapidly progressive syndrome of mental deterioration, lead pipe rigidity, myoclonus, aphasia, apraxia, and hallucinations.
- Normal pressure hydrocephalus: Gait apraxia, urinary incontinence, and dementia are present.
- Striatal nigral degeneration: Autonomic dysfunction and dystonia are present.
- Olivopontocerebellar atrophy: This condition is distinguished by inherited parkinsonism, progressive ataxia, dementia, difficulty with balance, and dysarthria.
- Multisystem atrophy: This includes olivopontocerebellar atrophy , striatal nigral degeneration, and Shy-Drager syndrome.
- Depression: Depression may be present in the early stages of Parkinson's disease.

Treatment: Drug therapy focuses on correcting the imbalance of dopamine and acetylcholine. Patients with mild disease with no interference with ADLs may not require treatment. When tremors and rigidity cause impairment of the patient's ability to perform ADLs, and disability level is mild to moderate, treatment may include amantadine, which is thought to augment dopamine release from presynaptic nerve terminals or to inhibit dopamine reuptake. Initial dose is usually 100 mg with breakfast. In 5 to 7 days, add amantadine,100 mg with lunch, then increase daily dose to 300 mg.

Patients with severe disability may require carbidopa and levodopa therapy alone to replenish the depleted dopamine in the brain by increasing the dopamine precursor levodopa to stimulate dopamine receptors. Carbidopa and levodopa can be started using Sinemet 25/100 (carbidopa 25 mg, levodopa 100 mg), 2 tablets once a day. The dosage can be increased by 2 tablets every 3 to 5 days until the total daily dosage is 3 doses of 2 tablets of Sinemet 25/100. Dopamine agonists include ropinirole, 0.25 mg three times daily; pergolide mesylate, 0.05 to 0.25 mg three times daily; and pramipexole, 0.125 mg three times daily. The catechol-*O*-methyltransferase inhibitors, entacapone, 200 mg with each dose of levodopa or 1600 mg daily, and Tolcapone, 100 mg three times daily (check liver function), are always used with levodopa. Blocking the 3-O-methylation of levodopa prolongs the actions of the levodopa dose. When the dosage of levodopa reaches 600 to 1000 mg (1 g) per day, an adjunct medication is recommended. Large doses of levodopa over time can contribute to the on-off phenomena and involuntary movements. The agonists may be used alone or may be used to extend the usefulness of levodopa, without increasing the dose.

Selegiline, a monoamine oxidase-B inhibitor, inhibits the enzyme responsible for inactivating dopamine. Adding selegiline, 5 mg/day (increasing to 10 mg/day within 1 week), can improve the wearing-off effect of levodopa. Deep brain stimulation has been approved for treatment of Parkinson symptoms in the United States. Stimulation of the thalamus is used for tremor-predominant Parkinson's disease, and stimulation of the globus pallidum and subthalamic nucleus is for bradykinesia, akinesia, dyskinesia and rigidity.

Follow-up: Ask the patient if any medications seem to be wearing off or if they have had any falls.

Sequelae: Because Parkinson's disease is chronic and progressive, the patient with advanced illness is susceptible to developing injury resulting from falls, infection, inanition related to problems with gastric motility, and respiratory complications such as pulmonary embolism. With the advancement of medical therapies, a patient with Parkinson's disease can have a normal life expectancy.

Prevention/prophylaxis: No preventive measures exist for idiopathic Parkinson's disease.

Referral: Refer to a neurologist any patients with unusual presentation or sustained complications of the illness and patients who do not respond to the initial medication regimen. Patients also may benefit from physical and occupational therapy to assist with adaptive equipment and techniques to enhance independence while maintaining a safe environment. Refer patients with voice changes or difficulty swallowing to a speech therapist. Patients receiving levodopa therapy may benefit from a dietary consultation.

Education: Provide patients and family members with written information about Parkinson's disease, including information about local support groups. The following are websites that patients and family may find beneficial:

www.parkinson.org
www.michaeljfox.org
www.pdf.org
www.wemove.org

The following list of national organizations can be contacted for educational resources:

American Parkinson's Disease Association, Staten Island, NY; 800-223-2732

National Parkinson's Foundation, Miami, FL; 800-327-4545

Parkinson's Disease Foundation, New York, NY; 800-457-6676

TRANSIENT ISCHEMIC ATTACK

SIGNAL SYMPTOMS temporary monocular blindness, weakness and numbness on one side of the body

Transient ischemic attack	ICD-9 CM: 435.9

Description: A TIA is a neurological impairment of presumed ischemic origin, lasting <24 hours. Attacks usually last <10 minutes.

Etiology: TIAs result from the temporary reduction in blood flow to a portion of the brain. Most TIAs are due to emboli of platelets and fibrin breaking from a vessel wall, usually the carotid artery, or originating from a cardiac lesion. Transient hypotension, in conjunction with significant carotid stenosis, also may cause a TIA.

Occurrence: In the United States, the prevalence of TIA is estimated between 1.6% and 4.1%, depending on age and gender. Because most TIAs are diagnosed by history only, and many more go unreported, the actual prevalence is probably considerably higher.

Age: TIAs can occur at any age, but risk increases exponentially with age.

Ethnicity: The incidence of reported TIA is almost equal among all ethnic groups in the United States, with a slight increase in African-Americans. Other minority groups also may be at slightly higher risk than white counterparts.

Gender: Sources are divided on the incidence of TIA among men and women. Because many episodes go unreported, the incidence is probably equal between the sexes.

Contributing factors: Risk factors for TIAs include advanced age, hypertension, diabetes, carotid stenosis, atrial fibrillation, hyperlipidemia, heart disease, sedentary lifestyle, smoking, alcohol abuse, obesity, and some infections (respiratory tract, periodontal disease). Additional risk factors include antiphospholipid antibody, hyperhomocystinemia, drug abuse, and hypercoagulability disorders.

Signs and symptoms: TIAs often are diagnosed on the basis of history alone because symptoms usually resolve before a patient can seek health care. Patients report a sudden onset of symptoms that can last 24 hours but usually last <10 minutes. TIAs can be divided into attacks indicating disease in the carotid circulation and attacks indicating disease in the vertebrobasilar area. Clues to carotid disease include monocular blindness, weakness or numbness on one side of the body, and disturbed speech. Vertebrobasilar disease is suggested by dizziness, vertigo, nausea and vomiting, paresthesia, ataxia, diplopia, dysarthria, generalized weakness, or loss of consciousness. Cardiac physical examination may reveal a carotid bruit, cardiac arrhythmia, or heart murmur during auscultation. Blood pressure may be elevated (Fig. 10–3).

Diagnostic tests: Selection of tests is not inclusive and is based on clinical judgment.

Test	Results Indicating Disorder	CPT Code
CBC	Rule out for hematological cause of symptoms	85031
PT PTT	Rule out coagulopathies	85610–85611 (PT) 85730–85732 (PTT)
Blood chemistries, including calcium, phosphorus, creatinine, and electrolyte levels	Rule out metabolic cause of symptoms	80048 (basic metabolic panel)
Toxicology screen (if indicated by history)	Rule out drug overdose, metabolic cause of symptoms	83015
ECG	Rule out arrhythmia	93000
Holter monitor	Rule out arrhythmia	93235
Carotid duplex studies	Reveal extracranial carotid disease	93880, 93882
Magnetic resonance angiography	Stenosis in extracranial or intracranial cerebral arteries	70496
MRI	Rule out infarction	70551–70553
CT scan	Rule out hemorrhage, infarction	70450–70470, 70496
Arteriography	Gold standard to evaluate condition of cerebral arteries	75600–75630

Because many TIA patients present after their symptoms have resolved, the goal of diagnostic testing is to exclude causes of TIA that require specific therapy and to assess modifiable risk factors. A CBC with differential and chemistry profile reveals hematological or metabolic causes of symptoms. PT and PTT rule out coagulopathies. ESR is a screen for inflammation and autoimmune disorders. All patients should receive an ECG and possibly a Holter monitor if arrhythmia is suspected. Carotid duplex studies reveal extracranial carotid disease. Magnetic resonance angiography detects stenosis in extracranial or intracranial cerebral arteries. Arteriography is the gold standard to evaluate the condition of cerebral arteries but is expensive and invasive. CT or MRI of the brain should be performed to detect silent or prior infarction, unsuspected hemorrhage, or tumor. EEG is helpful if a seizure is suspected.

Differential diagnoses:

- Focal seizures: Seizures are ruled out based on history, physical examination, MRI, and EEG.

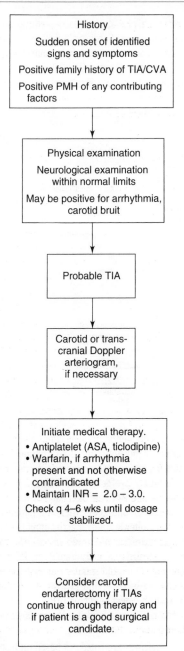

Figure 10–3. Transient ischemic attack.

- Migraine: Migraine is ruled out based on history and physical examination.
- Drug overdose: Overdose is ruled out based on history, physical examination, and toxicology screen.
- Cervical disc osteophyte: This is ruled out based on history, physical examination, and x-rays as indicated.
- Hyperventilation: Hyperventilation is ruled out based on history and physical examination.
- Carpal tunnel syndrome: This is ruled out based on history, physical examination, and x-rays as indicated.
- Hypoglycemia: Hypoglycemia is ruled out based on history, physical examination, and metabolic panel.
- Brain tumor: Tumor is ruled out based on history, physical examination, and brain imaging.

Treatment: Treatment for TIA focuses on prevention of stroke. Identify and control modifiable risk factors. Medical management begins with antiplatelet agents. Aspirin (50–325 mg) is a suitable choice for initial therapy; lower doses should be used in patients with dyspepsia. Aspirin with extended-release dipyridamole (Aggrenox) seems to lower risk of stroke more than aspirin alone, but side effects may not be tolerated. Ticlopidine (Ticlid) also has been shown to reduce the risk of stroke but has adverse effects that limit tolerance; rare instances of neutropenias make careful follow-up important. Ticlopidine should be reserved for patients who are aspirin intolerant or experience ischemic events while taking aspirin. Clopidogrel (Plavix) is chemically related to ticlodipine, but with a more favorable side effect profile. Many clinicians now utilize combinations of antiplatelets to inhibit platelet aggregation at multiple points on the clotting cascade. Anticoagulants (warfarin) are generally recommended for patients who continue to experience TIA's while taking antiplatelet agents or for those with atrial fibrillation. The risk for brain hemorrhage outweighs potential benefits if INR (international normalized ratio) exceeds 3.0, therefore a target INR of 2.5 is recommended. Simvastatin may be considered as an agent to reduce cholesterol if necessary, as it has demonstrated direct benefits in reducing the incidence of strokes in a high-risk population.

Surgical management (carotid endarterectomy) may be recommended for patients who have stenosis of 70% to 99% and a history of at least one TIA or minor stroke. Clinical features that influence stroke risk should be considered in the decision to pursue surgical management for patients with a less severe stenosis (50–69%).

Follow-up: Monitor patients periodically for continuation of symptoms, adequacy of antithrombotic therapy, and control of any comorbid illnesses.

Sequelae: About one third of patients who have a TIA go on to have a stroke. Of those, 50% have a stroke within 1 year after the TIA; 20% of strokes occur within 1 month. A higher risk of myocardial infarction also is noted in this population.

Prevention/prophylaxis: See under Treatment.

Referral: Patients who have drop attacks or vertigo or who have a focal neurological finding are referred to neurology for further workup. An ophthalmologist may be consulted for patients whose complaints include transient monocular blindness. Patients with any gross cardiac abnormalities should be referred to a cardiologist.

Education: Focus patient education on the cause of the TIA and explain the increased risk of stroke, appropriate prevention modalities, and modification of risk factors. The National Stroke Association has an informative website at www.stroke.org; the association also can be contacted at 1-800-STROKES (1-800-787-6537).

REFERENCES

General

American Medical Association: Current Procedural Terminology: CPT 2002, ed 4. AMA, Chicago, 2002.

Callahan, LF, and Jonas, BL: Arthritis. In Ham RJ, et al (eds): Primary Care Geriatrics: A Case-Based Approach, ed 4. Mosby, St Louis, 2002.

DeGowin, RL, and Brown, D: DeGowin's Diagnostic Examination, ed 7. McGraw-Hill, New York, 2000.

Goroll, A, and Mulley, AG: Primary Care Medicine: Office Evaluation and Management of the Adult Patient, ed 4. Lippincott Williams & Wilkins, Philadelphia, 2000.

Kennedy-Malone, L, et al: Management Guidelines for Gerontological Nurse Practitioners. FA Davis, Philadelphia, 1999.

Alzheimer's Disease and Related Disorders

Blackwell, J: Alzheimer's disease management. J Am Acad Nurse Practitioners 14:338, 2002.

Cummings, JL, and Frank, JC: Guidelines for managing Alzheimer's disease: Part II. Treatment. Am Fam Physician 65:2525, 2002.

Cummings, JL, et al: Guidelines for managing Alzheimer's disease: Part I. Assessment. Am Fam Physician 65:2263, 2002.

Erkinjuntti, et al: Efficacy of galantamine in probable vascular dementia and Alzheimer's disease combined with cerebrovascular disease: A randomized trial. Lancet 359:1238, 2002.

Hamdy, RC: Vascular dementia. South Med J 94:673, 2001.

Kennedy-Malone, LM, and Fletcher, K: Alzheimer's disease. Prim Care Pract 3:163, 1999.

Langbart, C: Diagnosing and treating Alzheimer's disease: A practitioner's overview. J Am Acad Nurse Practitioners 14:103, 2002.

Morris, M, et al: Vitamin E and cognitive decline in older persons. Arch Neurol 59:1125, 2002.

Reisberg, B, et al: Memantine in moderate-to-severe Alzheimer's disease. N Engl J Med 348:1333, 2003.

Solomon, PR, et al: Ginkgo for memory enhancement: A randomized trial. JAMA 288, 2002 Contact: http://jama.ama-assn.org/issues/v288n7/rfull/joc11334.html. Accessed August 26, 2002.

Solomon, PR, et al: A 7 minutes neurocognitive screening battery highly sensitive to Alzheimer's disease. Arch Neurol 55:349, 1998.

Brain Tumor

Jemal, A, et al: Cancer statistics, 2002. CA Cancer J Clin 52:23, 2002.

Jukich, PJ, et al: Trends in incidence of primary brain tumors in the United States, 1985–1994. Neuro-oncology 3:141, 2001.

Levin, VA, et al: Neoplasms of the central nervous system. In DeVita, VT, et al (eds): Cancer Principles of Practice and Oncology, vol 6. Lippincott Williams & Wilkins, Philadelphia, 2001.

Sugar, SM, and Israel, MA: Primary and metastatic tumors of the nervous system. In Braunwald, E, et al: Harrison's Principles of Internal Medicine, ed 15. McGraw-Hill,New York, 2001.

Cerebrovascular Accident (Stroke)

Goldstein, LB, et al: Primary prevention of ischemic stroke (American Heart Association Scientific Statement). Circulation 103:163, 2001.

Health Care Financing Administration: Stroke: National project overview. Contact: http://www.hcfa.gov/quality/11a6-a.htm.

National Stroke Association: Stroke: The First Hours: Guidelines for Acute Treatment Consensus Statement. National Stroke Association, Englewood, Colo., 2000.

Wolf, PA, et al: Preventing ischemic stroke in patients with prior stroke and transient ischemic attack (American Heart Association Scientific Statement). Stroke 30:1991, 1999.

Parkinson's Disease

Alder, CH, et al: Parkinson's disease: Progress along the continuum of care. Patient Care for Nurse Practitioners 3:26, 2000.

Kennedy-Malone, LM, and Loftus, SL: Parkinson's disease. Prim Care Pract 3:169, 1999.

Marjama-Lyons, JM, and Koller, WC: Parkinson's disease: Update in diagnosis and symptom management. Geriatrics 56:24, 2001.

Uitti, RJ: Medical treatment of essential tremor and Parkinson's disease. Geriatrics 53:46, 1998a.

Uitti, RJ: Tremor: How to determine if the patient has Parkinson's disease. Geriatrics 53:30, 1998b.

Transient Ischemic Attack

Albers, GW, et al: Supplement to the guidelines for the management of transient ischemic attack. Stroke 30:2502, 1999.

Wolf, PA, et al: Preventing ischemic stroke in patients with prior stroke and transient ischemic attack (American Heart Association Scientific Statement). Stroke 30:1991, 1999.

Chapter *11*
ENDOCRINE, METABOLIC, AND NUTRITIONAL DISORDERS

CHRONIC PANCREATITIS

SIGNAL SYMPTOMS▶ abdominal pain (right upper quadrant), maldigestion

Chronic pancreatitis	ICD-9 CM: 577.1

Description: Chronic pancreatitis is chronic inflammation of the pancreas associated with fibrotic changes and calcification, leading to functional and structural damage of the organ.

Etiology: Pancreatic insufficiency resulting from a long history of alcohol abuse (90%), vascular disease, pancreatic carcinoma, microlithiasis, and abdominal radiation therapy can result in chronic pancreatitis.

Occurrence: About 15 of 100,000 persons develop chronic pancreatitis.

Age: The prevalence of chronic pancreatitis is low in older adults because people with alcoholism usually do not live into old age. The peak age of occurrence of this disease is 35 to 45.

Ethnicity: Countries known to have high rates of alcoholism, such as the United States, Australia, and South Africa, have higher rates of chronic pancreatitis than other countries.

Gender: Chronic pancreatitis occurs equally in men and women.

Contributing factors: The most significant factor contributing to the development of chronic pancreatitis is alcoholism. Individuals who are addicted to narcotics are also susceptible to developing chronic pancreatitis. Elderly women with a history of cholelithiasis are at risk for recurring pancreatitis. Other conditions that may contribute to chronic pancreatitis are hyperparathyroidism; hyperlipidemia; cystic fibrosis;

peptic ulcer disease; obstruction of the main pancreatic duct because of carcinoma, stone, or stenosis; biliary tract disease; and systemic lupus erythematosus. Severe malnutrition is another cause of chronic pancreatitis.

Signs and symptoms: Signs and symptoms may be identical to acute pancreatitis. Of patients, 90% experience severe epigastric pain that may occur in the upper abdominal area, radiating to the back and left shoulder; the origin of the pain may be difficult to discern. The pain may be intermittent or continuous with fluctuations in intensity and often is induced by eating. By the first attack, the gland already is permanently damaged, and subsequent attacks usually are milder and short-lived. Older patients with chronic pancreatitis may or may not experience pain. Weight loss occurs because of either anorexia or malabsorption.

Physical examination may reveal mild fever, hypotension, tachycardia, and tachypnea. Auscultation of the lungs may indicate basilar atelectasis; the clinician should have the patient cough deeply and reassess to determine if the atelectasis is still present. Jaundice may be present. Bowel sounds may be diminished or absent. Epigastric tenderness may be elicited, and the abdomen may be rigid. The gallbladder is not usually palpable. If there is a bluish discoloration around the umbilicus (Cullen's sign) and at the flank (Turner's sign), hemorrhagic necrotizing pancreatitis should be suspected. Steatorrhea develops when lipase and protease secretions are reduced to <10% of normal. Islet cell destruction in the pancreas reduces insulin secretion and causes glucose intolerance.

Diagnostic tests:

Test	Results Indicating Disorder	CPT Code
Serum amylase	Elevated in the early stage of attack; returns to normal in a few days. Serum amylases can be normal in subsequent episodes of pancreatitis	82150
Serum lipase	Elevated in pancreatitis, usually longer than serum amylase and alkaline phosphatase	83690
Alkaline phosphatase	Elevated when bile flow is impaired Parallels with bilirubin	84075
Bilirubin	Elevated with common bile duct compression	82247 (total) 82248 (direct)
Aspartate aminotransferase	Elevated, especially in chronic alcoholism	84450
Lactic dehydrogenase	Elevated in cellular damage	83615
Calcium	Elevated in cellular damage	82310
Fecal fat analysis	Steatorrhea	89125
Abdominal x-rays	Pancreatic calcification	74240

(Continued on the following page)

Test	Results Indicating Disorder	CPT Code
Abdominal CT	Dilated ducts, rule out pseudocyst or pancreatic cancer, and enlarged pancreas	74150 (without contrast enhancement) 74160 (with contrast enhancement)
ERCP	Irregularly structured, dilated main pancreatic duct with beaded appearance	74330

CT, computed tomography; ERCP, endoscopic retrograde cholangiopancreatography.

Differential diagnosis:

- Choledocholithiasis
- Duodenal neoplasms
- Choledochal cyst
- Pancreatic pseudocyst
- Biliary tract stricture

These differential diagnoses all have in common signs and symptoms of left or right upper quadrant pain sometimes with radiation to the scapular or shoulder. There is local tenderness, abdominal pain, vomiting, and weight loss. There also may be fever and jaundice.

Treatment: Patients with chronic pancreatitis must avoid all alcoholic products. Pain control should be managed without the use of narcotics; non-narcotic analgesics can be tried unless contraindicated. Tricyclic antidepressants also are useful in controlling this type of pain. Potent pancreatic enzymes (recommended dose 30,000 U of lipase) can be used with each meal to treat chronic pain by inhibiting the release of cholecystokinin from the duodenal mucosa. This treatment is more successful with idiopathic pancreatitis than alcoholic pancreatitis. A low-fat and low-protein diet using small feedings should be prescribed. The use of H_2 blockers or antacids is increasing.

Refer patients with steatorrhea to a gastroenterologist for consideration of pancreatic supplements. Diabetes mellitus needs to be managed; patients may require insulin. Refer to a specialist patients who may benefit from surgical intervention to alleviate pain. If the main pancreatic duct is dilated, a lateral pancreaticojejunostomy (Puestow procedure) relieves pain in 70% to 80% of patients. If the main pancreatic duct not dilated, resection can be considered (a distal pancreatectomy, or Whipple operation). Denervation offers variable degrees of pain relief. When chronic pancreatitis can be attributed to cholelithiasis, hyperparathyroidism, peptic ulcer disease, or hyperlipidemia, these conditions should be treated, after which the symptoms from the pancreatic attacks should lessen or cease.

Follow-up: On return visits, ask patients about their diet, pain control, and compliance with abstaining from alcohol. Patients who have developed diabetes mellitus, hyperlipidemia, hyperparathyroidism, or peptic ulcer disease need continued evaluation.

Sequelae: Diabetes mellitus, pancreatic pseudocyst or abscess, peptic ulcer disease, and bile duct stricture may be complications of recurring pancreatitis.

Prevention/prophylaxis: Cessation of alcohol consumption is crucial to the prognosis of chronic pancreatitis. Patients are at increased risk for pancreatic cancer.

Referral: Refer patients with complicated chronic pancreatitis to a gastroenterologist. Surgical intervention also may be recommended. Refer any patient presenting with a severe pancreatic attack (i.e., patients who are dehydrated or febrile, have tachycardia, or have elevated amylase >1000 mg/dL) to a gastroenterologist for possible hospital admission.

Education: Instruct patients to eliminate all alcohol consumption. Recommend an alcohol treatment program, and provide the telephone number for the nearest chapter of Alcoholics Anonymous. Additional organizations that may be beneficial to patients with alcoholism include Secular Organization for Sobriety (301-821-8430) and Rational Recovery Systems (916-621-4374).

DIABETES MELLITUS

SIGNAL SYMPTOMS anorexia, paresthesias, proteinuria, chronic skin infections, blurred vision, nausea, gastroparesis, yeast vaginitis, impotence, fatigue, weight loss or gain

Type 1 diabetes mellitus:	ICD-9 CM: 250.0
Type 2 diabetes mellitus:	ICD-9 CM: 250.1

Description: Diabetes mellitus is to a chronic state of hyperglycemia that is divided primarily into two types: *type 1 diabetes* and *type 2 diabetes*. Formerly, type 1 diabetes was called *insulin-dependent diabetes* and type 2 diabetes was called *non–insulin-dependent diabetes mellitus* primarily to signify the age of onset of disease and whether or not insulin therapy was the required treatment.

Etiology: Type 1 diabetes most often occurs in childhood and is characterized by low or absent levels of insulin often resulting from an autoimmune response leading to pancreatic β-cell antibodies. Individuals with type 1 diabetes require insulin therapy for survival. Type 2 diabetes usually occurs in adulthood and is thought to be the result of insulin resistance and deficiency. Genetic predisposition for developing diabetes is more evident in type 2 diabetes. Hyperglycemic states that have not reached levels that warrant a type 2 diabetes diagnosis are identified as impaired glucose tolerance. Evidence indicates that individuals with impaired glucose tolerance have an increased risk of developing type 2 diabetes within 5 to 10 years of onset.

Occurrence: It is estimated that 15 million Americans are affected by diabetes, which is a leading cause of death, illness, and disability in the United States. Approximately 90% to 95% of individuals with diabetes have type 2 diabetes. Between 1990 and 2000, the Centers for Disease Control reported an increase in the number of people diagnosed with type 2 diabetes from 4.9% to 7.3% of the population. Morbidity includes blindness, end-stage renal disease, and lower extremity amputations. Macrovascular complications from diabetes substantially increase the risk of morbidity and death from coronary artery disease, stroke, and peripheral vascular disease. Complications may result from either type 1 diabetes or type 2 diabetes. Evidence indicates that the degree of severity with respect to microvascular, neuropathic, and possibly macrovascular complications seems to be related to the number of years an individual has had hyperglycemia and the magnitude of the glucose elevation.

Age: The onset of type 1 diabetes usually occurs in childhood with the major incidence of disease occurring in individuals <30 years old. The onset of type 2 diabetes usually occurs after age 40 years, with a mean age of 51. Age cannot be the only factor used to determine the classification of diabetes, however, because type 1 diabetes or type 2 diabetes can occur at any age.

Ethnicity: Type 1 diabetes primarily affects white Americans. The incidence of type 2 diabetes and subsequent microvascular and neuropathic complications are more prevalent among African-Americans, Native Americans, Asian-Americans, Pacific Islanders, and Hispanics.

Gender: Type 1 diabetes affects men and women equally. Type 2 diabetes affects women more frequently than men.

Contributing factors: Although the exact cause of type 1 diabetes is unknown, it has been linked to environmental, autoimmune, and viral toxins. A predisposition for acquiring type 1 diabetes has not been identified. Contributing factors for the development of type 2 diabetes have been associated strongly with obesity, sedentary lifestyle, and familial history. The following risk factors have been identified as significantly increasing an individual's risk of developing type 2 diabetes:

- Age ≥ 45 years
- Family history (parents or siblings with diabetes)
- High-density lipoprotein (HDL) cholesterol level ≤ 40 mg/dL and triglyceride level ≥ 250 mg/dL
- History of gestational diabetes or women delivering infants weighing ≥ 9 lb
- Hypertension (blood pressure $\geq 140/90$ mm Hg)
- Obesity ($\geq 20\%$ above ideal body weight or body mass index (BMI) ≥ 27 kg/m^2)

- History of impaired fasting glucose or impaired glucose tolerance
- Race/ethnicity: African-American, Hispanic, Native American, Asian-American, and Pacific Islander

The greater number of risk factors present increases the risk of development of the disease.

Signs and symptoms: Among adults ≥40 years old, diabetes often is discovered as an incidental finding during the workup for cardiovascular, renal, neurological, or infectious diseases. The primary presentation may be due to complications of the underlying and undiagnosed hyperglycemia in conditions such as stroke, myocardial infarction and ischemia, intermittent claudication, impotence, peripheral neuropathy, proteinuria, retinopathy, slow healing wound, and fatigue. Often the classic symptoms of polyuria, polydipsia, and polyphagia with weight loss are attributed to other disease entities and overlooked among older adults. It is prudent for the primary care practitioner periodically to screen for hyperglycemia among individuals >45 years old and repeat at 3-year intervals. More frequent screening is recommended for individuals with several risk factors. Periodic screening among adults >65 years old is warranted because these individuals rarely present with classic symptoms.

Diagnostic tests: The criterion for the diagnosis of diabetes is either two fasting blood glucose readings with results ≥126 mg/dL or two random blood glucose readings with values ≥200 mg/dL, if symptoms of diabetes are present. Oral glucose tolerance testing is no longer recommended in clinical practice. Hemoglobin A_{1c} (HbA_{1c}) measurement is not recommended as a screening test. An individual with a casual plasma glucose level ≥200 mg/dL but without symptoms should have fasting plasma glucose measured.

Status	Fasting Plasma Glucose (FPG)*†	Casual Plasma Glucose‡	CPT Code
Diabetes	FPG >126 mg/dL (7.0 mmol/L)	Casual plasma glucose ≥200 (11.1 mmol/L) plus symptoms	82947
Impaired glucose homeostatic	Impaired fasting glucose FPG ≥110 mg/dL; <126 mg/dL		82947
Normal	FPG <110 mg/dL		82947

* *Fasting* is defined as no caloric intake for at least 8 hours.

† FPG is the preferred test for diagnosis, but either of the listed is acceptable. In the absence of unequivocal disease, tests should be repeated at least once.

‡ *Casual* means any time of day, regardless of when last meal was taken.

When hyperglycemia has been established, a fasting urine for ketones should be performed to help differentiate between type 1 diabetes and type 2 diabetes and the need for insulin therapy.

Differential diagnosis: Includes drug toxicity and endocrine disorders that may affect glucose tolerance, interfere with insulin secretion, and induce insulin resistance.

Drugs associated with hyperglycemia include:

- Alcohol
- β-Adrenergic agents
- Calcium channel blockers
- Corticosteroids
- Lithium salts
- Pentamidine
- Rifampin
- Asparaginase
- Diazoxide
- Diuretics
- Glycerol
- Niacin
- Phenytoin
- Sympathomimetics

Drugs associated with hypoglycemia include:

- Anabolic steroids
- β-Adrenergic blockers
- Chloroquine
- Disopyramide
- Pentamidine
- Salicylates
- Chloramphenicol
- Warfarin
- Clofibrate
- Ethanol
- Phenylbutazone
- Sulfonamide

Endocrine disorders that may induce hyperglycemia include:

- Cushing's syndrome
- Glucagonoma
- Acromegaly
- Pheochromocytoma

The determination of whether or not the diabetes is type 1 or type 2 is based on ketonuria, age of onset, and BMI. Primarily, type 2 diabetes occurs in individuals who are ≥40 years old, have no or minimal ketonuria, and have a BMI of >27. In advanced age, frail individuals may present with type 2 diabetes, however.

Treatment: Establishing treatment goals for patients with type 2 diabetes centers around glycemic control, nutritional status with weight management, and exercise. Evidence shows that patients with type 2 diabetes benefit from maintaining near-normal glucose levels. The recommendations for fasting/preprandial glucose range are 80 to 140 mg/dL. Targets for HbA_{1c} are 6.5% to 8.5%. For patients with decreased life expectancies, comorbidities, and advanced age, strict glucose control may be unattainable and unwarranted. Individualized treatment plans are advisable.

Nonpharmacological

Nonpharmacological therapy is the recommended first-line therapy for newly diagnosed patients with mild-to-moderate hyperglycemia. If after 3 to 6 months nonpharmacological treatment fails or the hyperglycemia is severe (fasting plasma glucose 200 to 300 mg/dL or casual plasma glucose 250 to 350 mg/dL), oral agents may be added to the treatment regimen. Oral agents are never recommended to women during pregnancy or as a single agent to patients who have had diabetic ketoacidosis.

Pharmacological

Oral Agents

Sulfonylureas act by increasing pancreatic insulin secretion and include second-generation sulfonylureas such as glipizide (Glucotrol, Glucotrol XL), glyburide (DiaBeta, Micronase, Glynase), and glimepiride (Amaryl). The first-generation agents (chlorpropamide, tolazamide, or tolbutamide) for the most part are not recommended at the start of therapy and should be continued only in patients who are already adequately controlled on those medications. Side effects of this class of medications include weight gain, nausea, hypoglycemia, weakness, and photosensitivity. These agents should not be used in patients who have had diabetic ketoacidosis, are pregnant, or are lactating. Caution should be exercised in patients who are allergic to sulfonamides. The starting dose depends on the particular drug but should be a small dose and increased as tolerated.

Metformin (Glucophage, Glucophage XR) is a biguanide that acts by decreasing hepatic glucose production, decreasing glucose intestinal absorption, and increasing insulin sensitivity. This agent generally does not increase endogenous insulin production and has few hypoglycemic effects. In addition to glucose control, patients tend to lose weight and improve lipid profiles. Side effects include nausea, vomiting, diarrhea, abdominal pain, anorexia, and taste disturbances. A rare but potentially life-threatening reaction is the development of lactic acidosis. Metformin is contraindicated in patients with renal insufficiency (serum creatinine >1.4 mg/dL for women or >1.5 mg/dL for men), hepatic insufficiency, congestive heart failure, or elderly patients ≥75 years old. Care should be taken when patients who are taking metformin undergo intravenous contrast studies. It is important to withhold the medication for 1 to 2 days after the contrast agent has been administered to ensure normal renal function. Usually, metformin is started at 500 mg once a day given before the evening meal and increased gradually to a maximum dose of 2550 mg daily divided two to three times a day before meals. When given with food, the gastrointestinal side effects tend to be decreased.

Acarbose (Precose) and miglitol (Glyset) are α-glucosidases that act to decrease or delay glucose absorption and lower blood glucose levels. Serum triglycerides tend to be lowered. Side effects include flatulence, diarrhea, abdominal pain, and rash. α-Glucosidases are contraindicated in patients who have had ketoacidosis, inflammatory bowel disease, or intestinal obstruction and patients who have renal or hepatic impairment. Liver function tests should be done every 3 months for the first year. The patient should be instructed to take the medication with the first bite of each meal and tends to be better tolerated if titrated slowly.

Thiazolidinediones, which include pioglitazone (Actos) and rosiglitazone (Avandia), act by increasing sensitivity to insulin, decreasing hepatic glucose production, and increasing peripheral glucose uptake and use. Side effects include headache, weight gain, edema, and anemia. Serious reactions include liver toxicity and worsening congestive heart failure. Liver function tests should be monitored every 2 months for the first year of therapy. Caution should be used in administering these drugs to women who are taking oral contraceptives because of the resulting decrease in the effectiveness of the oral contraceptive.

Nateglinide (Starlix) and repaglinide (Prandin) act quickly to increase the endogenous release of insulin from the pancreas. Side effects include hypoglycemia, headache, upper respiratory infection, nausea, vomiting, constipation, diarrhea, muscle aches, and chest pain. Repaglinide and nateglinide are contraindicated in patients who have had ketoacidosis, renal insufficiency, or hepatic impairment.

The choice of an appropriate oral agent is a complex clinical decision; however, most guidelines agree that a sulfonylurea or biguanide (metformin) is a good first choice. For patients with severe obesity, treatment with a biguanide may be the best choice. If monotherapy with either of these agents is unsuccessful, combination therapy with the two oral agents together should be considered. The most common combinations are as follows: (1) adding sulfonylurea to metformin, (2) adding metformin to sulfonylurea, (3) adding thiazolidinedione to sulfonylurea or metformin, or (4) adding acarbose to sulfonylurea. When combination therapy fails, insulin therapy may be required either as a single agent or in combination with a sulfonylurea, metformin, or thiazolidinedione.

Insulin Therapy
Insulin therapy may be added when optimal glycemic control is not achieved with an oral regimen. Insulin always should be used as first-line therapy in type 1 diabetes or with patients who have had diabetic ketoacidosis. A variety of regimens are used in the administration of insulin

based on the time of onset of action, time of peak effects, and the duration of action. NPH or longer acting insulins can be added at bedtime to type 2 diabetics who are not controlled adequately with an oral regimen. When insulin is used as the primary agent, NPH and regular types frequently are mixed with a dose given before breakfast, then again before the evening meal. A premixed insulin such as 70/30 (70% NPH and 30% regular) can be used when patients have difficulty mixing the insulins because of poor eyesight or other disabilities.

Type of Insulin	Onset of Action (hr)	Peak Action (hr)	Duration of Action (hr)
NPH	1-2	6-12	18-24
Regular	0.5	2-4	6-8
Lente	1-3	6-12	18-24
Humulog	<0.5	0.5-1.5	<6
Lantus	1	No true peak	24

The frequency and timing of self-monitoring of blood glucose levels (SMBG) need to be individualized based on several factors, including age, ability to comply, and oral versus insulin therapies. For patients maintaining glucose levels by nonpharmacological means, SMBG is not recommended. For patients requiring oral medications who are incapable of SMBG, urine glycosuria testing once or twice weekly may be advantageous. Patients requiring oral medications who are capable of SMBG should test glucose levels two to three times per week, preferably before breakfast, the evening meal, and at bedtime. Patients receiving insulin therapy should perform SMBG at least two to three times daily. For all diabetics, SMBG monitoring should increase during illness, changes in diet and exercise, or a change in medications.

Follow-up: Patients with diabetes should be scheduled for appropriate follow-up to evaluate response, tolerability to therapy, goal reassessment, and management of acute and chronic complications. Older patients and patients on insulin therapy may need to be seen every 3 months. When there is a sudden change in health status or treatment regimen, follow-up of ≤ 1 month may be indicated. For stable patients who are able to maintain treatment goals, follow-up may be every 3 to 6 months.

The following evaluations are recommended at follow-up visits:

- Glycemia
- Foot complications
- Annual eye examination including dilation
- Routine urinalysis
- Blood pressure
- Serum creatinine levels
- Annual electrocardiogram and fasting lipid profile
- HgBA$_{1c}$ every 4 to 12 months

- Evaluation for neurovascular complications
- Self-management education
- Biannual oral examination
- Immunization update, including influenza and pneumococcal vaccines

Sequelae: Acute complications requiring immediate attention include diabetic ketoacidosis; recurring fasting hyperglycemia of >300 mg/dL; $HgBA_{1c}$ of $\geq 13\%$; or severe hypoglycemia with changes in sensorium, altered behavior, seizures, or coma. Complications resulting from prolonged hyperglycemia include renal failure, blindness, coronary artery disease, stroke, peripheral vascular disease, slow healing wounds, autonomic neuropathies, hypertension, sexual problems, and genitourinary system disorders. Macrovascular complications from diabetes substantially increase the risk of morbidity and death from coronary artery disease, stroke, and peripheral vascular disease. Complications may result from either type 1 diabetes or type 2 diabetes. Evidence indicates that the degree of severity with respect to microvascular, neuropathic, and possibly macrovascular complications seems to be related to the number of years a patient has had hyperglycemia and the magnitude of the glucose elevation.

Prevention/prophylaxis: The focus of prevention for developing type 2 diabetes is diet modification and exercise with subsequent weight loss. Weight loss of 10 to 20 lb can reduce glucose levels markedly. When a patient is diagnosed with type 2 diabetes, the maintenance of glucose levels at as near-normal levels as possible is extremely beneficial in preventing complications from the disease. Monitoring and controlling serum lipid levels and blood pressure can reduce greatly complications from coronary artery disease and stroke. Equally important is maintaining routine examinations recommended by the primary care provider.

Referral: Patients with type 2 diabetes should be referred when acute complications requiring hospitalization develop, such as ketoacidosis, severe hyperglycemia, or hypoglycemia. Patients with fasting glucose levels that are consistently >300 mg/dL or $HgBA_{1c}$ of ≥ 13 % also should be referred. Routine eye and oral examinations should be referred to appropriate providers. Patients with uncontrolled hypertension, hyperlipidemia, unmanageable skin disorders, or renal insufficiency should be referred to appropriate providers. Consider referring all patients interested in greater control of self-management of the disease to nutrition, exercise, and diabetes educators.

Education: The cornerstone of education for patients with diabetes is disease self-management. Assess the patient's knowledge and understanding of the disease, treatment goals, management, and response to complications. Include in the assessment barriers to treatment, which include cultural influences, health beliefs and behaviors, socioeconomic status, psychological factors, and education and skills deficits that may preclude the ability to self-manage diabetes adequately. Explicit instructions should be given to patients who participate in daily SMBG monitoring. For optimal results, families of patients with diabetes always should be included in the education and management of the disease. Information pertaining to diabetes can be obtained from the American Diabetes Association, 1701 North Beauregard Street, Alexandria, VA 22311, 1-800-DIABETES (1-800-342-2383), www.diabetes.org.

HYPERLIPIDEMIA

SIGNAL SYMPTOMS▶   severe obesity, central obesity, xanthelasma

Hyperlipidemia	ICD-9 CM: 272.4

Description: Elevated levels of circulating lipoproteins, or hyperlipidemia, can result from an increase in their synthesis owing to a diet high in saturated fats or from a genetically determined reduction in the amount removed from the circulation. This situation causes an increase in the concentration of cholesterol or triglycerides or both in the plasma. Slight reductions in lipid levels have been shown to be effective in primary and secondary prevention of cardiovascular disease.

According to the National Cholesterol Education Program Adult Treatment Panel III, lowering low-density lipoprotein (LDL) cholesterol and raising HDL cholesterol is the primary goal of therapy. Emphasis should be placed on identifying patients with multiple risk factors (e.g., the metabolic syndrome; see section on Obesity). Risk factor determination should be made for the presence of cardiovascular disease or diabetes, targeting these patients for intensive lifestyle changes along with the possible use of lipid-lowering agents. Diabetes now is viewed as a risk equivalent to known coronary heart disease; optimal LDL levels in diabetics should be <100 mg/dL.

Occurrence: The American Heart Association estimates that 100,870,000 American adults have a serum total cholesterol level of ≥200 mg/dL. It has been estimated further that about 40,600,000 American adults fall into the high-risk category, having a serum total cholesterol level of ≥240 mg/dL.

Age: Most common onset for hyperlipidemia is in the 60s.

Ethnicity: Hyperlipidemia is more common in whites than in African-Americans.

Gender: This condition is more prevalent in men than in women. Men may experience the onset of dyslipidemia 10 years before women.

Contributing factors: Factors contributing to development of hyperlipidemia are a high-fat diet, nephrotic syndrome, hypothyroidism, severe obesity (BMI ≥30 kg/m^2), central obesity (defined as a waist circumference ≥40 inches in men or ≥35 inches in women), diabetes mellitus, pancreatitis, hypertension, systemic lupus erythematosus, obstructive liver disease, excessive alcohol intake, renal failure, smoking, certain diuretics, anabolic steroids, sedentary lifestyle, and family history of coronary heart disease. Caffeine intake may increase cholesterol levels.

Signs and symptoms: Most patients do not present with physical complaints. Routine physical examination may reveal xanthomata, xanthelasma, arterial bruits, and evidence of claudication. Corneal arcus found in patients <50 years old often indicates hyperlipidemia.

Diagnostic tests: After the individual has been fasting for a minimum of 12 hours, a complete lipid profile should be done. If the opportunity for testing is limited to nonfasting, the total cholesterol and HDL cholesterol are usable. Thyroid-stimulating hormone (TSH) level should be measured if hypothyroidism is a suspected contributor to hyperlipidemia.

Differential diagnosis:

Test	Results Indicating Disorder	CPT Code
Clinical Indications of the Metabolic Syndrome*		
Triglycerides	150 mg/dL	84478
HDL cholesterol		83718
Men	<40 mg/dL	
Women	<50 mg/dL	
Blood pressure	130/85 mm Hg	
Fasting glucose	110 mg/dL	83718
Waist circumference		
Men	>102 cm (>40 inches)	401.9
Women	> 88 cm (>35 inches)	
Lipid Profile		
Total cholesterol	<200 mg/dL (desirable) 200–239 mg/dL (borderline high risk) 240 mg/dL (high risk)	82947
LDL cholesterol	<100 mg/dL (optimal) <130 mg/dL (desirable) 130–159 mg/dL (borderline high risk) 160 mg/dL (high risk) *Note:* An optimal LDL of <100 mg/dL in patients with diabetes or cardiovascular disease is the goal of therapy	82465
TSH	0.49–4.67 <0.49 (hypothyroidism)	80418, 80438–80440

* Three or more of the following values indicate the metabolic syndrome.

Treatment: Changing dietary habits is essential to lowering cholesterol level. Dietary restrictions of cholesterol (300 mg) and a restriction of foods with saturated fats to <10% of total calories daily are recommended to reduce LDL cholesterol. For the frail older adult, secondary measures, such as smoking cessation and control of hypertension, may be more advantageous because malnutrition may occur inadvertently if certain foods are restricted, which is often a problem in older adults with limited resources. Weight loss, aerobic exercise, and stress reduction also may be recommended for the stable, ambulatory older adult. Diet therapy with exercise and stress reduction should be initiated first for a 6-month trial before starting medications.

If a patient's LDL is >130 mg/dL and additional risk factors exist or the LDL is >160 mg/dL with or without additional risk factors, medication can be started. Lovastatin is recommended for use in older adults because of its few side effects. The initial dose is 20 mg with the evening meal, as tolerated. The dose may be increased, depending on the results of the follow-up cholesterol level, but should not be >80 mg/day. Liver function tests should be performed before the initial dose, then every 4 to 6 weeks during the first 12 to 15 months of treatment. Other HMG-CoA reductase agents include pravastatin (starting dose 10 mg) and simvastatin (starting dose 5 mg). Other cholesterol-lowering agents, such as bile acid sequestrants and nicotinic acid, which are costly, have been found to interact with many common medications, and require multiple doses throughout the day, are not recommended as first-line drug therapy in older adults. The newer sustained-release form of nicotinic acid, Niaspan, has less of the adverse effect of flushing. The addition of an aspirin with niacin has been shown to reduce flushing. Drug therapy may be contraindicated in advanced age and in debilitated patients.

Agents used to lower lipids are as follows:

Drug Class	Major Mechanism	Typical Dose	Efficacy	Adverse Effects
HMG CoA reductase inhibitors (statins): lovastatin	Enhanced LDL clearance by competitive inhibition of biosynthesis	20–80 mg/day	Significantly lowers LDL (18–55%) Increases HDL (5–10%) Lowers triglycerides (10–20%)	Myopathy Increased liver enzymes
Bile acid (sequestrants): cholestyramine	Increased gastrointestinal clearance	4–8 g two to three times daily	LDL lowered (10–25%)	Abdominal bloating, constipation, triglyceride elevation, multiple drug interactions

(Continued on following page)

Drug Class	Major Mechanism	Typical Dose	Efficacy	Adverse Effects
Nicotinic acid (niacin): Niaspan (sustained release)	Reduced fatty acid flux from adipose tissue	1–2 g/day	Triglyceride reduced (30–80%) LDL lowered (10–20%) Increased HDL (10–30%)	Flushing Rash Impaired glucose tolerance Hyper-uricemia Worsening peptic ulcer disease Acanthosis nigricans
Fibric acids (fibrates): gemfibrozil	Increases VLDL catabolism and increases HDL cholesterol content	600 mg twice daily	Mild lowering of LDL Triglycerides reduced (10–20%) HDL elevated (10–20%)	Dyspepsia Cholelithiasis Increase myopathy with statins

VLDL, very-low-density lipoprotein.

Follow-up: Inform patients and family members that medication therapy, laboratory testing, and lifestyle changes become a way of life after the diagnosis of hyperlipidemia. Dietary changes should be monitored with repeat blood work first in 4 and 6 weeks, then at 3 months. If no improvement is found, drug therapy should be added. Monitoring laboratory studies should be done at 6-week intervals for the first year of therapy and every 6 months thereafter.

Sequelae: If dietary and lifestyle changes are made and adhered to, prognosis is good for reduction of serum cholesterol. If drug therapy is used, results are just as promising. The major sequelae of hyperlipidemia are coronary heart disease and stroke.

Prevention/prophylaxis: Having lifelong dietary habits including <20 g of fat per day and following a moderate exercise regimen are the best prevention. The need for monitoring of total cholesterol levels throughout the patient's adult lifespan is emphasized.

Referral: Patients may benefit from a self-help group for dietary guidance, such as Weight Watchers or TOPS. Patients with diabetes who have suffered a major cardiac event (e.g., myocardial infarction or stroke) are at extremely high risk for death and may benefit from being referred to a lipid management clinic.

Education: The patient and family require dietary instruction, exercise parameters, and stress reduction information.

HYPERTHYROIDISM

Hyperthyroidism	ICD-9 CM: 242.90
Hyperthyroidism with goiter	ICD-9 CM: 242.0
Hyperthyroidism, multinodular	ICD-9 CM: 242.2
Hyperthyroidism, uninodular	ICD-9 CM: 242.3

Description: Hyperthyroidism is an excessive amount of thyroid hormone in the body tissue.

Etiology: The most common cause of new-onset hyperthyroidism in older adults is a toxic nodular goiter followed by Graves' disease and toxic adenoma. The multiple nodules of a toxic multinodular goiter are thought to produce thyroid hormone without TSH, resulting in thyrotoxicosis. Graves' disease is a familial autoimmune disease of unknown origin.

Occurrence: Of people in the United States, <5% have hyperthyroidism.

Age: Of all cases of hyperthyroidism, 15% to 25% occur in people ≥65 years old; of patients with hyperthyroidism, 10% to 15% are >60 years old.

Ethnicity: No significant evidence of ethnic prevalence exists.

Gender: Hyperthyroidism is more prevalent in women than in men. By age 70, the prevalence of the disease among men and women is almost equal.

Contributing factors: Patients with other autoimmune problems are at risk for developing hyperthyroidism. A familial tendency for developing hyperthyroidism exists. Patients taking amiodarone or radiographic contrast media can develop iodine-induced hyperthyroidism. Patients who are known to consume diets high in excess iodine are at risk for developing hyperthyroidism.

Signs and symptoms: Older patients may report weight loss, apathy, depression, heat intolerance, weakness, insomnia, palpitations, nervousness, and anxiety. Patients may report a new onset of angina. When questioned about their bowel habits, patients may report that they are no longer constipated. A reduction or increase in appetite may be revealed. Photophobia and blurred or double vision may be noted.

 Clinical Pearl: Onset of hyperthyroidism in older adults often has a subtle presentation, called *apathetic hyperthyroidism*. Lethargy is more common than hyperactivity

On physical examination, ophthalmologic changes, such as exophthalmos, are not as common in the elderly. Lid lag is a more common finding. An enlarged thyroid occurs only in 20% to 40% of patients ≥70

years old. The thyroid is found lower in the neck and substernal in older adults compared with younger individuals. Because cardiac findings are prevalent in older adults with hyperthyroidism, a thorough examination is essential. Tachycardia, atrial fibrillation, and congestive heart failure are common manifestations of untreated hyperthyroidism. A reduction in muscle mass may be detected (proximal weakness is common in hyperthyroidism), so muscle strength should be tested. Ask patients to stand up from a seated position. A coarse tremor may be evident. Assess for signs of anemia, such as pallor.

Diagnostic tests:

Test	Results Indicating Disorder	CPT Code
TSH	Decreased <0.1 U/L	80418, 80438–80440
Free T_4	Elevated, confirms diagnosis	84436–84439, 86360
Free T_3	Elevated, confirms diagnosis	84481, 84480 (total)
RAIU	Elevated	78000–78003
ECG	Evaluate any associated arrhythmias, cardiac abnormalities	93040 (tracing and evaluation) 93042 (rhythm evaluation)

T_4, thyroxine; T_3, triiodothyronine; RAIU, radioactive iodine uptake; ECG, electrocardiogram.

If the T_4 result is normal following a decreased TSH result, a serum T_3 test should be ordered. This value sometimes is increased, indicating T_3 toxicosis. If the T_3 result is also normal, the patient is said to have subclinical disease. RAIU is ordered to differentiate the cause of the thyrotoxicosis: This test usually is elevated in the presence of hyperthyroidism. There is a diffuse uptake of RAIU in Graves' disease, whereas there is focal uptake in toxic nodular thyroiditis.

Differential diagnosis:

- Anxiety
- Diabetes mellitus (normal fasting blood glucose)
- Certain endocrine malignancies (thyroid function studies are generally normal; fine-needle aspiration of nodule confirms diagnosis of malignancy)

Treatment: Hyperthyroidism needs immediate attention in older adults because it usually is associated with involvement of other organ systems, especially cardiac. Radioisotope therapy is the treatment of choice for toxic thyroid nodules and Graves' disease; however, patients should be in a euthyroid state before receiving radioactive iodine treatment. Patients may be treated with antithyroid agents initially. β-Blockers are indicated in the early treatment of hyperthyroidism to control the cardiac symptoms of palpitations and tachycardia. β-Blockers are not recommended for patients with bronchospasm, congestive heart failure, or insulin-dependent diabetes.

Clinical Pearl: Patients should be referred to an endocrinologist for treatment of hyperthyroidism.

Follow-up: Patients with hyperthyroidism require monitoring during treatment, including thyroid studies, cardiac status, and changes in mental status. The patient must be aware of changes to note impending hypothyroidism when treatment has been initiated. Diagnostic studies, usually ordered by the endocrinologist, include free T_4 and serum T_3 monitored every 6 to 8 weeks until a euthyroid state is achieved, then TSH levels every 3 months for the first year and twice yearly thereafter until the patient's condition is stable and he or she is asymptomatic for thyroid disease. Underlying anemia present when the patient was hyperthyroid needs re-evaluation.

Sequelae: Complications that can develop in patients with hyperthyroidism include underlying ischemic heart disease, angina, cardiac arrhythmia, myocardial infarction, and congestive heart failure. Bone density may decrease also, rendering the patient susceptible to the development of osteoporosis.

Prevention/prophylaxis: Hyperthyroidism is not known to be preventable. Because thyroid disease is prevalent in the elderly, regular screening for signs and symptoms of hyperthyroidism is essential for older adults, especially adults with a history of rheumatoid arthritis and other collagen diseases and diabetes mellitus.

Referral: Patients need to be referred to a radiotherapist for calculation of the dose of iodine-131. Patients with complicated hyperthyroidism should be treated by an endocrinologist, especially in the presence of atrial fibrillation and thyroid storm; these patients usually require hospitalization.

Education: Patients should note a change in their overall behavior after the initial treatment. Patients must realize that they need to take the prescribed medication daily and to continue with the radioactive iodine treatment. After patients have achieved the euthyroid state and received the radioactive iodine treatment, have them report to their health-care provider if they experience signs and symptoms of hypothyroidism or hyperthyroidism.

HYPOTHYROIDISM

SIGNAL SYMPTOMS ▶ weakness, cold intolerance, myalgias, depression, apathy, impaired memory, fatigue

Hypothyroidism	ICD-9 CM: 244.9

Description: Hypothyroidism occurs when the body tissues are subjected to subnormal amounts of thyroid hormone. Hypothyroidism is classified further as primary hypothyroidism, which is the failure of the thyroid glad to produce hormones; secondary hypothyroidism, which occurs when the pituitary gland fails to secrete an adequate amount of thyrotropin; and tertiary hypothyroidism, which is the failure of the thyroid to secrete thyrotropin-releasing-hormone.

Etiology: Autoimmune thyroiditis is the most common cause of hypothyroidism in older adults. Persons who have had prior thyroid surgery or ablation of the thyroid are also susceptible to hypothyroidism.

Occurrence: Of adults ≥65 years old, 6% have hypothyroidism; however, 20% have subclinical hypothyroidism.

Age: Hypothyroidism predominantly begins at age 40, although the age of onset can continue through old age. Women in their 70s are almost seven times more likely to develop hypothyroidism as women age 35.

Ethnicity: No significant evidence of ethnic prevalence exists.

Gender: Hypothyroidism is more prevalent in women than in men.

Contributing factors: Increased age and female gender are risk factors for developing hypothyroidism. Patients with previous thyroid dysfunction, Hashimoto's thyroiditis, and goiter may develop hypothyroidism. There is an association between leukotrichia and vitiligo and developing hypothyroidism. Patients who have had extensive neck surgery or radiation or prior thyroid surgery without proper follow-up often develop hypothyroidism. Hypothyroidism also can result from pituitary disease and certain infiltrative diseases, such as sarcoidosis and scleroderma. A relationship exists between contact with some environmental pollutants (e.g., fire retardation materials), fungicides, and coal conversion products and the development of hypothyroidism. Long-term lithium use and amiodarone use also can be a contributor to the disease. Patients with first-degree relatives with thyroid disease are at risk. Patients with insulin-dependent diabetes, rheumatoid arthritis, pseudogout, or Addison's disease should be screened routinely for thyroid disease. In patients with elevated lipids, consider hypothyroidism as an underlying condition.

Signs and symptoms: Patients often present with weakness, myalgias, arthralgias, fatigue, cold intolerance, constipation, hair loss, leg cramps, hoarseness, tinnitus, paresthesia, reported weight changes, and depression. Patients or family members may report impaired memory or the inability to concentrate. If the disease has progressed untreated, patients appear apathetic and debilitated, with possible psychosis. On physical examination, the overall appearance of the patient may reveal brittle nails, puffiness of the face and eyelids, thinning of the outer halves of the eyebrows, and dry skin.

During the thyroid examination, the examiner first should observe the thyroid while the patient swallows, then proceed to the hands-on examination. If the thyroid gland is tender to touch, the patient may have thyroiditis. A goiter may be present that feels rubbery, is not tender, and is possibly nodular. Thyroid nodules, which are common in older adults, are benign if they feel smooth and easy to manipulate, whereas malignant nodules are hard, irregular, fixed, and tender on palpation. Bradycardia and cardiac enlargement may be detected during the cardiac examination; the diastolic blood pressure may be elevated. Bowel sounds may be diminished. A change in reflexes may be present, notably normal upstroke with a delay in the relaxation phase. Nonpitting edema may be found in the lower extremities. Patients should be examined for signs of carpal tunnel disease and cerebellar dysfunction to check for ataxia. Patients with secondary hypothyroidism may have diminished body hair and postural hypotension. A screening mental status examination should be performed.

 Clinical Pearl: Patients may be asymptomatic, with hypothyroidism discovered only during diagnostic testing.

Diagnostic tests:

Test	Results Indicating Disorder	CPT Code
TSH	Elevation (>10 mU/L)	80418, 80438–80440
Free T$_4$	Decreased in clinical hypothyroidism. Normal in subclinical hypothyroidism	84436–84439, 86360
T$_3$ (order if T$_4$ is normal)	Low T$_3$ indicates severe hyperthyroidism	84481 (free) 84480 (total)
ECG	Bradycardia, prolonged QT intervals, conduction disturbances	93040 (tracing and evaluation) 93042 (rhythm evaluation)

The presence of thyroid antibodies is useful in the diagnosis of subclinical hypothyroidism or goiter and Hashimoto's thyroiditis. An ECG typically shows sinus bradycardia, prolonged QT intervals, and possibly atrioventricular block and conduction disturbances.

Differential diagnosis: In determining whether or not a patient has hypothyroidism, the first thing to consider is whether the disease is primary or secondary hypothyroidism. Hashimoto's thyroiditis, postirradiation disease, subacute thyroiditis, iodide deficiency, and subtotal thyroidectomy can cause primary hypothyroidism. People who have pituitary hyposecretion, pituitary tumors, and some infiltrative diseases (e.g., sarcoidosis) are susceptible to secondary hypothyroidism. In older adults, when there are numerous signs and symptoms of hypothyroidism, an increased number of these clinical findings points to thyroid disease.

- Dementia
- Anemia
- Depression

Treatment: Older adults with an underactive thyroid are prescribed levothyroxine for lifelong treatment. The starting dose in older adults is

25 µg/day; in some cases, however, the initial dose and the incremental dose may be 12.5 µg. Patients should be re-evaluated in 4 to 6 weeks for assessment of clinical presentation and TSH level. The dosage then can be adjusted upward by 12.5 µg increments every 4 to 6 weeks. The usual replacement dosage for older adults in the absence of cardiac disease eventually reaches 100 to 125 µg/day. Clinical presentation of hypothyroidism in older adults often mimics normal aging changes. Patients may continue to have increased TSH levels yet show signs of clinical improvement. Excessive doses of levothyroxine induce osteoporosis. Older adults with cardiac disease should receive ≤0.025 mg/day. A thorough medication history is necessary when prescribing levothyroxine; cholestyramine, ferrous sulfate, sucralfate, and antacids containing aluminum hydroxide can reduce the effectiveness of this medication. Phenytoin, carbamazepine, rifampin, and anticoagulants may increase drug metabolism. Patients taking any of these medications with levothyroxine should allow a 4- to 6-hour interval between the medications. Dietary fiber also can interfere with absorption, so levothyroxine should be taken on an empty stomach in the morning.

Follow-up: Patients should have a routine TSH evaluation every 6 to 12 months after stabilization. Patients with secondary hypothyroidism need a free T_4 test. Monitor clinical signs in all patients. Patients found to have subclinical hypothyroidism (TSH 5 to 10 mU/L) should be re-evaluated every 3 to 6 months to determine if hypothyroidism is clinically indicated at this time.

Sequelae: Patients with untreated hypothyroidism may develop coronary artery disease because of the increase in LDL and triglyceride levels associated with this disorder. Megacolon may occur in patients with a long history of untreated hypothyroidism. Myxedema coma with hypothermia and hypotension is a complication of severe untreated hypothyroidism.

Prevention/prophylaxis: Regular screening for thyroid disease is advocated for individuals ≥60 years old, especially patients with insulin-dependent diabetes, rheumatoid arthritis and other collagen-related disorders, and a family history of thyroid disease.

Referral: If the patient has numerous complications or is not responding to treatment despite compliance, refer him or her to an endocrinologist.

Education: Many drug interactions have been shown to interfere with thyroxine absorption, such as iron supplements, aluminum-containing antacids, and calcium carbonate. Tell patients not to increase their dosage even if they are experiencing symptoms of hypothyroidism; rather they should contact their health-care provider. Any unexplained weight gain of ≥5 lb should be reported. Encourage patients to increase their activity level. Alert patients to contact their health-care provider if they experience signs and symptoms of hypothyroidism or hyperthyroidism.

MALNUTRITION

SIGNAL SYMPTOMS▶ deficit in muscle mass, depleted visceral protein

Malnutrition, mild	ICD-9 CM 263.1
Malnutrition, severe	ICD-9 CM 261.0

Description: Protein-calorie malnutrition is diagnosed by a combination of indicators. Generally an unexplained involuntary weight loss and a drop in the serum albumin level to <3.5 g/dL are reliable indicators.

Etiology: Although many factors can lead to malnutrition in older adults, certain age-associated factors are precursors to malnutrition, including reduced food and micronutrient intake; decreased absorption of ingested food; and increased bodily demands for protein, calories, or micronutrients because of physiologic stressors. Decreases in metabolic rate, physical activity, and sensory input also can contribute to malnutrition. Malnutrition can take two forms: marasmus and kwashiorkor. In marasmus, the individual has a deficit in muscle mass and fat stores but retains visceral protein stores, and organ function is normal. Kwashiorkor occurs when the individual experiences further or acute stressors, which depletes visceral protein and is associated with edema.

Occurrence: Of older adults, >6 million are at high risk for malnutrition. Reports indicate that approximately 16% of community-dwelling elderly, 17% to 65% of acute care hospital patients, and 20% to 54% of nursing home residents experience undernutrition.

Age: Malnutrition can occur at any age. Frail older adults and adults >80 years old are at the highest risk for malnutrition.

Ethnicity: Because the reasons for malnutrition vary, no specific ethnic prevalence is known.

Gender: Malnutrition in people ≥ 85 years old is more prevalent in women because of the higher number of women than men in this age bracket.

Contributing factors: Several factors may contribute to malnutrition in older adults: poverty; decreased olfactory sensitivity; loss of taste buds; being edentulous; and certain chronic diseases, such as intestinal ischemia, hyperthyroidism, depression, chronic obstructive pulmonary disease, alcoholism, chronic impaction, malabsorption syndromes, dementia, obesity, and cholelithiasis. Hospitalization with a restricted diet, drug-nutrient interactions related to polypharmacy, and social isolation also may contribute to malnutrition.

Signs and symptoms: Identification of elders at risk for malnutrition is a complex process; however, unexplained weight loss is the best factor for predicting increased risk of malnutrition. Assessment of malnutrition is complex because it involves investigation of physiological, psychological, pathological, functional, and financial parameters to determine the possible causes of the malnutrition. In patients with suspected malnutrition, all risk factors for poor nutritional status should be assessed using objective measures as indicated (i.e., depression scales, mental status scales, functional status tests). Two screening tools have been validated as nutritional screening devices for the elderly; the Mini Nutritional Assessment, which can be found at www.mna-elderly.com, and the SCALES screening device (Table 11–1) have been cross-validated for use in the outpatient setting. The Clinical Guide to Prevent and Manage Malnutrition in Long-Term Care, which can be found at www.ltcnutrition.org, is a reliable tool for elderly nursing home residents because it incorporates the Resident Assessment Instrument and the mnemonic MEALS ON WHEELS (Box 11–1).

A thorough review of prescription and over-the-counter medications is indicated to determine if the patient is taking any substance that can cause anorexia, such as digoxin, quinidine, or hydralazine. During the physical examination, discern if the malnutrition is related to cardiac, respiratory, intestinal, endocrine, hepatic, neurological, or renal impairment. Look for specific signs of nutritional deficiencies, such as nail abnormalities, brittle hair, bruises, skin color (jaundice, pallor), cheilosis, glossitis, loss of subcutaneous body fat, muscle wasting, and edema. Explore any unexplained weight loss to rule out treatable causes of malnutrition. If a patient is found to be ≥15% below ideal body weight or had a recent loss of 10% below baseline weight, consider protein-calorie malnutrition (although dehydration should be ruled out). BMI is calculated using the formula weight (kg) divided by height (m^2). BMI is an effective measurement for obesity but is generally not as sensitive in indi-

Table 11–1 Scales Protocol for Evaluating Risk of Malnutrition in the Elderly

Item Evaluated	Assign 1 Point	Assign 2 Points
Sadness (as measured on the Geriatric Depression Scale)	10–14	≥ 15
Cholesterol level	< 160 mg/dL (< 4.15 mmol/L)	—
Albumin level	3.5–4 g/dL	< 3.5 g/dL
Loss of weight	1 kg (or 1/4-inch midarm circumference) in 1 mo	3 kg (or 1/2-inch midarm circumference) in 6 mo
Eating problems	Patient needs assistance	—
Shopping and food preparation problems	Patient needs assistance	—

A total score ≥3 indicates that the patient is at risk of malnutrition.
Modified from Morley JE, Miller DK: Malnutrition in the elderly. *Hospit Pract* 27:95–116, 1992.
From Beers, MH, and Berkow, R: The Merck Manual of Geriatrics, ed 3. Copyright 2000 by Merck & Co, Inc, Whitehouse Station, NJ.

Box 11–1

Reversible Causes of Protein-Energy Malnutrition in Nursing Homes: The "Meals on Wheels" Mnemonic

M	edications (digoxin, theophylline, antipsychotics)
E	motional problems (depression)
A	norexia tardive (nervosa/alcoholism)
L	ate-life paranoia
S	wallowing disorders
O	ral problems
N	osocomial infections (tuberculosis, *Helicobacter pylori*, *Clostridium difficile*)
W	andering and other dementia-related behaviors
H	yperthyroidism/hypercalcemia/hypoadrenalism
E	nteric problems (malabsorption)
E	ating problems
L	ow-salt, low-cholesterol diets
S	tones (cholelithiasis)

From Morley, JE, and Silver, AJ: Nutritional issues in nursing home care. *Ann Intern Med*, 123:850–859, 1995, with permission from Elsevier.

cating malnutrition. In the normal healthy older adult, the BMI should be 24 to 27 kg/m^2; BMI <21 kg/m^2 generally indicates a weight deficit and is used by the Council for Nutritional Clinical Strategies in Long-Term Care as an indication that nutritional intervention is required. In older adults, midarm circumference (MAC) and triceps skin fold (TSF) measurements are not accurate means for testing for malnutrition; however, as an estimate, a MAC or TSF measurement below the 10th percentile indicates poor nutritional status.

Diagnostic tests: There is no gold standard for diagnosis of malnutrition. Diagnostic studies help identify the severity and define the type of malnutrition.

Test	Results Indicating Disorder	CPT Code
Nutritional assessment/ counseling	Weight: involuntary weight loss in 30 days; 10% loss in ≤180 days; BMI <21; anthropometric variables of MAC and TSF <10th percentile	99387
Hemoglobin/hematocrit	Hemoglobin <12	83026
Serum albumin	<3.5 g/dL	82040
Lipid panel	Cholesterol <160 mg/dL	80061
Basic or complete metabolic panel	Multiple possibilities to identify reversible metabolic disorders	80048/ 80053

In screening for malnutrition, laboratory values should be considered only as an indirect measurement or as a tool to evaluate treatment. A complete blood count should be ordered to determine anemia and to rule out infection and immunocompromised status. Protein, iron, folate, and vitamin B_{12} deficiencies should be assessed for. Total lymphocyte counts <1500 cells/mm^3 are found in mild-to-moderate malnutrition; a total of <1000 cells/mm^3 is associated with immune paralysis. Serum albumin level <3.5 mg/dL and especially <3.0 mg/dL predicts protein depletion and is the most common biochemical parameter indicated when considering malnutrition. Serum albumin levels can be skewed, however, in patients experiencing urinary loss from the nephrotic syndrome or in patients receiving intravenous fluids. A dilutional effect on albumin also is seen when the patient is bedridden, which can produce a 0.5 mg/dL decrease. Because the half-life of albumin is 21 days, serum albumin levels rise slowly after nutritional supplementation. Prealbumin with an average life span of 2 to 3 days is highly dependent on iron levels and is not indicated as an evaluation tool unless the patient is hospitalized. A decrease in the serum transferrin levels also indicates malnutrition. In patients with coexisting iron-deficiency anemia, however, the results are misleading (normal to elevated serum transferrin).

 Clinical Pearl: If the elderly individual is not on a lipid-lowering agent, total cholesterol level <160 mg/dL is considered a marker for malnutrition and has been associated with increased mortality.

Differential diagnosis: When determining if a person has malnutrition, discern if any of the following conditions coexist:

- 783.0 Anorexia
- Dehydration
- Dementia—Alzheimer's disease related
- 291.2 Dementia—alcohol related
- 296.30 Depression—major
- 787.2 Dysphagia
- 307.5 Eating disorder
- 783.41 Failure to thrive
- 783.3 Feeding problem/elderly
- 269.9 Nutritional deficiency not otherwise specified

Treatment: Identifying the contributing factors to malnutrition in each patient is essential to treating this condition. When possible, a 3-day dietary intake should be obtained to determine the severity of the nutritional deprivation. All medications that can cause drug-induced malnutrition should be discontinued or reconsidered, or an alternative should be used. Fecal impaction should be identified and removed. Because not all factors, such as alterations in sensory input, can be treated, dietary consultation should be ordered to assist in the diagnosis of malnutrition and planning of diet supplementation. An older person experiencing a physiological stressor, such as surgery, infection, or trauma, requires an increase in protein, calories, and micronutrients. If the patient is diagnosed with protein-energy malnutrition, nutritional support depends on the patient's medical condition and the degree of the protein-energy malnutrition. Enteral nutritional support is considered when the patient's nutritional intake is inadequate to meet physiological requirements for >7 days or when the weight loss is >10% of the patient's pre-illness weight.

Follow-up: Patients who are hospitalized for malnutrition or who develop malnutrition secondary to an acute-care hospitalization should be monitored daily for response to the nutritional supplementation. The patient's weight should be monitored weekly until the malnutrition has been corrected. If a psychosocial factor contributed to the malnutrition, periodic review of the patient's improvement is warranted. Community-dwelling older adults may benefit from a nurse case manager to follow their progress in the home.

Sequelae: An older person's initial reaction to prescribed nutrient supplements may result in electrolyte abnormalities, hyperglycemia, hypotension, and aspiration pneumonia. Long-term malnutrition increases the risk of morbidity and mortality. Careful assessment is necessary to determine if a patient is experiencing failure to thrive.

Prevention/prophylaxis: Given the number of older adults who are at risk for malnutrition, the health-care provider must screen patients periodically for nutritional deficits. A two-step approach for identifying malnutrition is suggested using the Mini-Nutritional Assessment Tool (MNA). A shortened version of the MNA (MNA-SF) has been studied and approved as an initial screening tool when undernutrition is suspected in the geriatric population (Table 11–2). The MNA-SF is highly correlated with the MNA, with a diagnostic accuracy of 98.7% for predicting undernutrition. The six-item MNA-SF can be used easily in the first step of the process because it does not require anthropometric testing. For the second-level screening, the MNA is considered the most reliable and

Table 11–2   Six-Item Mini-Nutritional Assessment Tool (MNA-SF)

1. Body mass index (BMI) (weight/kg/height [m^2]): $<19 = 0, 19–20.9 = 1, 21–22.9 = 2, 23+ = 3$
2. Recent weight loss (<3 mo)? >3 kg = 0, don't know = 1, 1– 3 kg = 2, no weight loss = 3
3. Acute disease or stress over the last 3 mo?   yes = 0, no = 2
4. Mobility: bed/chair = 0, at home = 1, can leave home = 2
5. Dementia/depression: severe = 0, mild = 1, no = 2
6. Loss of appetite over the last 3 mo?   severe = 0, mild = 1, no = 2

From Salva, A. et al; Nutrition and aging screening for malnutrition in dwelling elderly. *Public Health Nutrition* 4:1377; 2001.

validated nutritional tool. It is appropriate for use in the outpatient and nursing home settings. It does not require invasive laboratory testing and is cost-effective. The tool consists of an anthropometric assessment, general assessment, dietary assessment, and a self-assessment that engages the elderly person to assess their nutritional status. International studies have validated that subjects with an MNA score between 17 and 23.5 are at risk of malnutrition and intervention is indicated.

Referral: Referring patients who are malnourished to a specialist depends on the identifiable cause of the nutrition depletion. A dietitian should be consulted for a nutritional support evaluation. Refer patients who need long-term enteral support to a gastroenterologist for consideration of a percutaneous endoscopic gastrostomy or, in some cases, a feeding jejunostomy. Arrangements can be made for the community-dwelling older adult to receive Meals on Wheels. Provide information on the location of centers for congregate meals sites. For the patient diagnosed with a terminal illness, discuss the patient's and family's decision on nutritional support before beginning any intervention. If social isolation, low income, or functional status contributed to the development of malnutrition, the patient should be referred for social services or discharge planning.

Education: For the alert ambulatory older adult, review the Dietary Guidelines for Americans and the Food Pyramid. Teach family members caring for cognitively impaired or physically disabled older adults about dietary requirements and nutritional supplementation. Caregivers and elderly persons can improve nutritional status by simple measures, such as preparation of an adequate diet, hand feeding, adequate fitting dentures and oral hygiene, and adding liquid nutritional supplements between meals.

OBESITY

SIGNAL SYMPTOMS▶   elevated BMI, central obesity

Generalized obesity	ICD-9 CM: 278.0

Description: Screening for generalized obesity is determined by the calculation of a BMI (weight [kg] divided by height [m^2]). When the BMI is ≥ 30 kg/m^2, the individual is classified as obese. Obesity is associated strongly with increased morbidity and mortality. Individuals who lose weight reduce their risk for chronic diseases such as diabetes and cardiovascular disease.

Etiology: The etiology of obesity is unknown. Obesity is highly familial and hereditary, involving constitutional, lifestyle, and psychological factors.

Occurrence: Obesity is the most common nutritional disorder in the

United States. In the United States, 34 million people are obese, and 13 million are morbidly obese.

Age: Obesity rarely begins in the older adult; it is usually a lifelong process.

Ethnicity: African-American women have more of a tendency to be obese than do white women.

Gender: Obesity is more prevalent in women than in men.

Contributing factors: Familial tendency, sedentary lifestyle, lack of dietary instruction, social impetus to eat, mood and hormone fluctuation, environmental stressors, metabolism, endocrine disorders, boredom, medications, and preexisting diseases may contribute to the development of obesity.

Signs and symptoms: Obesity is recognized when an individual's BMI is $\geq$30 kg/m^2. A thorough nutritional assessment is warranted when an individual meets the overweight category: BMI $\geq$25 kg/m^2. Symptoms resulting from obesity include arthralgia, lethargy, headaches, urinary frequency, and alopecia. As part of the physical examination, determine the degree and distribution of the patient's body fat. Look for secondary causes of obesity, such as hypothyroidism or Cushing's syndrome.

Diagnostic tests:

Test	Results Indicating Disorder	CPT Code
*Clinical Indications of Metabolic Syndrome**		
Triglycerides	150 mg/dL	84478
HDL cholesterol		83718
Men	<40 mg/dL	
Women	<50 mg/dL	
Blood pressure	130/85 mm Hg	
Fasting glucose	110 mg/dL	401.9
Waist circumference		
Men	>102 cm (>40 inches)	
Women	>88 cm (>35 inches)	
Lipid Profile		
Total cholesterol	<200 mg/dL (desirable) 200–239 mg/dL (borderline high risk) 240 mg/dL (high risk)	82465
LDL cholesterol	<100 mg/dL (optimal) <130 mg/dL (desirable) 130–159 mg/dL (borderline high risk) 160 mg/dL (high risk) *Note:* The goal of therapy in patients with diabetes is an optimal LDL <100 mg/dL	84443
TSH	0.49–4.67 μIU/mL <0.49 μIU/mL (hypothyroidism)	80418, 80438–80440

* Three or more of the following values indicate the metabolic syndrome.

Obese individuals should be screened for the components of the metabolic syndrome (central obesity, hypertriglyceridemia, low HDL cholesterol, hypertension). Lipid profile, fasting glucose levels, and waist circumference should be obtained for all obese patients.

 Clinical Pearl: Individuals who are at a normal BMI but have central obesity still may be at risk for chronic illnesses and in need of diet and exercise prescriptions.

Waist circumference for adults is the best indirect measurement of fat distribution because compared with studies using imaging techniques, it is least affected by gender, race, or overall level of adiposity. The National Heart, Lung and Blood Institute (NHLBI, 1998) recommended waist circumference as a comparable measurement of central obesity. Taken with the subject standing, waist circumference is measured from the uppermost lateral border of the iliac crest. Adults ≥18 years old are considered to have central obesity if waist circumference is >102 cm (40 inches) for men and 88 cm (35 inches) for women (NHLBI, 1998). Waist circumference cut points can be standardized across all adult ethnic populations except for individuals <5 feet tall or individuals with a BMI >35. The NHLBI recommends that waist circumference in these cases be adjusted by age and BMI.

If an endocrine disorder is suspected, TSH levels should be ordered to rule out hypothyroidism. Dexamethasone suppression testing is suggested to determine presence of Cushing's syndrome.

Differential diagnosis: Determine the BMI:

$$BMI = (weight\ [lb] \times 703)/(height^2\ [inches])$$

Definition of Obesity in Adults

BMI	Definition
<18.5	Underweight
18.5–24.9	Normal
25.0–29.9	Overweight
30.0–34.9	Class I obesity
35.0–39.9	Class II obesity
≥40.0	Class III extreme obesity

From National Heart, Lung and Blood Institute/The National Institute of Diabetes and Digestive and Kidney Diseases: The evidence report: Clinical guidelines on the identification, evaluation, and treatment of overweight and obesity in adults. NIH Publication No. 98-4083. National Institutes of Health, Bethesda, Md., 1998.

BMI has been the traditional measurement to detect the presence of obesity. It has been widely theorized that an elevated BMI leads to an array of metabolic risk factors for chronic diseases. Researchers and practitioners alike have been puzzled, however, by the different constellations of metabolic findings in individuals with the same BMI. More recently, central obesity has been described as an independent correlate of cardiovascular risk in adults. Android fat patterns in adults have been associated more closely with the components of the metabolic syndrome than generalized obesity. When screening obese individuals, assess specifically for the clustering of symptoms that comprise the metabolic syndrome because it is highly associated with increased cardiovascular risk.

Treatment: Weight loss, with reductions of salt, fat, and carbohydrates in the diet, is recommended. Patients should increase their activity level and participate in group therapy or self-help groups (i.e., Weight Watchers, TOPS, Diet Center). Diet suppressants generally are not recommended for older adults.

Follow-up: Return visits should occur as often as needed to monitor weight reduction and achieve the goal set for the patient.

Sequelae: Coronary artery disease, diabetes, and hypertension are all much more prevalent in obese individuals.

Prevention/prophylaxis: A low-fat, nutritionally adequate diet and regular exercise help prevent and treat obesity.

Referral: Morbidly obese patients may require surgical intervention, but most obese persons can be treated by primary-care practitioners. Patients may be referred to the local Weight Watchers or TOPS organization.

Education: Teach patients and significant others meal preparation, calorie counts, and fat gram calculation. Elimination of alcohol and fatty foods is essential. Encourage patients to begin a safe exercise regimen. Educate regarding the need to maintain a normal waist circumference.

PANCREATIC CANCER

SIGNAL SYMPTOMS ▶ lesions of pancreatic head: painless jaundice, acholic stools, nausea and vomiting, lesions of the pancreatic body and tail: weight loss, vague abdominal or back pain

Pancreatic cancer ICD-9 CM: 159.9 (malignant neoplasms–gastrointestinal tract NOS)

Description: Pancreatic cancer, found primarily in older adults, is one of the leading causes of death in this population. Of exocrine neoplasms of the pancreas, 80% occur in the head of the pancreas, with the remaining 20% occurring in the body and tail. The types of pancreatic cancer are as follows:

Ductal cell adenocarcinoma accounts for 75% to 96% of all types of pancreatic cancers.

Giant cell carcinoma (also called *carcinosarcoma*) is a highly malignant lesion with early distant metastases.

Adenosquamous carcinoma is more common in men and in patients with a history of radiation treatment.

Cystadenocarcinoma has the best prognosis with only 20% metastasizing by surgery.

Etiology: Although the etiology of pancreatic cancer is unknown, many predisposing factors, such as cigarette smoking, carcinogens in the environment (e.g., coal tar derivatives), diabetes mellitus, and heredity, may be precursors to pancreatic cancer.

Occurrence: Pancreatic cancer is the fifth most common cause of death from cancer, accounting for 13% of gastrointestinal malignancies. It is the second most common gastrointestinal cancer, with about 29,000 new cases per year; 20,000 of these cases occur in patients >65 years old. The incidence increases with age and is 10 times greater in men >75 years old. The incidence of pancreatic cancer seems to be highest in people from urban areas and in lower socioeconomic classes.

Age: Pancreatic cancer usually occurs in persons age 60 to 80, with the peak time of onset in the 80s.

Ethnicity: Exocrine pancreatic cancer is higher in African-Americans and in people of Hawaiian descent than in whites.

Gender: Pancreatic cancer is more prevalent in men than in women.

Contributing factors: Pancreatic cancer is more common in heavy cigarette smokers than in nonsmokers. Persons with a history of familial colorectal cancer, polyposis syndrome, diet high in animal fat, chronic pancreatitis, and diabetes mellitus are susceptible to pancreatic cancer.

Signs and symptoms: Older adults with pancreatic cancer often present with anorexia, weight loss, anxiety, diarrhea, and depression and may report that these symptoms have existed for the past 3 to 6 months. In 70% to 80% of patients with ductal cell adenocarcinoma, metastatic spread is evident at diagnosis. Complaints of epigastric pain radiating to the back, unexplained weight loss, and in some cases steatorrhea are common. Jaundice appears with progression of the disease, and patients may complain of itching. Symptoms of diabetes may appear or worsen. During the abdominal examination, supraclavicular lymphadenopathy may be noted. You also may find a palpable gallbladder (Courvoisier's sign), hepatomegaly, overall abdominal tenderness, and possibly evidence of ascites. Thrombophlebitis occurs in a few patients.

Diagnostic tests:

Test	Results Indicating Disorder	CPT Code
Complete blood count	Mild anemia	85031
Fasting blood glucose	Glycosuria	80422–80424, 80430–80435
Liver function tests		80076
Serum amylase	May be elevated	82150

Test	Results Indicating Disorder	CPT Code
Abdominal CT followed by a CT-guided needle aspiration	Confirmation of pancreatic cancer cells	74150 (without contrast enhancement) 74160 (with contrast enhancement) 76360 (needle biopsy)
ERCP	Useful if the mass is located at the pancreaticobiliary junction	74330

Differential diagnosis:
- Choledocholithiasis
- Pancreatitis
- Duodenal neoplasms
- Choledochal cyst
- Pancreatic pseudocyst
- Biliary tract stricture

Treatment: Given the poor prognosis of pancreatic cancer combined with the advanced age of the patient, treatment usually is limited to palliative measures. For patients with nonmetastatic lesions located in the head of the pancreas, pancreatoduodenectomy (Whipple's procedure) may be recommended. In some cases, a specialist may recommend use of a biliary stent to reduce the jaundice and itching. Control of pain is essential; analgesics and oral narcotics should be ordered. An antihistamine can be prescribed to control pruritus. Chemotherapy yields little response and no long-term benefit; if used, however, 5-fluorouracil is the most widely used drug and has a response rate of 15% in the elderly and is tolerated relatively well.

Follow-up: Emotional support and pain control are crucial for patients with pancreatic cancer. Because the progression of the disease can be rapid, patients and their families may need assistance in preparing for end-of-life decisions.

Sequelae: The prognosis of pancreatic cancer in older adults is grim. The mortality rate for adenocarcinoma of the pancreas is high shortly after diagnosis.

Prevention/prophylaxis: Cessation of alcohol consumption and cigarette smoking is recommended.

Referral: Refer to an oncologist when the diagnosis of pancreatic cancer is suspected. Contact local hospice care services for the patient and family.

Education: For their nutritional needs, advise patients to consume six small meals a day instead of the usual three. Patients may prefer nutritional supplements in place of one or more of these meals each day. When the disease has reached the terminal stage, assure the patient that you will collaborate with the hospice agency to provide for the patient's comfort throughout the disease process.

REFERENCES

General

American Medical Association: Current Procedural Terminology: CPT 2002, ed 4. AMA Press, Chicago, 2002.

DeGowin, RL, and Brown, D: DeGowin's Diagnostic Examination, ed 7. McGraw-Hill, New York, 2000.

Goroll, A, and Mulley, AG: Primary Care Medicine: Office Evaluation and Management of the Adult Patient, ed 4. Lippincott Williams, & Wilkins, Philadelphia, 2000.

Kennedy-Malone, L, et al: Management Guidelines for Gerontological Nurse Practitioners. FA Davis, Philadelphia, 1999.

Chronic Pancreatitis

Etemad, B, and Whitcomb, DC: Chronic pancreatitis: Diagnosis, classification, and new genetic development. Gastroenterology 11:682, 2000.

Hutchins, RR, et al: Long-term results of distal pancreatectomy for chronic pancreatitis in 90 patients. Ann Surg 236:612, 2002.

Pennachio, D: The latest approaches to pancreatic disease. Patient Care 35:55, 2001.

Diabetes Mellitus

American Academy of Family Physicians: Benefits and risks of controlling blood glucose levels in patients with type 2 diabetes mellitus. J Fam Pract 49:453, 2000.

American Diabetes Association: Standards of medical care for patients with diabetes mellitus. Diabetes Care 24:S33, 2001.

Mokdad, AH, et al: The continuing epidemics of obesity and diabetes in the United States. JAMA 286:1195, 2001.

Mokdad, AH, et al: Diabetes trends in the U.S.: 1990–1998. Diabetes Care 23:1278, 2001.

Hyperlipidemia

American Heart Association: Heart and Stroke Statistical Update 2000. American Heart Association, Dallas, 2001.

Bartol, T: Endocrine and metabolic health. In Meredith, P, and Horan, N (eds): Adult Primary Care. WB Saunders, Philadelphia, 2000.

Expert Panel: Summary of the third report of the National Cholesterol Education Program (NCEP) Expert Panel on Detection, Evaluation, and Treatment of High Blood Cholesterol in Adults (Adult treatment panel III). JAMA 285:2486, 2001.

Grundy, SM: Metabolic complications of obesity. Endocrine 13:155, 2000.

Juhan-Vague, I, and Alessi, MC: PAI-1, obesity, insulin resistance and risk of cardiovascular events. Thromb Haemost 78:656, 1997.

Lemieux, I, et al: Hyper triglyceridemic waist: A marker of atherogenic metabolic triad (hyperinsulinemia; hyperapolipoprotein B; small dense LDL) in men? Circulation 102:179, 2000.

National Heart, Lung and Blood Institute/The National Institute of Diabetes and Digestive and Kidney Diseases: The evidence report: Clinical guidelines on the identification, evaluation, and treatment of overweight and obesity in adults. NIH Publication No. 98-4083. National Institute of Health, Bethesda, Md., 1998.

Reaven, GM: Banting lecture 1988: Role of insulin resistance in human disease. Diabetes 37:1597, 1988.

Hyperthyroidism

Canaris, GJ, et al: Managing geriatric endocrine disorders. Patient Care 35:43, 2001.

Fisher, J: Management of thyrotoxicosis. South Med J 95:493, 2002.

Fowler, MJ, et al: Pitfalls to avoid while interpreting thyroid function tests: Five illustrative cases. South Med J 95:486, 2002. Contact: http://www.medscape.com/viewarticle/433853_print. Accessed June 18, 2002.

Levine, N, and Wallace, K: Thyroid dysfunction: How to manage overt and subclinical disease in older patients. Geriatrics 53:32, 1998.

LoBuono, C: Managing geriatric endocrine disorders. Patient Care for the Nurse Practitioner 4:26, 2001.

Shrier, DK, and Burman, KD: Subclinical hyperthyroidism: Controversies in management. Am Acad Fam Physicians 65:431, 2002. Contact: http://www.aafp.org/afp/20020201/431.html. Accessed June 28, 2002.

Supit, EJ, and Peiris, A: Interpretation of laboratory thyroid function tests for the primary care physician. South Med J 95:481, 2002.

Hypothyroidism

Canaris, GJ, et al: Managing geriatric endocrine disorders. Patient Care 35:43, 2001.

Fowler, MJ, et al: Pitfalls to avoid while interpreting thyroid function tests: Five illustrative cases. South Med J 95:486, 2002. Contact: http://www.medscape.com/viewarticle/433853_print. Accessed June 18, 2002.

Levine, N, and Wallace, K: Thyroid dysfunction: How to manage overt and subclinical disease in older patients. Geriatrics 53:32, 1998.

LoBuono, C: Managing geriatric endocrine disorders. Patient Care for the Nurse Practitioner 4:26, 2001.

Supit, EJ, and Peiris, A: Interpretation of laboratory thyroid function tests for the primary care physician. South Med J 95:481, 2002.

Guha, B, et al: The diagnosis and management of hypothyroidism. South Med J 95:475, 2002.

Hueston, WJ: Treatment of hypothyroidism. Am Fam Physician 64:1717, 2001.

Michalek, AM, et al: Hypothyroidism and diabetes mellitus in an American Indian population. J Fam Pract 49:638, 2000. Contact: http://www.jfponline.com/content/2000/07/jfp_0700_06380.asp. Accessed March 18, 2002.

Orlander, PR, and Woodhouse, WR: Hypothyroidism. eMedicine Journal 3, 2002. Contact: http://www.emedicine.com/med/topic1145.htm. Accessed March 20, 2002.

Malnutrition

Ennis, BW, et al: Diagnosing malnutrition in the elderly. Nurse Practitioner 26:52, 2001.

Kamel, H, et al: Nutritional deficiencies in long-term care: Part II. Management of protein energy malnutrition and dehydration. Ann Long-Term Care 6:250, 1998.

Morley, JE, et al: Nutritional deficiencies in long-term care: Part I. Detection and diagnosis. Ann Long-Term Care 6:183, 1998.

Morley, JE, and Silver, AJ: Nutritional issues in nursing home care. Ann Intern Med 123: 850, 1998.

Obesity

Bray, GA: Contemporary Diagnosis and Management of Obesity. Handbooks in Healthcare. Newton, Pa., 1998.

Despres, J, et al: Treatment of obesity: Need to focus on high risk abdominally obese patients. BMJ 322:716, 2001.

Expert Panel: Summary of the third report of the National Cholesterol Education Program (NCEP) Expert Panel on Detection, Evaluation, and Treatment of High Blood Cholesterol in Adults (Adult treatment Panel III). JAMA 285:2486, 2001.

Grundy, SM: Metabolic complications of obesity. Endocrine 13:155, 2000.

Harris, M, et al: Associations of fat distribution and obesity with hypertension in a bi-ethnic population: The ARIC Study. Obes Res 8:516, 2000.

Katzmarzyk, P, et al: Familial risk of obesity and central adipose tissue distribution general Canadian population. Am J Epidemiol 149:933, 1999.

Kelley, D, et al: Subdivisions of subcutaneous abdominal adipose tissue and insulin resistance. Am J Endocrinol Metab 278:E941, 2000.

Lean, M, et al: Waist circumference as a measure for indicating need for weight management. BMJ 311:158, 1995.

Lemieux, I, et al: Hyper triglyceridemic waist: A marker of atherogenic metabolic triad (hyperinsulinemia; hyperapolipoprotein B; small dense LDL) in men? Circulation 102:179, 2000.

National Heart, Lung and Blood Institute/The National Institute of Diabetes and Digestive and Kidney Diseases: The evidence report: Clinical guidelines on the identification, evaluation, and treatment of overweight and obesity in adults. NIH Publication No. 98-4083. National Institute of Health, Bethesda, Md., 1998.

Okosun, I, et al: Abdominal adiposity in the United States: Prevalence and attributable risk of hypertension. J Hum Hypertens 13:425, 1999.

Okosun, I, et al: Abdominal adiposity values associated with established body mass indexes in white, black and Hispanic Americans: A study from the third National Health and Nutrition Examination Survey. Int J Obes Rel Metab Disord 24:1279, 2000.

Reaven, GM: Banting Lecture 1988: Role of insulin resistance in human disease. Diabetes 37:1597, 1988.

Tremblay, A, et al: The treatment of obesity in the elderly patient. Ann Long-Term Care 10:58, 2002.

Vague, J: The degree of masculine differentiation of obesities: A factor determining predisposition to diabetes, atherosclerosis, gout, and uric calculous disease. Am J Clin Nutr 4:20, 1956.

Pancreatic Cancer

Klein, AP, et al: Evidence for a major gene influencing the risk of pancreatic cancer. Genet Epidemiol 23:133, 2002.

Pennachio, D: The latest approaches to pancreatic disease. Patient Care 35:55, 2001.

Chapter 12
HEMATOLOGICAL AND IMMUNE SYSTEM DISORDERS

ANEMIA OF CHRONIC DISEASE

SIGNAL SYMPTOMS ▶ minimal to none; patients with cardiopulmonary decompensation or combined anemia of chronic disease and iron deficiency anemia may experience the following: easy fatigability, headache, irritability, dyspnea, tachycardia, palpitations

| Anemia of chronic disease (ACD) | ICD-9-CM: 285.2 |

Description: Anemia is defined as a decline in red blood cell (RBC) mass to below the expected laboratory norms for age and gender. Three underlying mechanisms are responsible for anemia: bleeding, inadequate production of RBCs, and excessive destruction of RBCs. ACD is anemia in the presence of a chronic condition, such as inflammatory or autoimmune disorders, chronic infection, malignancy, or protein-calorie malnutrition. It is generally normocytic and normochromic, although about 25% to 35% may be microcytic in advanced stages; it coexists with iron-deficiency anemia (IDA) in some older persons. Anemia in patients with renal, hepatic, or endocrine disorders is categorized separately because it manifests with a different hematological profile.

Etiology: The exact mechanism is poorly understood. Inflammatory cytokines suppress erythropoietin production and may interfere with the proliferation of erythroid progenitor cells. There is decreased production of RBCs and a shorter than normal RBC life span. The iron that is produced is sequestered in the reticuloendothelial system and so is not available for use. This results in normal or high bone marrow iron stores, decreased serum iron and total iron-binding capacity (TIBC), and normal to increased serum ferritin.

Occurrence: ACD is the most common anemia in older adults.

Age: ACD is most frequent in older adults.

Ethnicity: No ethnic groups are more prone to ACD.

Gender: More women than men have anemia; this is not specific to ACD.

Contributing factors: Presence of one or more chronic conditions, such as cancer, chronic infection, chronic inflammation, or autoimmune conditions.

Signs and symptoms: Usually none. Signs may be discovered incidentally through laboratory work; symptoms may be those of the underlying condition as well as easy fatigability, myalgias, weight loss, and poor appetite.

Diagnostic tests:

Test	Results Indicating Disorder	CPT Code
CBC	Hemoglobin <12 g/dL (120 g/L) women <13 g/dL (130 g/L) men Rarely <10 g/dL (100g/L) Hematocrit high 20s to mid-30s Rarely <25% (suggests additional cause) Mean corpuscular volume 80–96 μm^3 (normocytic) 70–80 μm^3 (microcytic) RBC distribution width normal	85031
Reticulocyte production index	<2	85044–85046
TIBC	Low/decreased	83550
Serum iron	Low/decreased	83540
Transferrin saturation	Decreased	84466
Serum ferritin	Normal to increased	82728

CBC, complete blood count.

See section on IDA for comparison of laboratory findings in ACD, IDA, and coexisting IDA with ACD.

Differential diagnosis: Early or partially treated IDA.

Treatment: Treat underlying cause; if anemia is severe or underlying disease is resistant to treatment, treatment with epoetin alfa (Epogen, Procrit) or transfusion may be indicated; if IDA and ACD coexist, initiate a trial of iron therapy (see section on IDA).

Follow-up: Follow-up is individualized depending on underlying cause and extent of anemia.

Sequelae: Variable depending on underlying condition.

Prevention/prophylaxis: Early education in healthy lifestyle may prevent or delay onset of some chronic conditions.

Referral: Referral is indicated for progression of anemia and need for transfusion and exacerbation of chronic condition requiring specialty evaluation.

Education: Teach patient and family about the importance of management of the underlying condition; individualize education.

HUMAN IMMUNODEFICIENCY VIRUS

SIGNAL SYMPTOMS none, initially; fever, fatigue, sore throat, weight loss, myalgias, decreased physical endurance, declining mental capacity

Human immunodeficiency virus (HIV) ICD-9 CM: 042 (symptomatic), V08 (infection)

Description: HIV, a human retrovirus, is the infectious agent that causes acquired immunodeficiency syndrome (AIDS). Two types of HIV have been identified: HIV-1 and HIV-2. Although the viruses share similar epidemiological traits, they are serologically and geographically distinct. HIV-1, the more pathogenic of the two, is found worldwide, with infection being most prevalent in the sub-Saharan regions of Africa, the Americas, Western Europe, and South and Southeast Asia. The HIV-2 virus resides primarily in West Africa; cases in other areas have been linked epidemiologically to West Africa.

Etiology: HIV, the etiological agent for AIDS, is spread by contact with parenteral and body fluids. The three known modes of transmission are:

- Contact with blood and blood products: needle sharing, transfusions
- Sexual transmission: anal, oral, or vaginal intercourse
- Perinatal transmission: in utero, during delivery, through breast-feeding

Traditionally the primary mode of transmission was men having sex with men; however, heterosexual contact is the most rapidly increasing mode of transmission.

Occurrence: HIV occurs worldwide; the World Health Organization estimates that >40 million people have HIV. The United States has reported the largest number of cases, with a cumulative total of 807,075 adult/adolescent AIDS cases as of December 2001; 462,653 (57%) of these patients have died. An estimated 159,000 adults and adolescents in the United States are infected with HIV but have not developed AIDS.

Age: HIV occurs in all age groups; 11% of all AIDS cases reported to the Centers for Disease Control and Prevention (CDC) have involved patients >50 years old, with 3% of these patients >60 years old. As of December 2001, a cumulative total of 11,555 AIDS cases were reported in the ≥65 years old age group; 12,898 were reported in the 60- to 64-year-old group. Older patients with AIDS are likely to die sooner from the disease; however, this is changing with the advent of highly active antiretroviral therapy (HAART).

Ethnicity: African-Americans have the highest rate of HIV and AIDS in the United States; Hispanics have the second highest rate.

Gender: More men than women have HIV; however, the largest rate of increase in reported AIDS cases is currently in women.

Contributing factors: High-risk behaviors, such as engaging in unprotected heterosexual or homosexual sex, can lead to HIV infection. The older patient is much less likely to use a condom because there is no fear of pregnancy. Ignorance about the disease and its consequences also contributes to risky behavior. The frequency of sexual contact and number of sexual partners affect an individual's risk for getting HIV. Postmenopausal women are more likely to have lesions of vaginal mucus membranes, owing to atrophic changes. Intravenous drug use is a risk factor, particularly with shared needles. Blood transfusion with contaminated blood is no longer a significant factor because the Red Cross screens blood for HIV. Possibly the immune system changes that occur with aging may render older patients more susceptible to contracting HIV once they have encountered it. Health-care providers do not routinely ask older patients about sexual behaviors and HIV risk factors; this leads to a delay in detection and treatment.

Signs and symptoms: In the initial asymptomatic phase of HIV infection, the patient does not have any symptoms. In the older patient, the first sign may be confusion or AIDS-related dementia. Vague signs and symptoms, such as weight loss, dehydration, ataxic gait, fatigue, or withdrawal, may go unnoticed or be attributed to other illnesses. Because the index of suspicion is generally low in the older patient, the diagnosis may never be made. A sexual history is crucial in exposing risk factors. When the possibility has been established, permission for diagnostic testing should be obtained. The presence of disseminated herpes zoster, vaginal or oral candidiasis, tuberculosis, or pneumonia should raise the index of suspicion for HIV.

Diagnostic tests:

Test	Results Indicating Disorder	CPT Code
ELISA	Positive	87390 (HIV-1) 87391 (HIV-2)
Confirmatory Western blot	Positive	86689
CD4+ T-cell count	Low; $<350/mm^3$ is one factor used to consider treatment	86360
Plasma HIV RNA (viral load)	High; $>55,000$ copies/mL is one factor used to consider treatment	87536

ELISA, enzyme-linked immunosorbent assay.

HIV diagnosis requires a positive ELISA test result, followed by a confirmatory positive Western blot test. When the diagnosis has been confirmed, a pretreatment plasma HIV RNA level and a CD4+ T-cell count should be obtained.

Differential diagnosis: Differential diagnosis in the older patient with

HIV includes Alzheimer's dementia, influenza, depression, malabsorption, malnutrition, occult malignancy, tuberculosis, and pneumonia.

Treatment: For best outcomes, patients should be referred to an HIV specialty center or HIV specialists. No specific guidelines exist at present for treatment specific to older adults with HIV. Adult and adolescent guidelines are used. The most salient issues with older adults are ignorance of risk, attributing symptoms to other comorbidities or age leading to delay in seeking care, and advanced disease before seeking treatment. The recommended treatment is a combination drug treatment with three or more HIV drugs (HAART).

Before treatment, obtain HIV RNA level (baseline viral load set-point) and a CD4+ T-cell count, preferably on two different occasions, using the same laboratory both times to ensure accuracy and consistency. Patients presenting with advanced disease should be treated after the initial measurement. If the patient is not treated, HIV RNA levels should continue to be measured every 3 to 4 months; CD4+ T cells should be measured every 3 to 6 months.

Patients are divided into two categories for discussion: asymptomatic infection or symptomatic disease including AIDS. All patients with symptomatic disease should be offered antiretroviral therapy. Treatment of asymptomatic patients presents a complex situation. Studies have shown that antiretroviral therapy is clinically beneficial to HIV-infected patients with advanced disease and immunosuppression. The treatment options available that offer the maximum benefit are medically complex, however, with a high incidence of side effects, interactions, and potential drug resistance. The challenge is achieving patient compliance. The HIV specialist and the patient must consider many factors before deciding on treatment during this asymptomatic stage. (Complete guidelines for further information in this area can be found on the CDC website.)

When a decision has been made to initiate therapy in either category, the following studies should be performed:

- Complete history and physical examination
- CBC, chemistry profile, including lipid profile and serum transaminases
- CD4+ T-lymphocyte count
- Plasma HIV RNA measurement (viral load)

Routine studies pertinent to prevention of opportunistic infections include:

- Venereal Disease Research Laboratory test or rapid plasma reagin
- Purified protein derivative
- Toxoplasma IgG
- Pap smear and gynecological examination for women

Other tests as clinically indicated may include:

- Chest x-ray examination
- Hepatitis C serology

- Ophthalmologic examination
- Cytomegalovirus serology
- Hepatitis B serology

For older patients, perform liver function and creatinine clearance studies.

Treatment for Asymptomatic Patients

Aggressive

Give early treatment, based on awareness of the progressive nature of HIV. Begin treatment before development of significant immunosuppression, and treat to achieve undetectable viremia. Treatment decision is determined by considering CD4+ T-cell count and plasma HIV RNA (viral load), clinical picture, and willingness of patient to commit to treatment regimen. Therapy is begun with a regimen that reduces viral replication to undetectable levels.

Conservative

Delay therapy because low risk of clinically significant progression and other factors weigh in favor of observation and delay.

Starting Therapy in Patients with Advanced HIV

Advanced HIV is any condition that meets the 1993 CDC definition of AIDS. These patients require treatment with antiretroviral agents (Table 12–1), despite plasma viral levels, as do patients who have symptomatic HIV without AIDS, defined by presence of thrush or unexplained fever. Although many of these patients have opportunistic infections, malignancy, wasting, or dementia when initially diagnosed, drug therapy still is needed. The provider must consider the whole picture, including drug toxicity, treatment compliance, drug interactions, and laboratory findings, before beginning treatment with a powerful and efficacious regimen such as HAART. Strict criteria for discontinuation of therapy should be adhered to, despite acute situations; problems with drug toxicity, intolerance, or interactions are valid considerations. The complexity of the drug treatment regimen and the potential for drug interactions and toxicities are impressive. Additionally, the protease inhibitors (PIs) and non-nucleoside reverse transcriptase inhibitors (NNRTIs) involve the cytochrome P-450 enzymatic pathway. Interactive communication about drug treatment and avoidance of over-the-counter and other drugs without first consulting the HIV specialist are essential. If interruption of antiretroviral drug therapy is necessary, all agents should be discontinued simultaneously to minimize the development of resistant strains.

The health-care provider must distinguish between drug failure and drug toxicity causing a need to change therapy. A multiplicity of factors must be considered before making a change, including plasma HIV RNA levels measured on two different occasions, CD4+ T-lymphocyte count,

Table 12–1   Classes of Antiretroviral Agents Used in HIV/AIDs Treatment

Protease Inhibitors
Indinavir (Crixivan)
Saquinavir (Invirase, Fortovase)
Amprenavir (Agenerase)
Nelfinavir (Viracept)
Ritonavir (Norvir)
Ritonavir/lopinavir (Kaletra)

Non-Nucleoside Reverse Transcriptase Inhibitors
Nevirapine (Viramune)
Delavirdine (Rescriptor)
Efavirenz (Sustiva)

Nucleoside/Nucleotide Reverse Transcriptase Inhibitors
Didanosine (ddI) (Videx)
Lamivudine (*3TC) (Epivir)
Stavudine (d4T) (Zerit)
Zidovudine (AZT, ZDV) (Retrovir)
Zalcitabine (ddC) (Hivid)
Tenofovir (Viread)
Zidovudine/lamivudine (Combivir)
Zidovudine/lamivudine/abacavir (Trizivir)

treatment options, compliance and complexity of regimen, mental health issues, pharmacokinetics, patient education, and toxicity.

The goal of antiretroviral therapy is improvement of length and quality of life by maximal suppression of viral replication to undetectable levels (<50 copies/mL) early enough to preserve immune function. If this goal is not accomplished with one regimen, a change is indicated. Plasma HIV RNA level is the key parameter indicating response to therapy. (See References for sources of more in-depth information in this area.)

Follow-up: Planned follow-up by the HIV specialist includes plasma HIV RNA and CD4+ T-cell counts as specified earlier, self-monitoring, and development of good self-care habits. If a patient's sexual contact is the source of the infection, encourage that person to undergo testing. Report disease to proper the public health authority within confidentiality guidelines and state regulations. Close monitoring of the patient for medication side effects and toxicity is especially needed with older patients. Older patients are more compliant with treatment than younger ones, but the importance of adherence in preventing drug resistance must be emphasized.

Sequelae: HIV has many possible complications, including opportunistic infections; poor adherence can result in drug resistance and treatment failure. HAART side effects may include hyperlipidemia, diabetes, lipodystrophy syndrome, increased bleeding in hemophiliacs, osteonecrosis, osteopenia, osteoporosis, hepatotoxicity, lactic acidosis, hepatic steatosis, and skin rash.

Prevention/prophylaxis: Patients can prevent HIV infection through avoidance of unprotected sex and intravenous drug use and by considering autologous blood transfusion for any planned surgery. Health-care providers should inquire about sexual activity at each visit and target healthy older adult groups such as widow/widower/divorce support groups for risk factor education. Immunization of HIV-positive individuals with pneumococcal and influenza vaccines is indicated, unless the patient is allergic to these vaccines. Health-care personnel should use universal precautions and proper handling and disposal of contaminated needles and blood collection equipment.

Referral: On diagnosis, refer patients to an HIV specialty nurse practitioner or other health-care specialist in HIV; whenever possible, management should be done by an HIV specialist. Collaborative management is indicated during stable periods. Refer patients to a nutritionist for dietary guidance for weight loss or wasting. Refer community-dwelling older adults to home health services when appropriate. Refer to support group if patient desires.

Education: Teach patient and family or caregivers about disease transmission, precautions, treatment options, self-care measures, and safe sex to prevent transmission to others. Teach patient not to take any other medications or over-the-counter preparations without first clearing it with the health-care provider because of the potential for interactions with cytochrome P-450 drugs.

Resources:

- www.hivatis.org
- www.cdc.gov
- www.actis.org
- www.avert.org
- www.hivinsite.ucsf.edu
- www.unaids.org

IRON-DEFICIENCY ANEMIA

SIGNAL SYMPTOMS ▶ vague or absent symptoms in early stage, easy fatigability, dizziness, tachycardia, palpitations, exertional dyspnea

Iron-deficiency anemia	ICD-9 CM: 280.9

Description: IDA is a microcytic anemia caused by reduced iron stores. The onset may be acute, reflecting rapid blood loss, or chronic with slow blood loss and poor nutrition. IDA can be normocytic in the early stages.

Etiology: Potential causes of IDA include inadequate ingestion and increased requirements, decreased absorption or use, or blood loss. The etiology may be multifactorial. In older adults, slow gastrointestinal blood loss frequently is identified.

Occurrence: IDA is the second most common type of anemia in the older adult; ACD is the most common in older adults.

Age: IDA affects all ages. It is the second most common anemia in the older adult.

Ethnicity: Not significant.

Gender: More women than men are affected.

Contributing factors: In the older patient, decreased oral intake, partial gastrectomy, malabsorption syndromes, low socioeconomic status, medications including non-steroidal anti-inflammatory drugs, combination of medication and alcohol, and chronic blood loss (most frequently from the gastrointestinal tract), are contributing factors for IDA. Some gastrointestinal causes include peptic ulcer disease, gastritis, hiatal hernia with mucosal ulceration, neoplasms, angiodysplasia, and diverticular disease. In patients with prosthetic heart valves, intravascular hemolysis may lead to IDA related to increased hemosiderin loss in the urine. Chronic blood loss from genitourinary cancer is a less frequent cause.

Signs and symptoms: The presentation of IDA is vague, frequently going unnoticed in older patients. It may be an incidental blood study finding, prompting further investigation. Fatigue, weakness, lethargy, tachycardia, palpitations, dyspnea on exertion, headache, irritability, inability to concentrate, neuralgia, sore tongue, paresthesias, and susceptibility to infection are possible as hemoglobin decreases to <8 g/dL. Dizziness, faintness, claudication, exercise intolerance, or angina also may present. Mental confusion, disorientation, loss of memory, or depression can occur in older adults. In some cases, symptoms may reflect the underlying cause (e.g., stomach discomfort with peptic ulcer disease).

Physical examination may be unremarkable. Pallor, common in patients with significant anemia, is also common with aging and may be discounted as a normal age-related finding. Conjunctival pallor, bluish discoloration of the sclerae, cheilosis, glossitis, brittle ridged nails, or spoon nails (koilonychia) may be present.

Cardiovascular and respiratory examination may reveal tachycardia, systolic murmur, or signs of congestive heart failure. In some patients, splenomegaly may be present owing to hemolysis of iron-deficient RBCs.

Diagnostic tests:

Test	Results Indicating Disorder	CPT Code
CBC	Hemoglobin <12 g/dL (120 g/L) RBC distribution width increased	85031
Reticulocyte production index	<2	85044–85046
TIBC	High/increased	83550
Serum iron	Low/decreased	83540
Transferrin saturation	Decreased	84466
Serum ferritin	Decreased	82728

Diagnostic tests: CBC done initially reveals a low hemoglobin (<12 g/dL). RBCs are normocytic and normochromic at this point. Serum ferritin is the first value to change (<30 μg/L) and is the most reliable test to distinguish IDA from ACD. Serum ferritin is an acute phase reactant for liver damage and some types of tumors and so may not be accurate if these conditions exist. As iron deficiency progresses, peripheral smear shows microcytosis, poikilocytosis, and hypochromia (usually at hemoglobin <8 g/dL). Bone marrow iron stain is usually unnecessary, unless there are confounding factors. Diagnostic studies related to the possible cause of the iron deficiency also must be done. See Table 12–2 for comparison of diagnostic test results in IDA, ACD, and concomitant IDA and ACD.

Differential diagnosis:
- ACD (both are normocytic in early stage)
- Sideroblastic anemia R/T toxic effects of isoniazid or pyrazinamide therapy for tuberculosis (in patients with tuberculosis)
- Mild thalassemia

Treatment: Besides relieving symptoms, treatment must address the underlying disorder whenever possible. Transfusion with packed RBCs may be necessary initially, if blood loss threatens to damage vital organs. Oral iron supplementation should be instituted with ferrous sulfate, 325 mg orally three times daily for 6 months, on an empty stomach, if tolerated. Ascorbic acid taken with the medication enhances absorption. If follow-up laboratory studies fail to show increases in hematocrit after 4 to 8 weeks, re-evaluate the patient for noncompliance, malabsorption, ongoing bleeding, or missed diagnosis.

Medication therapy may cause significant gastrointestinal side effects in 20% to 25% of patients, including constipation, diarrhea, nausea, or abdominal cramping. Ferrous gluconate or fumarate may be tolerated better; alternatively, consider a reduction in ferrous sulfate dosage to once daily over a 1-year period. In some cases, taking the medication with food may be necessary. Milk, antacids, and tetracycline should not be administered within 2 hours of oral iron therapy. Caffeinated bever-

Table 12–2   Comparison of Diagnostic Test Results in Iron-Deficiency Anemia (IDA), Anemia of Chronic Disease (ACD), and Concomitant IDA and ACD

Test	Results in IDA	Results in ACD	Results in IDA with ACD
Serum iron	Decreased	Decreased	Decreased
TIBC	Increased	Decreased	Decreased
Serum ferritin	Decreased	Normal to increased	Decreased
Transferrin saturation	Decreased	Decreased	Decreased

TIBC, total iron-binding capacity.

ages, especially tea, can reduce iron absorption; proton-pump inhibitors and H_2-receptor blockers reduce absorption. Enteric-coated preparations do not act on the site for maximal absorption. For patients who are unable to take oral iron preparations, parenteral therapy with iron dextran must be considered. This costly alternative, associated with a high incidence of tissue toxicity, requires individualization of dosage. Dietary measures to treat iron deficiency include addition of meat, beans, and green, leafy vegetables. An increase in dietary fiber may help to prevent constipation from oral iron therapy. Patient activity levels should be adjusted as tolerated for safety.

Follow-up: Reticulocyte count should be done within 5 to 10 days, followed by hemoglobin after 4 weeks of therapy; if the reticulocyte count increases but the hemoglobin does not, poor iron absorption or continued bleeding must be suspected, and further evaluation is indicated.

All patients should be seen to reassess symptoms or side effects from the treatment regimen. Emphasize the need to continue treatment. If the patient is stable, re-evaluate in 3 to 6 months. A serum ferritin of 50 µg/L usually indicates satisfactory iron replacement. Depending on the cause, maintenance therapy of ferrous sulfate, 325 mg once daily, may be indicated.

Sequelae: Possible complications include failure to identify an occult bleeding source, especially a bleeding malignancy.

Prevention/prophylaxis: Following good nutrition guidelines, with adequate iron intake, can prevent some IDA.

Referral: Refer patients with complex conditions to a specialist (e.g., a gastroenterologist for diagnostic studies, a hematologist or oncologist if malignancy is suspected). Collaborative management is appropriate if many confounding factors are present or medication regimen is complex. Refer patients to a nutritionist for evaluation of dietary inadequacies and assistance with meal planning or with congregate or home-delivered meals.

Education: Teach the patient about the mechanism of anemia, its possible causes, and the need for workup. Patients need to continue their medication regimen until discontinued by the health-care provider. Instruction should include dietary sources of iron.

REFERENCES

Altschuler J, Katz AD: Countertransference reactions toward older adults facing HIV and AIDS. Clin Gerontol 23:99, 2001.

Ansell, JE: Cardinal manifestations of hematologic disease, anemias, and related conditions. In Noble, J (ed): Textbook of Primary Care Medicine, ed 3. Mosby, St. Louis, 2001.

Brill, JR, and Baumgardner, DJ: Normocytic anemia. Am Fam Physician 62:2255, 2000.

Centers for Disease Control and Prevention: HIV/AIDS Surveillance Report 2001

13(2). Contact: http://www.cdc.gov/hiv/stats/hasr1302.htm. Accessed October 5, 2002.

Demangone, D, and Schrader, B: HIV infection: Diagnosis and treatment. In Bosker, G (ed): Primary and Acute Care Medicine. American Health Consultants, Atlanta, 2002.

Desai, SP, and Isa-Pratt, S: Clinician's Guide to Laboratory Medicine, ed 2. Lexi-Comp, Hudson, Ohio, 2002.

Emlet, CA, and Farkas, KJ: Correlates of service utilization among midlife and older adults with HIV/AIDS: The role of age in the equation. J Aging Health 14:315, 2002.

Heckman, TG, et al: Depressive symptomatology, daily stressors, and ways of coping among middle-age and older adults living with HIV disease. J Ment Health Aging 5:311, 1999.

HIV/AIDS Treatment Information Service: HIV and Its Treatment: What You Should Know, ed 2. 2002. Contact: www.hivatis.org. Accessed October 10, 2002.

Hollander, H, and Katz, MH: HIV infection. In Tierney, LM, et al (eds): Current Medical Diagnosis and Treatment 2001. Lange Medical Books/McGraw-Hill, New York, 2001.

Holcomb, SS: Anemia: Pointing the way to a deeper problem. Nursing 31:36, 2001.

Jordan, R, et al: Systematic review and meta-analysis of evidence for increasing numbers of drugs in antiretroviral combination therapy. BMJ 324:757, 2002.

Karon, JM, et al: HIV in the United States at the turn of the century: An epidemic in transition. Am J Public Health 91:1060, 2001.

Little, DR: Ambulatory management of common forms of anemia. Am Fam Physician 59:1598, 1999.

Little, DR: Anemia. In Bosker, G (ed): Primary and Acute Care Medicine. American Health Consultants, Atlanta, 2002.

Linker, CA: Blood. In Tierney, LM, et al (eds): Current Medical Diagnosis and Treatment 2001. Lange Medical Books/McGraw-Hill, New York, 2001.

McKnight, JT, and Eklund, EA: Hematology. In Rakel RE (ed): Textbook of Family Medicine, ed 6. WB Saunders, Philadelphia, 2002.

Morey, SS: Practice guidelines: HHS updates guidelines for antiretroviral therapy in HIV infection. Am Fam Physician 62, 2000. Contact: http://www.aafp.org/afp/20000801/practice.html. Accessed September 25, 2002

Panel on Clinical Practices for the Treatment of HIV Infection: Guidelines for the use of antiretroviral agents in HIV-infected adults and adolescents. 2002. Contact: http://www.hivatis.org/guidelines/adult/May23_02/AAMay23.pdf. Accessed September 20, 2002.

Sacher, RA, and McPherson, RA: Widmann's Clinical Interpretation of Laboratory Tests, ed 11. FA Davis, Philadelphia, 2000.

Siegel, K, et al: Symptom interpretation: implications for delay in HIV testing and care among HIV-infected late middle-aged and older adults. AIDS Care 11:525, 1999.

Skiest DJ, and Keiser P: Human immunodeficiency virus infection in patients older than 50 years: A survey of primary care physicians' beliefs, practices, and knowledge. Arch Fam Med 6:289, 1997.

Smith, DL: Anemia in the elderly. Am Fam Physician 62:1565, 2000.

Szirony, TA: Infection with HIV in the elderly population. J Gerontol Nurs 25:25, 1999.

Tabnak, F: Need for HIV/AIDS early identification and preventive measures among middle-aged and elderly women. Am J Public Health 90:287, 2000.

Trachtenberg, JD, and Sande, MA: Emerging resistance to nonnucleoside reverse transcriptase inhibitors: A warning and a challenge. JAMA 288:239, 2002.

Wians, FH, et al: Discriminating between iron deficiency anemia and anemia of chronic disease using traditional indices of iron status vs transferrin receptor concentration. Am J Clin Pathol 115:112, 2001.

Wink, D, et al: Adult anemia: determine clinical significance. Nurse Practitioner 27:38, 2002.

Wooten-Bielski, K: HIV and AIDS in older adults. Geriatr Nurs 20:268, 1999.

Chapter 13
PSYCHOSOCIAL DISORDERS

ALCOHOL ABUSE

SIGNAL SYMPTOMS▶ may be none; falls, transient confusion, insomnia, anxiety, gastrointestinal problems

Alcoholism	ICD-9-CM: 303.9 + 5th digit
Intoxication, acute	ICD-9-CM: 305.0 + 5th digit
Dependence	ICD-9-CM: 303.0 + 5th digit

Description: Alcohol abuse is a pathological pattern of alcohol use involving social, occupational, or functional impairment that has persisted for at least 1 month or recurred repeatedly over a long period. Older adults with alcohol problems often do not meet the *Diagnostic and Statistical Manual of Mental Disorders* (DSM-IV) criteria for alcohol abuse but are impaired nonetheless.

Etiology: Four models are viewed as explanations for alcohol abuse. The *biogenetic model* posits that genetic factors influence the metabolism of alcohol, producing changes in the neurotransmitters and receptors. The *sociocultural model* suggests that external factors, such as poverty, social isolation, loss, and culture, predispose an older adult to alcohol abuse. The *learning theory or behavioral model* supports alcohol abuse as a learned behavior that can be reversed. The *psychological-psychodynamic model* views alcohol abuse as a manifestation of underlying psychopathology.

Occurrence: About 16% of older adults are heavy alcohol users.

Age: More middle-aged adults are currently at risk for developing alcohol-related problems because alcohol use throughout life has been greater in this cohort than in previous cohorts.

Ethnicity: Not significant.

Gender: Men > women.

Contributing factors: Male gender, major life changes, and losses are contributing factors. Concerns about alcohol consumption in the older adult are directed primarily toward the physiological changes that accompany aging and the problems posed by regular alcohol consumption. Chemical breakdown of alcohol does not seem to change with aging; however, the changes associated with aging may increase the concentration of alcohol in the blood. These age-related changes include decreased lean muscle mass, decreased amount of body water, changes in liver function, and increased nervous system sensitivity to alcohol. After drinking 1 oz. of 80-proof alcohol, a 60-year-old would have a 20% higher blood alcohol level than a 20-year-old, and a 90-year-old would have a 50% higher blood alcohol level than a 20-year-old. Another major concern associated with alcohol abuse in the older adult is the increased occurrence of drug-alcohol interactions. The decreased metabolism of drugs by the liver in older adults yields significantly higher than normal drug levels, and alcohol increases this effect. Alcohol diminishes the effect of oral hypoglycemics, anticoagulants, and anticonvulsants and unpredictably strengthens the effects of sedatives.

Signs and symptoms: Alcohol abuse often is overlooked in older adults because medical problems, psychosocial problems, and medication use may obscure the signs of alcoholism. In addition, many older adults are solitary, so the drinking is hidden. One way that alcohol abuse comes to light is when elders are brought to the emergency department. One study found that Medicare is billed for alcohol-related hospitalizations more commonly than for acute myocardial infarction in older people. Patterns of alcohol dependence in older adults have been divided into two categories: early onset, which occurs before age 60, and late onset, which occurs after age 60. Early-onset alcohol abusers have a family history of alcoholism, are less well adjusted, and may have experienced alcohol-related legal problems; this category is predominantly men. It is thought that late-onset alcohol abuse is related to the stresses and losses of aging and may respond more favorably to treatment; there are more women in this category. Complaints that may suggest alcohol abuse include the following:

- Inconsistent mild hypertension
- Insomnia or anxiety
- Confusion
- Falls
- History of pancreatitis without stones
- Paranoid ideation

Diagnostic and screening tests: Diagnostic assessment depends on a thorough history. The CAGE questions, the screening test of choice for early detection, should be part of every health history (Box 13–1).

Other alcohol use screening tools include the Alcohol Use Disorders Identification Test (AUDIT); Brief Michigan Alcohol Screening Test (BMAST)–Geriatric Version; and TWEAK, an alcohol screening test

> **Box 13–1**
> *CAGE Alcohol Use Screening Instrument*
>
> *Questions*
> Have you ever felt the
>   need to **C**ut down
>   on drinking?
> Have you ever felt
>   **A**nnoyed by criticism
>   of drinking?
> Have you ever had **G**uilty
>   feelings about drinking?
> Have you ever taken a
>   morning **E**ye opener?
>
> *Expected Result with Condition*
> A positive response to one ques-
>   tion should prompt further
>   inquiry
> Two or more positive responses
>   are highly suspicious of alcohol
>   abuse

developed for women. Another approach that may elicit more accurate alcohol-related information is to ask, "Have you ever had a drinking problem?" and "When was your last drink?" Standard questions such as, "How much do you drink?" and "How often do you drink?" often result in dishonesty. A psychosocial assessment that includes a mental status examination and a geriatric depression scale should be performed. Also, consider a cultural assessment, if appropriate.

Test	Expected Result with Condition	CPT Code
Complete blood count	Increased MCV with normal hemoglobin, possible decreased hemoglobin	85022–85025
Aspartate aminotransferase-to-alanine aminotransferase ratio	>2 suggests alcoholic liver disease	84450–84460
Gamma glutamyltransferase	Increased in all liver disease including alcoholic; may remain increased for weeks after cessation of chronic alcohol intake	82977
Electrocardiogram	Cardiomyopathy	93005

Physical findings may include hepatomegaly, ascites (late stage), jaundice (with pancreatitis), and spider angiomata; men may have gynecomastia, testicular atrophy, and loss of pubic and axillary hair. A complete neurological examination that includes cranial nerves, gait, sensory, motor, reflexes, Romberg's sign, and tandem walking should be included.

Differential diagnoses:

- Abuse of other psychoactive substances such as opiates
- Hypnotics and sedatives can cause symptoms similar to those of alcohol abuse
- Dementia
- Cerebrovascular accident
- Urinary tract infection

- Gastritis
- Pancreatitis should also be considered

Treatment: The goal of treatment is sobriety or total abstinence from alcohol. Patients with symptoms of alcohol withdrawal should be hospitalized. Uncomplicated alcohol abuse can be treated in the outpatient setting. Alcoholics Anonymous (AA) is the most successful group in encouraging ongoing sobriety; however, the self-sufficient spirit often characteristic of older adults reduces the probability of participation. An AA volunteer of the same gender and of an age comparable to the patient's age is usually available to meet with an individual at the clinic site and can assume the role of the patient's sponsor, reducing fear and providing the support that may encourage group participation. For older adults, people who are important in their lives need to be instructed by counselors in ways to encourage the treatment process and decrease behaviors that enable the older adult to abuse alcohol. After consultation with a physician, naltrexone may be given to help maintain abstinence in healthy patients; because of side effects, disulfiram (Antabuse) is not recommended. Another drug, acamprosate, is currently in use outside the United States and may be available soon. For chronic alcoholism, the diet should be supplemented with multivitamins containing folic acid and thiamine, 100 mg/day. The patient should be evaluated for electrolyte problems and anemia.

Follow-up: Initially the older adult should be seen weekly to provide continuity in the practitioner-patient relationship and to monitor treatment effectiveness. When the patient is participating in the treatment protocol, monthly visits should be adequate to monitor progress.

Sequelae: Alcohol abuse can lead to gastrointestinal bleeding, especially if the patient is taking aspirin or arthritis medications. More than two alcoholic drinks daily can contribute to hypertension. Gait disturbances, peripheral neuropathy, and decreased functional ability are consequences of alcohol abuse. Malnutrition, cirrhosis, urinary incontinence, decline in cognitive status, insomnia, anxiety, addiction, and tolerance with concomitant withdrawal symptoms may occur. Depression and suicide increase with alcohol use.

Prevention/prophylaxis: Taking a brief drinking history with the yearly evaluation and administering the CAGE or other screening tool provides the practitioner with an opportunity for patient education. If a problem is suspected, brief interventional counseling at each visit is warranted. Education of patients on definition of "a drink" is helpful (see Education).

Referral: Specialty physician referral is warranted for suspected complications. Consider for inpatient detoxification program if indicated. Refer to mental health professional as indicated. Refer to community-based, peer mentoring program such as AA.

Education: Patients must be encouraged to continue participation in a treatment program, and family members should participate in a support group. Early intervention with family members who mistakenly believe that "a few drinks can't hurt" may prevent progression. Educate patients on possible consequences of continued use. Dietary supplements should be taken as ordered. Providers and patients must be educated about what constitutes "a standard drink," as follows: 1.5 oz. of 80-proof distilled spirits, 12 oz. of beer or wine cooler, or 5 oz. of wine. The National Institute of Alcohol Abuse and Alcoholism considers one drink per day to be the maximum amount for moderate use by adults ≥65 years old.

Resources:

- http://www.aa.org/
- http://www.asam.org/
- http://caas.caas.biomed.brown.edu/
- http://www.hazelden.org/
- http://www.johnsoninstitute.com/
- http://www.health.org/
- http://www.niaaa.nih.gov/

ANXIETY

SIGNAL SYMPTOMS excessive worrying, feelings of impending doom, restlessness, edginess, difficulty concentrating, sleep problems

Anxiety, generalized	ICD-9-CM: 300.02

Description: Anxiety is a symptom as well as a group of disorders. *Generalized anxiety disorder,* according to the DSM-IV, is excessive anxiety and worry occurring more days than not for at least 6 months. It is one of several anxiety disorders; in older adults, it frequently occurs with depression and other comorbid physical conditions. Symptoms are experienced to a much greater degree than warranted by the life situation.

Etiology: Anxiety tends to occur without conscious stimulus. Many anxiety-producing events occur in the lives of older adults when their mastery and control of changes are diminished. Neurobiologically, there is disruption of multiple neurotransmitters and brain structures. Autonomic hyperreactivity is characteristic of generalized anxiety disorder and panic disorders.

Occurrence: About 10% to 15% of older adults seek medical treatment for anxiety.

Age: Anxiety can occur at all ages; however, anxiety states may be more incapacitating to older adults than to persons of other ages.

Ethnicity: Not significant.

Gender: The distribution of anxiety in older adults is slightly higher in women than in men.

Contributing factors: Contributing factors include prior history of anxiety or related psychosocial problem; physical dependence; lack of control; change in daily routine; environmental change; fear of death; chronic illness, such as thyroid disease, hypoglycemia, hyperparathyroidism, chronic obstructive pulmonary disease, arrhythmias, and seizure disorders; lack of social support; high caffeine intake; alcohol or drug use; use of β-adrenergic agonists, theophylline, corticosteroids, thyroid hormones, and sympathomimetics; and depression.

Signs and symptoms: Anxiety is divided into four categories in the DSM-IV:

- Motor tension (shakiness, jumpiness, trembling, inability to relax)
- Autonomic hyperactivity (sweating, palpitations, dry mouth, dizziness, hot or cold spells, frequent urination, or diarrhea)
- Apprehensive expectation (worry or anticipation of personal misfortune)
- Vigilance and scanning (distractibility, poor concentration, insomnia, edginess)

The patient must manifest symptoms in at least three of the four categories, and these symptoms should persist for at least 6 months.

Diagnostic tests: Obtain a complete history, including a careful drug profile that encompasses current and recently discontinued medications, caffeine and alcohol intake, and over-the-counter (OTC) medications. Most laboratory studies are to rule out physical illness that can cause symptoms. A complete blood count to rule out anemia, metabolic profile to rule out diabetes or electrolyte imbalance, thyroid studies to rule out hyperthyroidism, and electrocardiogram to rule out arrhythmias may be indicated. A psychosocial assessment that includes a mental status examination and a depression scale aids in the evaluation of psychiatric disorders.

Differential diagnoses: The differential diagnosis may include hyperthyroidism, excessive caffeine intake, unstable angina, substance abuse, dementia, delirium, depression, hypertension, chronic obstructive pulmonary disease exacerbation, nutritional insufficiency, and drug side effect.

Treatment: Management requires a strong practitioner-patient relationship, counseling, family support, and appropriate medication. Psychotherapeutic approaches may be useful in alleviating generalized anxiety, especially if it is related to the bereavement process. Cognitive behavioral therapy is helpful for specific phobias and panic attacks seen in the older adult.

Pharmacological therapy requires careful evaluation of health/disease status and existing medications, including OTC and herbal. Although the advice to "start low and go slow" applies, studies have shown that under-treatment by primary-care providers accounts for treatment failure in anxiety and depression. Initial treatment with short-acting benzodi-azepines such as lorazepam (Ativan), alprazolam (Xanax), or oxazepam (Serax) for symptom control is warranted unless the patient has a prior history of substance abuse issues. The antianxiety drug buspirone (BuSpar) can be initiated in this time period and the benzodiazepine can be withdrawn in 4 to 6 weeks when the buspirone has taken effect. Venlafaxine (Effexor), a newer antidepressant, has been used success-fully for treating anxiety. If the patient has a mixed disorder, other anti-depressants may be indicated. The combination of agitation and anxiety seen in dementia may require an anxiolytic and antipsychotic.

Follow-up: Return visit should be scheduled for 1 week and as often as necessary to continue supportive therapy and pharmacologic treatment.

Sequelae: Reduced quality of life and impaired social interaction pat-terns are sequelae.

Prevention: Prevention strategies include management of stress, aug-mentation of social supports, maintenance of daily routines when possi-ble, and patient participation in decision affecting care.

Referral: Patients with evidence of underlying organic or other disease state, including manifestation of a symptom not consistent with general-ized anxiety, should be referred to a physician. Mental health referral is indicated if there is evidence of depressant drug abuse, the presenting symptoms are long-standing and not related to a current crisis, and symptoms persist after 2 weeks of treatment.

Education: Health-care providers need to be educated to consider pos-sibilities of anxiety and depression in conjunction with other comorbidi-ties. Many patients are reluctant to seek treatment; education regarding the biological basis of anxiety disorder may help.

DEPRESSION

SIGNAL SYMPTOMS ▶ irritability, anxiety, somatic symptoms, insomnia, poor appetite and weight loss, self-reproach, fatigue, pain

Depression	ICD-9-CM: 311
Depression, acute	ICD-9-CM: 296.2
Depression, with agitation	ICD-9-CM: 296.2
Recurrent episode	ICD-9-CM: 296.3

Description: Depression encompasses several disorders, including major depression, dysthymic disorder, bipolar disorder, psychotic depression, adjustment disorder, and mood disorder secondary to a medical condition. *Major depressive disorder* is defined by DSM-IV as at least five of the following symptoms present almost every day during the same 2-week period, signifying a change from prior functioning, and at least one of the symptoms is number 1 or 2:

1. Depressed mood by subjective account or observation by others
2. Markedly diminished interest or pleasure in almost all activities
3. Significant weight loss or weight gain or decrease or increase in appetite
4. Insomnia or hypersomnia
5. Psychomotor agitation or retardation
6. Fatigue or loss of energy
7. Feelings of worthlessness or inappropriate guilt
8. Diminished ability to think or concentrate
9. Recurrent thoughts of death or suicide

Major depressive disorder is less common in the elderly without a prior history of depression.

Etiology: No single cause of depression has been given. Many theories exist related to the biological etiology of depression. Most theories postulate problems with neurotransmitters, such as impaired synthesis, lack of neurotransmitter, increased uptake, and increased metabolism or breakdown. In older adults, cerebral white matter lesions on magnetic resonance imaging are thought to represent vascular abnormalities associated with depression. A psychosocial theory of the etiology of depression also has been proposed. According to cognitive theory, depression is a result of habitual reinforcement of negative ideas about oneself, others, and the future. Finally, environmental and social factors contribute to depression when major stressors such as losses occur and social support systems are inadequate.

Occurrence: The prevalence of depression ranges from 8% to 15% of the older adult population; however, the incidence of depression rises to 12% of hospitalized elderly persons and to 30% of elderly nursing home residents.

Age: Major depression tends to occur more in younger adulthood; the diagnosis of primary depression after age 50 is uncommon. The risk for suicide is highest for elderly white men, however.

Ethnicity: Native Americans have high rates of depression. Asian-Americans have high suicide rates. Elderly white men have the highest suicide rate.

Gender: Depression is more common in women than in men.

Contributing factors: In older adults, factors that contribute to the development of depression in later life include a change in the environment or admission to a health-care facility; stressful losses, including loss of autonomy, privacy, functional status, a body part, or friend or family member; alcohol or substance abuse; and a history of attempted suicide or psychiatric hospitalizations. A personal or family history of depression also contributes to the onset of depression. Several medical conditions predispose a person to depression, including Alzheimer's dementia, arthritis, vitamin deficiencies, Parkinson's disease, cerebrovascular accident, Huntington's disease, progressive supranuclear palsy, heart disease, hypothyroidism, anemia, chronic obstructive pulmonary disease, and malignancies, especially pancreatic. Medications associated with a high risk of depression include corticosteroids, antihypertensives, antipsychotics, benzodiazepines, β-blockers, H_2 blockers, narcotic analgesics, sedative/hypnotics, and alcohol.

Signs and symptoms: Patients who are experiencing depression may be able to tell you if there was a precipitating event before the depression began and what symptoms they have been experiencing. Older adults may present with a sense of hopelessness, excessive worry, persistent sadness, anxiety, irritability, constipation, and social withdrawal. Clinical examination may reveal a patient with inattention to personal appearance, tearfulness or poor eye contact, and slowed speech and movements. Patients may exhibit hand wringing and pacing. Patients or family members may report social withdrawal or isolation.

Physical examination to check for any secondary causes of depression is recommended. The neurological examination should focus on ruling out neurological causes of depression (e.g., dementia or Parkinson's disease). A standardized depression screening tool, such as the Geriatric Depression Rating Scale, can be administered to patients at risk. A score of ≥11 suggests the need for referral for a more detailed evaluation. If the patient seems confused, a mental status examination should be administered.

Diagnostic tests: There are no diagnostic tests for depression. The Geriatric Depression Scale has been used widely to assess depression in older adults; a score ≥11 is significant for depression. When medical causes for depression are suspected, laboratory tests may be indicated to confirm or rule out these medical conditions.

Differential diagnosis: Consider the following presentations in the workup of depression in older adults: organic mood disorders secondary to drugs or illness, schizophrenia, grief, substance abuse, hypochondriasis, somatization disorder, sleep disorder, pseudodementia, and dementia. Also, discern if the patient is experiencing melancholic depression or nonmelancholic depression. Symptoms of melancholic depression include marked loss of pleasure, psychomotor retardation, weight loss, and insomnia. Knowing whether the patient is having a psychotic or a nonpsychotic episode also helps determine the treatment plan.

Treatment: The initial step in treating depression in older adults is to evaluate the present medication regimen and remove or change any medications that contribute to depression. Treat any metabolic or systemic disorder that may have predisposed the patient to depression. Ensure that the patient's nutrition, elimination, sleep, and physical comfort are considered in the treatment plan.

Pharmacological

Pharmacotherapy is indicated when the symptoms of depression are moderately severe or when patterns of melancholic or endogenous depression are manifested. Antidepressant medications are recommended considering the patient's age and coexisting medical conditions and medications, the drug's side-effect profile, and prior response to or failure of a particular drug. Start at a low dosage, and monitor response. Agents with little or no anticholinergic effects are recommended. Selective serotonin reuptake inhibitors are the mainstay of treatment, although some tricyclics are still prescribed. The newer atypical antidepressants, including bupropion (Wellbutrin), venlafaxine (Effexor), mirtazapine (Remeron), and nefazodone (Serzone), are also used.

Psychotherapy

Psychotherapy, often used in conjunction with pharmacotherapy, tends to be more beneficial to patients with nonmelancholic depression. If the patient is delusional or the condition is rapidly deteriorating, consult a psychiatrist because electroconvulsive therapy may be indicated.

Follow-up: Older adults who present without suicidal ideation should be seen in 2 weeks to evaluate therapeutic response and the possible need to increase medication dosage, then again 6 weeks after the initial trial of medications. If psychotherapy was ordered, re-evaluate in 6 to 8 weeks to determine if at least partial improvement has occurred and there is symptom relief. By 10 to 12 weeks, a full response to treatment should be expected. If there is no noticeable improvement, a new treatment can be ordered. Then patients should be followed every 4 to 6 months. Antidepressant medications can be discontinued when no longer needed.

Sequelae: The most critical complication of depression in older adults is suicide. Social isolation, personal neglect, and malnutrition also may occur.

Prevention/prophylaxis: For primary prevention, avoid medications that tend to contribute to depression in older adults, especially for patients with a history of depression. Support patients through times of great loss and stressors by providing information about community resources and other educational materials. For patients in long-term care facilities, especially for the newly admitted, arrange for participation in group activities, such as reminiscence, music, or movement therapy, and if they have a history of having domestic animals, pet therapy if available. For anyone who has had a change or loss in physical functioning, arrange for physical or occupational therapy to assist with enhancement of independence as much as possible.

Referral: Patients with major depression; suicidal ideation; history of substance abuse; or severe, recurrent, or psychotic depression should be referred to a geriatric psychiatrist. Patients with problems refractory to treatment also should be referred.

Education: Patients need to be informed that the medication will not work right away and that a change in mood may not occur for some time after initiating therapy. Explain to the patient that understanding the cause of the depression (if known) would be beneficial. Emphasize the need to avoid alcohol as a means of alleviating the depressed mood, and explain that alcohol is contraindicated when taking antidepressant medications. Provide information about community resources for older adults.

ELDER ABUSE

SIGNAL SYMPTOMS ▶ difficult to assess because of unintentional bruising and falls by frail older adults; unexplained or frequent fractures, including skull fracture, sprains; broken eyeglasses; bruises, welts, restraint marks; older adult's report of being hit, kicked, or mistreated; caregiver refusal to allow others to see elder alone; bruises or blood around genital area (sexual abuse); behavioral change such as agitation, withdrawal, or fearfulness (psychological abuse); unkempt appearance, signs of dehydration or malnutrition (neglect)

Adult, physical	ICD-9-CM: 995.81
Emotional	ICD-9-CM: 995.82
Multiple forms	ICD-9-CM: 995.85
Neglect (nutritional)	ICD-9-CM: 995.84
Sexual	ICD-9-CM: 995.83

Description: Elder mistreatment, defined as the abuse and neglect of older persons, includes physical, psychological or emotional, and sexual abuse; caregiver neglect and self-neglect; abandonment; and financial or material exploitation. *Physical abuse* includes striking, beating, shaking, restraining, or feeding improperly. *Psychological abuse* inflicts emotional stress or injury through verbal abuse. *Sexual abuse* is a form of sexual intimacy without consent or by force or threat of force. *Financial or material abuse* is the misuse or exploitation of an older adult's possessions or financial assets. *Neglect* is the unintentional or intentional failure to provide essentials such as food, personal care, or medications. *Abandonment* is desertion by someone who has assumed responsibility to care for the elder. *Self-neglect* is failure to care for oneself adequately to maintain physical and mental health.

Etiology: The major etiological theories that surface in the literature are (1) abuser psychopathology, (2) stress, (3) transgenerational violence, and (4) dependency. The theory of *abuser psychopathology* suggests that the abuser has been hospitalized repeatedly for serious psychiatric disorders and may abuse alcohol or drugs or both. The *stress* theory posits that external stresses superimposed on the psychological and physical caregiving demands are expressed through violent acts. *Transgenerational violence* theory indicates that violence is a learned response to difficult life experiences and a learned method of expressing anger and frustration. The *dependency* theory states that physical or mental impairment poses a greater risk for abuse.

Occurrence: Slightly less common than child abuse. Estimated prevalence of elder mistreatment ranges from 700,000 to 2.5 million annually.

Age: Elder abuse is most prevalent in persons >75 years old.

Ethnicity: A greater incidence exists among whites.

Gender: Noncontributory.

Contributing factors: Abuse occurs in all socioeconomic groups; however, it is more likely to occur among the lower class. The typical victim is female, has a cognitive impairment, and is dependent. Aggressive behavior, wandering, verbal outbursts, or embarrassing behavior can provoke abuse. Social isolation facilitates abuse, as does a shared living arrangement of abuser and victim. Characteristics of the abuser are also significant, including financial or emotional dependence on the elder, a history of psychiatric problems, substance abuse, or legal problems.

Sign and symptoms: The health-care provider must exercise clinical judgment in identifying elder abuse. The following indicators are suspicious:

- Medication misuse
- Pattern of missed appointments or cancellations
- Frequent change in health-care providers
- Poor hygiene, unkempt appearance
- Malnutrition, dehydration
- Unexplained injuries, recurrent fractures
- Bruises with a characteristic shape (e.g., belt, iron, handprints on both wrists)
- Burns in unusual places, bruises
- Pain, discharge, bleeding, lacerations in rectum or vagina
- Untreated pressure ulcers
- Depression, fearfulness, sleep problems, mood changes
- Missing prosthetic devices (dentures, hearing aids, eyeglasses)

Diagnostic tests: The individual's history and physical examination findings dictate which diagnostic tests to perform. The history is key; the patient, caregiver, and other significant people should each be interviewed individually. A thorough physical examination, mental status assessment, and mood assessment should be conducted.

Differential diagnosis: Differential diagnosis includes unintended injury and poverty that may preclude access to food, appropriate shelter, and health care.

Treatment: Elder abuse is a multidisciplinary issue that includes health-care providers, social workers, lawyers, law enforcement officers, and psychiatrists. The following interventions should be considered:

Determine if the victim is in immediate danger. If mistreatment results in life-threatening conditions or if urgent medical or psychiatric care is needed, obtain necessary legal protection orders for treatment. Hospital admission, court-ordered protection from abuse, or relocation to a safe environment may be indicated.

Report to adult protective services (APS) or other public agency, as mandated by the law. APS must investigate reported elder mistreatment cases by interviewing victims, despite the victim's wishes, and others who may be knowledgeable about the case.

Perform a full, private, comprehensive assessment, including functional assessment. Elicit detailed information on any physical injury and record including inconsistencies. Photos or drawings should be used for accurate and specific documentation.

Administer a complete mental status examination to determine if the older adult is a competent consenting victim, a competent nonconsenting victim, or an incompetent victim.

Record accurately, including the patient's own words when possible, because this documentation may become part of a court case.

Coordinate approach with APS as mandated by state law.

Follow-up: Monitor the outcome of all cases of abuse and neglect.

Sequelae: Elder abuse can result in unnecessary injury, psychological trauma, enforced long-term care placement, and death. Abusers may become involved in legal proceedings (for intentional cases) and alienation from the elder and other family members.

Prevention/prophylaxis: Prevention of abuse comes from an increased understanding of the complex needs of a dependent older adult and the support available to the caregiving family. Preventive interventions may include family/caregiver support groups, stress management education, respite care, home health, adult day care, and other community services.

Referral: Refer to community and social service resources and caregiver support groups.

Education: Educate providers to recognize risk factors for elder abuse and signs of elder mistreatment and to intervene early, preventively if possible. Educate the public about the problem. Educate caregivers about stresses, strategies for management, and caregiver relief resources. Educate policy makers about the need for legislative changes to support families and patients with long-term dependency needs.

GRIEF

Grief	ICD-9-CM: None
Bereavement	ICD-9-CM: V62.82
As adjustment disorders	ICD-9-CM: 309.0

Description: Grief is a normal emotional response to loss; when the patient is unable to work through it, physical or psychological illness may occur.

Etiology: Loss or change perceived as loss.

Occurrence: Approximately 50% of women >65 years old are widows; 13% of men >65 years old are widowers.

Age: Grief may occur at any age.

Ethnicity: Not significant.

Gender: Grief affects more women than men.

Contributing factors: Length of illness, amount of suffering, relationship quality, survivor guilt, financial burden of illness, caregiver burden, personality attributes of deceased and survivor, and cultural expectations all may be related to the variety of grief responses. Studies have not found a positive correlation between anticipatory grief and adaptation to the loss of a spouse, alerting practitioners to notice varied grief reactions despite the expectancy of death. Widows and widowers with recent disabilities, few friends, and poor relationships with their children were more apt to require counseling. Current studies are re-evaluating the helpfulness of the stages model and citing individual responses as the norm. Length of time for grieving also is being reconceptualized as variable and individual.

Signs and symptoms: Grief is characterized by feelings of depression with associated symptoms of poor appetite and weight loss or compulsive eating and weight gain, sleep disturbance, tearfulness, lack of interest, withdrawal and isolation, emptiness, indecisiveness, and guilt feelings; some grieving individuals may respond by making dramatic changes in a short time to avoid dealing with feelings.

Diagnostic tests: None.

Differential diagnoses: Social phobia, depression, adjustment reaction.

Treatment: Provide emotional support, allowing the older adult to express feelings. Reminiscence is helpful to many. Encourage patients to return to their normal routine as soon as possible. Daily physical exercise can help patients cope with the depression that accompanies grief. Referral to a bereavement support group may help some individuals.

Follow-up: Once a month or more often depending on patient needs.

Prevention/prophylaxis: The goal is to encourage and support the patient in the normal grieving process and prevent dysfunctional grieving. Bereavement groups, activation of social and spiritual support networks, discussion of anticipated loss by participants, and involvement in group activities may be helpful.

Sequelae: In the first 3 months after the death of a spouse for adults >65 years old, the mortality rate increases 48% in men and 22% in women. Practitioners must be alert to older adults who do not improve in 3 months after the loss. Additionally, a major depressive syndrome that occurs for ≥2 weeks early in the course of bereavement should be taken seriously and managed accordingly.

Referral: Older adults experiencing abnormal grieving may benefit from a mental health referral. Referral to support groups, such as Widow-to-Widow, may be helpful in the grieving process.

Education: Make patients and their support networks aware of the variability of normal grieving; alert them to signs of dysfunctional grieving and resources for help.

INSOMNIA

SIGNAL SYMPTOMS▶ patient report of not sleeping, excessive daytime sleepiness, loud snoring (sleep apnea), complaint of restless legs, difficulty falling asleep and staying asleep, irritability, difficulty concentrating

Insomnia	ICD-9-CM: 780.52
With sleep apnea	ICD-9-CM: 780.51
Subjective complaint	ICD-9-CM: 307.49

Description: Insomnia is difficulty falling asleep or staying asleep despite the desire to do so.

Etiology: Insomnia can have several etiologies, including medical, behavioral, circadian, or psychiatric. Sleeping states and sleep schedules change with age. Sleep efficiency (time actually sleeping versus time in bed) is <80% in older adults, and time to fall asleep is extended. The most important age-related changes in sleep include:

- Decreased continuity of sleep with an increase in the number of arousals
- Tendency for the major period of sleep and rapid eye movement (REM) sleep to occur earlier in the night
- Decrease in the deepest parts of nonrapid eye movement (NREM) sleep
- Increased napping during the day
- Tendency to spend more time in bed

Transient insomnia, which lasts a few nights, is related to situational stress and usually resolves without medical intervention when the older adult adapts to the change or removes it.

Short-term insomnia, which is similar to transient insomnia, lasts <1 month and is related to an acute medical or psychological condition or to persistent situational stress.

Chronic insomnia lasts >1 month and results from age-related changes in sleep and chronic stressors.

Occurrence: Approximately 35% of people >60 years old experience and regularly complain of poor sleep quality.

Age: Insomnia can occur at any age; however, older adults have greater difficulty falling asleep and staying asleep.

Ethnicity: Not significant.

Gender: Older men show poorer sleep maintenance than do older women.

Contributing factors: Factors that may contribute to insomnia include:

- Restless syndrome
- Periodic limb movement disorder
- Sleep apnea
- Dementia
- Depression
- Drugs, including caffeine, alcohol, antipsychotics, β-blockers, stimulant decongestants, sedative-hypnotics, sympathomimetic bronchodilators, diuretics, carbidopa-levodopa, H_2 blockers, and centrally acting α-agonist antihypertensives
- Many chronic medical conditions, including musculoskeletal, cardiac, respiratory, gastrointestinal, renal, endocrine, and neurological

Signs and symptoms: A complete history should reveal a full description of the problems. Patients may complain about difficulty falling asleep and staying asleep, frequent awakenings, early morning awakening and inability to return to sleep, daytime fatigue with unwanted naps, irritability, or difficulty concentrating. Additionally an older adult may spend 10 to 12 hours in bed at night trying to sleep. A pertinent physical examination should evaluate the systems associated with any medical conditions listed here. A mental status examination is useful in detecting psychiatric disease.

Diagnostic tests: None, unless indicated by history and physical examination.

Differential diagnosis:

- Anxiety
- Inadequate sleep hygiene
- Medical problems
- Medication-related sleep disorder

- Depression
- Alcohol-related sleep disorder or primary sleep disorder

Treatment: Patients should avoid caffeine for 12 hours before bedtime and discontinue alcohol and unnecessary sleep-interrupting drugs. For transient or short-term insomnia, initiate a short-acting sedative-hypnotic, such as zolpidem (Ambien) or zaleplon (Sonata), before desired bedtime for ≤1 week. If a benzodiazepine is used, temazepam (Restoril) is relatively short-acting. If this is ineffective, re-evaluate diagnosis, and restructure treatment modalities. For chronic insomnia, the treatment is more complex. The patient should keep a sleep diary and bring it to the next office visit. If the patient has a bed partner, this person should be interviewed as well. Cognitive behavioral therapy focused on reducing time in bed, correcting false beliefs and expectations regarding sleep, and decreasing exposure to stimuli that deter sleep has been shown to be superior and long-lasting compared with short-term sedative-hypnotic use. Medications should be evaluated in light of ability to interfere with sleep, and modifications should be made where possible. Small increases in activity level should be encouraged. Treat underlying or coexisting disorders. If sleep apnea is suspected, refer for polysomnography.

Follow-up: Patients should return in 2 weeks. Examine the patient's sleep diary and evaluate the effectiveness of the treatment. If indicated, re-evaluate diagnosis and restructure treatment.

Sequelae: Sequelae are reduced quality of life, depression, increased risk for falls/injury, and potential for drug dependence or drug interactions resulting from use of OTC sleep aids.

Prevention/prophylaxis: Sleep hygiene suggestions may include the following:

Establish a regular bedtime and wake-up time.
Set aside a time each evening for relaxation and thinking.
Avoid caffeine, alcohol, and nicotine because they all interrupt sleep.
Minimize awake time in bed, reserving bed for sleep and sexual activity.
Create an optimal sleep environment.
Establish regular eating habits because hunger can interrupt sleep.
Avoid napping.
Exercise daily to extent possible, but avoid exercise just before bedtime.
Maximize daytime exposure to bright light.

Referral: If therapy brings no improvement and other underlying causes have been eliminated, refer the patient to a sleep laboratory for evaluation.

Education: Explain age-related sleep changes to patient and family. Teach the patient to follow the guidelines listed under Prevention/prophylaxis.

WANDERING

Wandering	ICD-9-CM: None

Description: Wandering is one of the behavioral problems seen with dementia. It is characterized by excessive ambulation by the patient with little regard for safety or environmental barriers. Wandering has been viewed as a form of agenda behavior that is directed toward meeting perceived social, emotional, or physical needs. Agenda behavior may be a method for the wanderer to regain feelings of safety and belonging that provided satisfaction in the past.

Etiology: Factors that have been identified with wandering include:

- Cognitive impairment
- Confusion
- Darkened or unfamiliar environment
- Diseases of the central nervous system
- Stress
- Tension
- Anxiety
- Lack of control
- Lack of exercise
- Boredom

Nocturnal wandering that accompanies sundowning appears to be associated with the onset of darkness and related to the individual's loss of spatial relationships in the dark.

Age: Dementia affects 5% to 10% of persons >65 years old and approximately 30% of persons >85 years old.

Occurrence: The most common type of dementia is Alzheimer's disease, which accounts for 50% to 60% of cases of dementia. Because a positive correlation exists between the frequency of wandering and severity of dementia, the more severe the dementia, the greater the probability the person will exhibit wandering behavior.

Ethnicity: Not significant.

Gender: Because Alzheimer's disease is twice as common in women as in men, wandering may be more prevalent in women.

Contributing factors: Wandering can be affected by individual factors, environmental factors, or both. Physiological factors that may contribute to wandering include:

- Medication interactions or use of psychotropic agents or both
- Physical discomfort caused by pain, thirst, or hunger
- Need for toileting
- Desire to exercise

Psychological factors suggest wandering may stem from loneliness and separation and may serve to dissipate stress. Environmental factors may include an impoverished social climate, restrictive surroundings, an overstimulating climate, or new and unfamiliar situations.

Signs and symptoms: Wanderers may have greater overall impairment of basic cognitive skills, such as memory, orientation, and concentration, and impairment of higher order cognitive skills, including abstract thinking, judgment, language, and spatial skills. Language impairment seems to distinguish wanderers from nonwanderers. Behaviors associated with wandering include:

- Pacing
- Agitation
- Aggressiveness
- Incontinence

Diagnostic tests: There are no diagnostic tests specific to wandering. Most patients already have diagnosed dementia. Obtain a complete history, including a careful drug profile that encompasses current and recently discontinued medications, caffeine and alcohol intake, and OTC medications. Perform a psychosocial assessment that includes a mental status examination. Assess for medical causes with attention directed toward disorders associated with wandering; assess for depression and anxiety. Suggested screening tools include the Mini-Mental State Examination, Geriatric Depression Scale short version, Algase Wandering Scale, Memory and Behavior Problems Checklist, and Cohen-Mansfield Agitation Inventory.

Differential diagnosis:

- Medication interactions
- Inappropriate psychotropic medication use
- Physical discomfort caused by pain
- Nutritional deficiency
- Cardiac decompensation
- Diseases of the central nervous system
- Urinary tract infection or incontinence

Treatment: Management strategies include environmental modifications, caregiver and staff education and support, physical and psychosocial interventions, and technological interfaces for safety and monitoring. Pharmacotherapeutic measures should be part of a comprehensive dementia management plan but not a first-line treatment for wandering. Strategies that are directed toward physiological, psychological, and environmental factors are shown in Table 13–1.

Follow-up: Follow-up visits are scheduled as indicated by the environment in which the wanderer resides. If the patient lives at home and cannot be managed by his or her family, more intense follow-up may be indicated; the patient may need placement in a more secure environment.

Table 13–1 Wandering Management Guidelines

Factor	Strategies
Physiological	
Medications	Re-evaluate, discontinue or substitute drug with more favorable side-effect profile
Pain	Assess for physical sources and treat; if complex, refer for pain management
Nutritional deficiencies	Dietary consult; supplements as appropriate
Incontinence	Regular toileting program; frequent assessment of skin particularly if continence management pads or pants are used; skin protection program
Mobility impairment	Evaluate cause and correct or refer as necessary
Psychological	
Social skills deficit	Structured activity program, use of distraction, tasks within abilities of wanderer
Environmental	
Falls	Proper lighting, clear pathways; secure hazardous materials
Elopement	Door alarms/locks; camouflage exit doors. Exit door to safe area, such as enclosed courtyard

Sequelae: Death may ensue if the patient wanders out in temperature extremes or encounters someone with criminal intent. Other sequelae include injury, such as falls and fractures, related to cognitive impairment and gait disturbance; weight loss related to high expenditure of calories and inability to stay sedentary long enough to consume a meal; behavior problems, such as agitation; and caregiver fatigue related to need for constant monitoring of wanderer.

Referral: Because wandering often is associated with negative outcomes for the patient and the caregiver, a referral for home health support or long-term care placement may be indicated. Evidence of underlying organic or other disease state, including manifestation of a symptom not consistent with wandering, may require physician consultation.

Education: Educate the caregiver and the staff in the residential care facility within the contextual world of the wandering individual.

REFERENCES

Alcohol Abuse

Adams, WL: The aging male patient: Alcohol and the health of aging men. Med Clin North Am 83:1195, 1999.

Adams, WL: (1998). Alcohol and substance abuse. In Duthie (ed): Practice of Geriatrics, ed 3. WB Saunders, Philadelphia, 1998, pp 307–316.

American College of Emergency Room Physicians: Alcohol screening and brief interventions in the ED resource kit information. Contact: http://www.acep.org/1,4688,0.html. Accessed December 9, 2002.

Barrick, C, and Conners, GJ: Relapse prevention and maintaining abstinence in older adults with alcohol-use disorders. Drugs Aging 19:583, 2002.

Beers, MH, and Berkow, R (eds): The Merck Manual of Geriatrics, ed 3. Merck Research Laboratories, Whitehouse Station, N.J., 2000, pp 333–340.

Cherpite, CJ: Brief screening instruments for alcoholism. Alcohol Health Research World 21, 1997. Contact: http://www.niaaa.nih.gov/publications/arh21-4/348.pdf. Accessed December 9, 2002.

Clark, WD: Alcohol problems: Effective interviews with moderate, at-risk, and dependent drinkers. In Noble, J (ed): Textbook of Primary Care Medicine, ed 3. Mosby, St. Louis, 2001, pp 429–437.

Epperly, TD: Health issues in men: Part II. Common psychosocial disorders. Am Fam Physician 62:117, 2000.

Fingerhood, M: Substance abuse in older people. J Am Geriatr Soc 48:985, 2000.

Isaacson, JH: Screening for alcohol problems in primary care. Med Clin North Am 83:1547, 1999.

Menninger, JA: Assessment and treatment of alcoholism and substance-related disorders in the elderly. Bull Menn Clin 66:166, 2001.

Rigler, SK: Alcoholism in the elderly. Am Fam Physician 61:1710, 2000.

Sedlak, CA, et al: Alcohol use in women 65 years of age and older. Health Care Women Int 21:567, 2000.

Sherin, K, and Kaiser, G: Alcohol abuse. In Rakel, RE (ed): Textbook of Family Practice, ed 6. WB Saunders, Philadelphia, 2002, p 428.

Anxiety

Beers, MH, and Berkow, R (eds): The Merck Manual of Geriatrics, ed 3. Merck Research Laboratories, Whitehouse Station, N.J., 2000, pp 322–327.

Benedek, DM, and Engel, CC: (2001). Anxiety and anxiety disorders. In Noble, J (ed): Textbook of Primary Care Medicine, ed 3. Mosby, St. Louis, 2001, pp 413–421.

Crabtree, HL: The Comorbidity Symptom Scale: a combined disease inventory and assessment of symptom severity. J Am Geriatr Soc 48:1674, 2000.

Cummings, JL: Guidelines for managing Alzheimer's disease: part I. Assessment. Am Fam Physician 65:2263, 2002.

Cutson, TM: Management of pain in the older adult. Clin Fam Pract 3:667, 2001.

Dada, F: Generalized Anxiety Disorder in the Elderly. Psychiatr Clin North Am 24:155, 2001.

Fortner, BV, and Neimeyer, RA: Death anxiety in older adults: A quantitative review. Death Studies 23:387, 1999.

Goldstein, MZ: Depression and anxiety in older women. Prim Care 29:69, 2002.

Gurvich, T: Appropriate use of psychotropic drugs in nursing homes. Am Fam Physician 61:1437, 2000.

Howell, HB: Generalized Anxiety Disorder in Women. Psychiatr Clin North Am 24:165, 2001.

Lang, AJ, and Stein, MB: Anxiety disorders: How to recognize and treat the medical symptoms of emotional illness. Geriatrics for Midlife and Beyond 56:24, 2001.

Lagomasino, I: Medical assessment of patients presenting with psychiatric symptoms in the emergency setting. Psychiatr Clin North Am 22:819, 1999.

Marx, J, et al: Rosen's Emergency Medicine: Concepts and Clinical Practice, ed 5. Mosby, St Louis, 2002.

Penninx, BW: The protective effect of emotional vitality on adverse health outcomes in disabled older women. J Am Geriatr Soc 48:1359, 2000.

Velez, L: Managing behavioral problems in long-term care. Clin Fam Pract 3:561, 2001.

Worthington, JJ III, and Rauch, SG: Approach to the patient with anxiety. In Gorroll, AH, and Mulley, AG (eds): Primary Care Medicine: Office Evaluation and Management of the Adult Patient, ed 4. Lippincott Williams & Wilkins, Philadelphia, 2000, pp 1147–1157.

Depression

American Psychiatric Association. Diagnostic and Statistical Manual of Mental Disorders, Fourth Edition Text Revision. American Psychiatric Association, Washington, DC, 2000.

Bains, J, et al: The efficacy of antidepressants in the treatment of depression in dementia. Cochrane Dementia and Cognitive Improvement Group. Cochrane Database of Systematic Reviews 4, 2002.

Battaglia, BA: Depression in older adults. Cross Cultural Connection 5:1, 2000.

Benjamin, D, and Battaglia, BA: Depression in older adults... second article in the next issue of the Cross Cultural Connection will address causes of depression and treatment. Cross Cultural Connection 5:2, 2000.

Bookwala, J, et al: (2000). Pharmacotherapy of geriatric depression: Taking the long-view. In Williams GM, et al (eds): Physical Illness and Depression in Older Adults: A Handbook of Theory, Research and Practice. Kluwer Academic/Plenum Publishers, New York, 2000, pp 93–131.

Boyd, J, et al: Early-onset and late-onset depression in older adults: Psychological perspectives. Rev Clin Gerontol 10:149, 2000.

Brautigan, R, and Reno, B: Depression in older adults. In Leggen, AS, et al (eds): NGNA core curriculum for gerontological advanced practice. Sage, Thousand Oaks, Calif., 1998, pp 495–503.

Bruce, MB: (2001). Depression and disability in late-life: Directions for future research. Am J Geriatr Psychiatry 9:102, 2001.

DeGroot, JC, et al: Cerebral white matter lesions and depressive symptoms in elderly patients. Arch Gen Psychiatry 57:1071, 2000.

Dyer, CB, et al: (2000). The high prevalence of depression and dementia in elder abuse or neglect. J Am Geriatr Soc 48:205, 2000.

Faison, WE, and Steffens DC: Prevalence and treatment of depression in the elderly. Clin Geriatr 9:46, 2001.

Forlenza, OV, et al: Antidepressant efficacy and safety of low-dose sertraline and standard-dose imipramine for the treatment of depression in older adults: Results from a double-blind, randomized, controlled clinical trial. Int Psychogeriatr 13:75, 2001.

Gallo, JJ: Depression without sadness: alternative presentations of depression in late life. Am Fam Physician 60:820, 1999.

Goldstein, MZ: Women's mental health depression and anxiety in older women. Prim Care Clin Office Pract 29:69, 2002.

Goodwin, PE, and Smyer, MA: Accuracy of recognition and diagnosis of comorbid depression in the nursing home. Aging Ment Health 3:340, 1999.

Gottschalk, LA: Commentary on "shame and community: social components in depression:" On shame, shame-depression, and other depressions. Psychiatry 64:225, 2001.

Hay, DP, et al: Novel uses of selective serotonin reuptake inhibitors in older patients. Ann Long Term Care 6:221, 1998.

Hedelin, B, and Strandmark, M: The meaning of depression from the life-world perspective of elderly women. Issues in Mental Health Nursing 22:401, 2001.

Kanga, K, et al: Comorbidity of depression with other medical diseases in the elderly. Biol Psychiatry 52:559, 2002.

Lenze, EJ, et al: Anxiety symptoms in elderly patients with depression: What is the best approach to treatment? Drugs Aging 19:753, 2002.

Montgomery, P, and Dennis, J: Bright light therapy for sleep problems in adults aged 60+. Cochrane Developmental, Psychosocial and Learning Problems Group Cochrane Database of Systematic Reviews 4, 2002.

Montgomery, P, and Dennis, J: Cognitive behavioural interventions for sleep problems in adults aged 60+. Cochrane Developmental, Psychosocial and Learning Problems Group Cochrane Database of Systematic Reviews 4, 2002.

Moore, KA, and Blumenthal, JA: Exercise training as an alternative treatment for depression among older adults. Altern Ther Health Med 4:48, 1998.

Musil, CM, et al: Stress, health, and depressive symptoms in older adults at three time points over 18 months. Issues in Mental Health Nursing 19:207, 1999.

Reynolds, CF, et al: Pharmacotherapy of geriatric depression: Taking the Longview. In Williams GM, Shaffer DR, Parmlee PA (eds): Physical Illness and Depression in Older Adults: A Handbook of Theory, Research and Practice. Kluwer Academic/Plenum Publishers, New York, 2000, pp 277–294.

Ryden, MB, et al: Nursing interventions for depression in newly admitted nursing home residents. J Gerontol Nurs 25:20, 1999.

Unützer, J, et al: Care for depression in HMO patients aged 65 and older. J Am Geriatr Soc 48:871, 2000.

van der Wurff, F, et al: Electroconvulsive therapy for depressed elderly. Cochrane Depression, Anxiety and Neurosis Group Cochrane Database of Systematic Reviews 4, 2002.

Velez, L, and Peggs, J: Long-term care in geriatrics: Managing behavioral problems in long-term care. Clin Fam Pract 3: 561, 2001.

Watt, LM, and Cappeliez, P: Integrative and instrumental reminiscence therapies for depression in older adults: Intervention strategies and treatment effectiveness. Aging Ment Health 4:166, 2000.

Zylstra, RG, and Steitz, JA: Physician and public knowledge of depression among older adults. Gerontol Geriatr Educ 21:13, 2001.

Elder Abuse

Beers, MH, and Berkow, R (eds): The Merck Manual of Geriatrics, ed 3. Merck Research Laboratories, Whitehouse Station, N.J., 2000.

Clarke, ME, and Pierson, W: Management of elder abuse in the emergency department. Emerg Med Clin N Am 17:631, 1999.

Collins, KA, et al, and the Autopsy Committee of the College of American Pathologists Autopsy and Medicine: Elder abuse and neglect. Arch Intern Med 160: 1567, 2000.

Cummings, JL: Guidelines for managing Alzheimer's disease: Part II. Treatment. Am Fam Physician 65:2525, 2002.

Dyer, CB, et al: The high prevalence of depression and dementia in elder abuse or neglect. J Am Geriatr Soc 48:205, 2000.

Goldstein, MZ: Elder abuse, neglect and exploitation. In Kaplan and Sadock's Comprehensive Textbook of Psychiatry. Lippincott Williams & Wilkins, Philadelphia, 2000, p 179.

Goldstein, MZ: Depression and anxiety in older women. Prim Care 29:69, 2002.

Jogerst, GJ, et al: Community characteristics associated with elder abuse. J Am Geriatr Soc 48:513, 2000.

Levine, SA, and Barry, PP: (2001). Geriatric patients. In Noble, J (ed): Textbook of Primary Care Medicine, ed 3. Mosby, St. Louis, 2001, pp 87–88.

Medline Plus: Elder abuse. 2002. Contact: http://www.nlm.nih.gov/medlineplus/elderabuse.html. Accessed December 12, 2002.

National Center on Elder Abuse at the American Public Human Services Association: The national elder abuse incidence study: final report. 1998. Contact: www.aoa.gov/abuse/report/default.htm. Accessed December 12, 2002.

National Center on Elder Abuse: The basics. 2002. Contact: http://www.elderabusecenter.org/. Accessed December 12, 2002.

Parks, SM: A practical guide to caring for caregivers. Am Fam Physician 62:2613, 2000.

Swagerty, DL, Jr: Elder mistreatment. Am Fam Physician 59:2804, 1999.

U.S. Department of Health and Human Services Administration on Aging: Elder abuse prevention. 2001. Contact: http://www.aoa.dhhs.gov/Factsheets/abuse.html. Accessed December 12, 2002.

Wolf, RS: Suspected abuse in an elderly patient. Am Fam Physician 59:1319, 1999.

Grief

Gilbert, KR: Taking a narrative approach to grief research: Finding meaning in stories. Death Studies 25:223, 2002.

Ott, CH, and Lueger, RJ: Patterns of change in mental health status during the first two years of spousal bereavement. Death Studies 25:387, 2002.

Sable, P: Attachment, loss of spouse, and grief in elderly adults. Omega: The Journal of Death and Dying 23, 2002.

Sklar, F, and Hartley, SF: Close friends as survivors: Bereavement patterns in a "hidden" population. Omega: The Journal of Death and Dying 21, 2002.

Van Baarsen, B, et al: Patterns of adjustment to partner loss in old age: The widowhood adaptation longitudinal study. Omega 44:5, 2002.

Insomnia

Anonymous: Behaviorial therapy effective for long-term management of insomnia. Geriatrics 54:52, 1999.

Anonymous: Trend watch: Insomnia in the elderly. Clin Geriatr 9:48, 2001.

Barthlen, GM: Obstructive sleep apnea syndrome, restless legs syndrome, and insomnia in geriatric patients. Geriatrics 57:34, 2002.

Beers, MH, and Berkow, R (eds): The Merck Manual of Geriatrics, ed 3. Merck Research Laboratories, Whitehouse Station, N.J., 2000.

Montgomery, P, and Dennis, J: Cognitive behavioural interventions for sleep problems in adults aged 60+. Cochrane Developmental, Psychosocial and Learning Problems Group Cochrane Database of Systematic Reviews 4, 2002.

Montgomery, P, and Dennis, J: Bright light therapy for sleep problems in adults aged 60+. Cochrane Developmental, Psychosocial and Learning Problems Group Cochrane Database of Systematic Reviews 4, 2002

Reynolds, CF, et al: Treating insomnia in older adults: Taking a long-term view. JAMA 281:1034, 1999.

Ring, D: Management of chronic insomnia in the elderly. Clinical Excellence for Nurse Practitioners 5:13, 2001.

Wroble, R, et al: Insomnia in the elderly: Assessment and management in a primary care setting. J Clinical Outcomes Management 7:50, 2000.

Vignola, A: Effects of chronic insomnia and use of benzodiazepines on daytime performance in older adults. J Gerontol 55B:P54, 2000.

Wandering

Cohen-Mansfield, J, and Werner, P: Outdoor wandering parks for persons with dementia: A survey of characteristics and use. Alzheimer Dis Assoc Disord 13:109, 1999.

Cummings, JL: Guidelines for managing Alzheimer's disease: part I. Assessment. Am Fam Physician 65:2263, 2002.

Cummings, JL: Guidelines for managing Alzheimer's disease: Part II. Treatment. Am Fam Physician 65:2525, 2002.

Hughes, CM: The impact of legislation on psychotropic drug use in nursing homes: a cross-national perspective. J Am Geriatr Soc 48:931, 2000.

McCallion, P: An evaluation of a family visit education program. J Am Geriatr Soc 47:203, 1999.

McCurry, SM: Treatment of sleep disturbance in Alzheimer's disease. Sleep Med Rev 4:603, 2000.

Roberts, C: Research in brief: The management of wandering in older people with dementia. J Clin Nurs 8:322, 1999.

Rubenstein, L: The epidemiology of falls and syncope. Clin Geriatr Med 18:141, 2002.

Shaw, F: Falls in cognitive impairment and dementia. Clin Geriatr Med 18:159, 2002.

Steinberg, M, et al: Falls in the institutionalized elderly with dementia: A pilot study. Ann Long Term Care 6:153, 1998.

Sullivan-Marx, EM: Predictors of continued physical restraint use in nursing home residents following restraint reduction efforts. J Am Geriatr Soc 47:342, 1999.

Teri, L: Nonpharmacologic treatment of behavioral disturbance in dementia. Med Clin North Am 86:641, 2002.

University of Iowa Gerontological Nursing Interventions Research Center: Evidence based protocol. wandering. complete summary. 2002. Contact: http://www.ngc.org. Retrieved December 10, 2002.

Velez, L: Managing behavioral problems in long-term care. Clin Fam Pract 3:561, 2001.

Zanetti, O: Contrasting results between caregiver's report and direct assessment of activities of daily living in patients affected by mild and very mild dementia: the contribution of the caregiver's personal characteristics. J Am Geriatr Soc 47:196, 1999.

PHYSIOLOGICAL INFLUENCES OF THE AGING PROCESS

Age-Related Change	Appearance or Functional Change	Implication
	Integumentary System	
Loss of dermal and epidermal thickness	Paper-thin skin	Prone to skin breakdown and injury
Flattening of papillae	Shearing and friction force more readily peels off the epidermis	
	Diminished cell-mediated immunity in the skin	
Atrophy of the sweat glands	Decreased sweating	Frequent pruritus
Decreased vascularity	Slower recruitment of sweat glands by thermal stimulation	Alteration in thermoregularity response
		Fluid requirements may change seasonally
	Decreased body odor	Loss of skin water
	Decreased heat loss	Increased risk of heat stroke
	Dryness	
Collagen cross-linking	Increased wrinkling	Potential effect on one's morale and feeling of self-worth
Elastin regression	Laxity of skin	
Loss of subcutaneous fat	Intraosseous atrophy, especially to back of hands and face	Loss of fat tissue on soles of feet—trauma of walking increases foot problems
Decreased elasticity		
Loss of subcutaneous tissue	Purpuric patches after minor surgery	Reduced insulation against cold temperatures; *prone to hypothermia*
		Check why injury is occurring; be alert— potential abuse or falls
Decreased number of melanocytes	Loss of pigment	Teach importance of using sun block creams; refer to dermatologist as needed
	Pigment plaque appears	

Age-Related Change	Appearance or Functional Change	Implication
Decline in fibroblast proliferation	Decreased epidermal growth rate Slower re-epithelialization Decreased vitamin D production and synthesis	Decreased tissue repair response
Decreased hair follicle density	Loss of body hair	
Decreased growth phase of individual fibers	Thin, short villus hairs predominate Slower hair growth	
Loss of melanocytes from the hair bulb	Graying of the hair	Potential effect on self-esteem
Alternating hyperplasia and hypoplasia of nail matrix	Longitudinal ridges Thinner nails of the fingers Thickened, curled toenails	Nails prone to splitting Advise patient to wear gloves, keep nails short, avoid nail polish remover (cause dryness); refer to podiatrist May cause discomfort
	Respiratory System	
Decreased lung tissue elasticity	Decreased vital capacity Increased residual volume Decreased maximum breath capacity	Reduced overall efficiency of ventilatory exchange
Thoracic wall calcification	Increased anteroposterior diameter of chest	Obscuration of heart and lung sounds Displacement of apical impulse
Cilia atrophy	Change in mucociliary transport	Increased susceptibility to infection
Decreased respiratory muscle strength	Reduced ability to handle secretions and reduced effectiveness against noxious foreign particles Partial inflation of lungs at rest	Prone to atelectasis
	Cardiovascular System	
Heart valves fibrose and thicken	Reduced stroke volume, cardiac output; may be altered Slight left ventricular hypertrophy	Decreased responsiveness to stress Increased incidence of murmurs, *particularly aortic stenosis and mitral regurgitation*
Mucoid degeneration of mitral valve	S_4 commonly heard Valve less dense; mitral leaflet stretches with intrathoracic pressure	
Fibroelastic thickening of the sinoatrial node; decreased number of pacemaker cells Increased subpericardial fat Collagen accumulation around heart muscle	Slower heart rate Irregular heart rate	Increased prevalence of arrhythmias

Age-Related Change	Appearance or Functional Change	Implication
Elongation of tortuosity and calcification of arteries	Increased rigidity of arterial wall	Aneurysms may form
Elastin and collagen cause progressive thickening and loss of arterial wall resiliency	Increased peripheral vascular resistance	Decreased blood flow to body organs Altered distribution of blood flow
Loss of elasticity of the aorta dilation		Increased systolic blood pressure, contributing to coronary artery disease
Increased lipid content in artery wall	Lipid deposits form	Increased incidence of atherosclerotic events, such as *angina pectoris*, stroke, gangrene
Decreased baroreceptor sensitivity (stretch receptors)	Decreased sensitivity to change in blood pressure	Prone to loss of balance—potential for falls
	Decreased baroreceptor mediation to straining	Valsalva maneuver may cause sudden drop in blood pressure

	Gastrointestinal System	
Liver becomes smaller	Decreased storage capacity	
Less efficient cholesterol stabilization absorption	Increased evidence of gallstones	
Dental enamel thins	Staining of tooth surface occurs	Tooth and gum decay; tooth loss
Gums recede	Teeth deprived of nutrients	
Fibrosis and atrophy of salivary glands	Prone to dry mucous membranes	Shift to mouth breathing is common
	Decreased salivary ptyalin	Membrane more susceptible to injury and infection May interfere with breakdown of starches
Atrophy and decrease in number of taste buds	Decreased taste sensation	Altered ability to taste sweet, sour, and bitter Change in nutritional intake Excessive seasoning of foods
Delay in esophageal emptying	Decline in esophageal peristalsis Esophagus slightly dilated	Occasional discomfort as food stays in esophagus longer

Age-Related Change	Appearance or Functional Change	Implication
	Gastrointestinal System	
Decreased hydrochloric acid secretion Decrease in gastric acid secretion	Reduction in amount of iron and vitamin B_{12} that can be absorbed	Possible delay in vitamin and drug absorption, *especially calcium and iron* Altered drug effect Fewer cases of gastric ulcers
Decreased muscle tone Atrophy of mucosal lining	Altered motility Decreased colonic peristalsis	Prone to constipation, functional bowel syndrome, esophageal spasm, diverticular disease
	Decreased hunger sensations and emptying time	
Decreased proportion of dietary calcium absorbed	Altered bone formation, muscle contractility, hormone activity, enzyme activation, clotting time, immune response	Symptoms more marked in women than in men
Decreased basal metabolic rate (rate at which fuel is converted into energy)		May need fewer calories Possible effect on life span
	Genitourinary and Reproductive Systems	
Reduced renal mass	Decreased sodium conserving ability	Administration and dosage of drugs may need to be modified
Loss of glomeruli	Decreased glomerular filtration rate	
	Decreased creatinine clearance Increased blood urea nitrogen concentration	
Histological changes in small vessel walls Sclerosis of supportive circulatory system	Decreased renal blood flow	
Decline in number of functioning nephrons	Decreased ability to dilute urine concentrate	Altered response to reduced fluid load or increased fluid volume
Reduced bladder muscular tone	Decreased bladder capacity or increased residual urine	Sensation of urge to urinate may not occur until bladder is full
Atrophy and fibrosis of cervical and uterine walls	Menopause; decline in fertility	Urination at night may increase
Reduced number and viability of oocytes in the aging ovary	Narrowing of cervical canal	
Decreased vaginal wall elasticity	Vaginal lining thin, pale, friable Narrowing of vaginal canal	Potential for discomfort in sexual intercourse
Decreased levels of circulating hormones	Reduced lubrication during arousal state	Increased frequency of sexual dysfunction
Degeneration of seminiferous tubules	Decreased seminal fluid volume Decreased force of ejaculation Reduced elevation of testes	

Age-Related Change	Appearance or Functional Change	Implication
Proliferation of stromal and glandular tissue	Prostatic hypertrophy	Potentially compromised genitourinary function; *urinary frequency, and increased risk of malignancy*
Involution of mammary gland tissue	Connective tissue replaced by adipose tissue	Easier to assess breast lesions
	Neuromuscular System	
Decreased muscle mass	Decreased muscle strength	Decreased tendon jerks Increased muscle cramping
	Tendons shrink and sclerose	
Decreased myosin adenosine triphosphatase activity	Prolonged contraction time, latency period, relaxation period	Decreased motor function and overall strength
Deterioration of joint cartilage	Bone makes contact with bone	Potential for pain, crepitation, and limitation of movement
Loss of water from the cartilage	Narrowing of joint spaces	Loss of height
Decreased bone mass Decreased osteoblastic activity Osteoclasts resorb bone	Decreased bone formation and increased bone resorption, leading to osteoporosis Hormonal changes	More rapid and earlier changes in women Greater risk of fractures Gait and posture accommodate to changes
Increased proportion of body fat Regional changes in fat distribution	Centripetal distribution of fat and invasion of fat in large muscle groups	Anthropometric measurements required Increased relative adiposity
Thickened leptomeninges in spinal cord	Loss of anterior horn cells in the lumbosacral area	Leg weakness may be correlated
Accumulation of lipofuscin	Altered RNA function and resultant cell death	
Loss of neurons and nerve fibers	Decreased processing speed and vibration sense Altered pain response Decreased deep tendon, Achilles tendon	Increased time to perform and learn Possible postural hypotension Safety hazard
Decreased conduction of nerve fibers Few neuritic plaques	Decreased psychomotor performance	Alteration in pain response Possible cognitive and memory changes
Neurofibrillary tangles in hippocampal neurons		Heavy tangle formation and neuritic plaques in cortex of patients with Alzheimer's disease

Age-Related Change	Appearance or Functional Change	Implication
	Neuromuscular System	
Changes in sleep-wake cycle	Decreased stage 4, stage 3, and rapid eye movement phases	Increased or decreased time spent sleeping
	Deterioration of circadian organization	Increased nighttime awakenings
		Changed hormonal activity
Slower stimulus identification and registration	Delayed reaction time	Prone to falls
Decreased brain weight and volume		May be present in absence of mental impairments
	Sensory System	
Morphological changes in choroid, epithelium, retina	Decreased visual acuity	Corrective lenses required
	Visual field narrows	Increased possibility of disorientation and social isolation
Decreased rod and cone function		Slower light and dark adaptation
Pigment accumulation		
Decreased speed of eye movements	Difficulty in gazing upward and maintaining convergence	
Sclerosis of pupil sphincter	Difficulty in adapting to lighting changes	Glare may pose an environmental hazard
	Increased threshold for light perception	Dark rooms may be hazardous
Increased intraocular pressure		Increased incidence of glaucoma
Distorted depth perception		Incorrect assessment of height of curbs and steps; potential for falls
Ciliary muscle atrophy	Altered refractive powers	Corrective lenses often required
Nuclear sclerosis (*lens*)	Presbyopia	Near work and reading may become difficult
Reduced accommodation	Hyperopia	
Increased lens size	Myopia	
Accumulation of lens fibers		
Lens yellows	Color vision may be impaired	Less able to differentiate lower color tones: blues, greens, violets
Diminished tear secretion	Dullness and dryness of the eyes	Irritation and discomfort may result
		Intactness of corneal surface jeopardized
Loss of auditory neurons	Decreased tone discrimination and voice localization	Suspiciousness may be increased because of paranoid dimensions secondary to hearing loss
	High frequency sounds lost first	Social isolation

Age-Related Change	Appearance or Functional Change	Implication
Angiosclerosis calcification of inner ear membrane	Progressive hearing loss, especially at high frequency Presbycusis	Difficulty hearing, particularly under certain conditions such as *background noise, rapid speech, poor acoustics*
Decreased number of olfactory nerve fibers Alteration in taste sensation	Decreased sensitivity to odors	May not detect harmful odors Potential safety hazard Possible changes in food preferences and eating patterns
Reduced tactile sensation	Decreased ability to sense pressure, pain, temperature	Misperceptions of environment and safety risk
Endocrine System		
Decline in secretion of testosterone, growth hormone, insulin, adrenal androgens, aldosterone, thyroid hormone	Decreased hormone clearance rates	Increased mortality associated with certain stresses (burns, surgery)
Defects in thermoregulation	Shivering less intense	Susceptibility to temperature extremes (*hypothermia/ hyperthermia*)
Reduction of febrile responses	Poor perceptions of changes in ambient temperature Reduced sweating; increased threshold for the onset of sweating Fever not always present with infectious process	Unrecognized infectious process operative
Alteration in tissue sensitivity to hormones	Decreased insulin response, glucose tolerance, and sensitivity of renal tubules to antidiuretic hormone	
Enhanced sympathetic responsivity Increased nodularity and fibrosis of thyroid		Increased frequency of thyroid disease
Decreased basal metabolic rate	Alteration in carbohydrate tolerance	Increased incidence of obesity
Hematological System		
Decreased percentage of marrow space occupied by hematopoietic tissue	Ineffective erythropoiesis	Risky for patient who loses blood

Age-Related Change	Appearance or Functional Change	Implication
	Immune System	
Thymic involution and decreased serum thymic hormone activity	Decreased number of T cells Production of antiself reactive T cells	Less vigorous and/or delayed hypersensitivity reactions
Decreased T-cell function	Impairment in cell-mediated immune responses	Increased risk mortality
Appearance of autoantibodies	Decreased cyclic adenosine monophosphate and glucose monophosphate	Increased incidence of infection
	Decreased ability to reject foreign tissue	Reactivation of latent infectious diseases
	Increased laboratory autoimmune parameters	Increased prevalence of autoimmune disorders
Redistribution of lymphocytes	Impaired immune reactivity	
Changes in serum immunoglobulin	Increased immunoglobulin A levels	Increased prevalence of infection
	Decreased immunoglobulin G levels	

LABORATORY VALUES IN THE OLDER ADULT

Laboratory Test	Normal Values	Changes with Age	Comments
		Urinalysis	
Protein	0–5 mg/100 mL	Rises slightly	May be due to kidney changes with age, urinary tract infection, renal pathology
Glucose	0–15 mg/100 mL	Declines slightly	Glycosuria appears after high plasma level; unreliable
Specific gravity	1.005–1.020	Lower maximum in elderly 1.016–1.022	Decline in nephrons impairs ability to concentrate urine
		Hematology	
Erythrocyte sedimentation rate	Men: 0–20 Women: 0–30	Significant increase	Neither sensitive nor specific in aged
Iron	50–160 µg/dL	Slight decrease	
Iron binding	230–410 µg/dL	Decrease	
Hemoglobin	Men: 13–18 g/100 mL Women: 12–16 g/100 mL	Men: 10–17 g/mL Women: none noted	Anemia common in the elderly
Hematocrit	Men: 45–52% Women: 37–48%	Slight decrease speculated	Decline in hematopoiesis
Leukocytes	4300–10,800/mm³	Drop to 3100–9000/mm³	Decrease may be due to drugs or sepsis and should not be attributed immediately to age
Lymphocytes	500–2400 T cells/mm³ 50–200 B cells/mm³	T-cell and B-cell levels fall	Infection risk higher; immunization encouraged
Platelets	150,000–350,000/mm³	No change in number	
		Blood Chemistry	
Albumin	3.5–5.0/100 mL	Decline	Related to decrease in liver size and enzymes; protein energy malnutrition common

Laboratory Test	Normal Values	Changes with Age	Comments
		Blood Chemistry	
Globulin	2.3–3.5 g/100 mL	Slight increase	
Total serum protein	6.0–8.4 g/100 mL	No change	Decreases may indicate malnutrition, infection, liver disease
Blood urea nitrogen	Men: 10–25 mg/100 mL Women: 8–20 mg/100 mL	Increases significantly up to 69 mg/100 mL	Decline in glomerular filtration rate; decreased cardiac output
Creatinine	0.6–1.5 mg/100 mL	Increases to 1.9 mg/100 mL seen	Related to lean body mass decrease
Creatinine clearance	104–124 mL/min	Decreases 10%/decade after 40 years of age	Used for prescribing medications for drugs excreted by kidney
Glucose tolerance	62–110 mg/dL after fasting; < 120 mg/dL after 2 hours post-prandial	Slight increase of 10 mg/dL/decade after 30 years of age	Diabetes increasingly prevalent; drugs may cause glucose intolerance
Triglycerides	40–150 mg/100 mL	20–200 mg/100 mL	
Cholesterol	120–220 mg/100 mL	Men: increase to 50 mg/100 mL, then decrease Women: increase post-menopausally	Risk of cardiovascular disease
Thyroxine	4.5–13.5 µg/100 mL	No change	Changes suggest thyroid disease; may be seen in euthyroid patients with acute or chronic illness or caloric deficiencies
Triiodo-thyronine	90–220 ng/100 mL	Decrease 25%	
Thyroid-stimulating hormone	0.5–5.0 µg/mL	Slight increase	Sensitive indicator for diagnosing thyroid disease
Alkaline phosphatase	13–39 IU/L	Increase by 8–10 IU/L	Elevations > 20% usually due to disease; elevations may be found with bone abnormalities, drugs (e.g., narcotics), and eating a fatty meal

Appendix *C*
COMMON TESTS AND THEIR ASSOCIATIONS WITH DISEASES AND CONDITIONS

Laboratory Test	Increase	Decrease
Acid phosphatase	Prostate cancer, prostatic massage, prostatitis, myocardial infarction, excess platelet destruction, bone disease, liver disease	—
Alanine amino-transferase	Hepatitis, cirrhosis, liver metastases, obstructive jaundice, infectious mononucleosis, hepatic congestion, pancreatitis, renal disease, alcohol ingestion	Pyridoxine (vitamin B_6) deficiency
Albumin	Dehydration, diabetes insipidus	Overhydration, malnutrition, malabsorption, nephrosis, hepatic failure, burns, multiple myeloma, metastatic carcinomias, acute illness
Alkaline phosphatase	Bone growth, bone metastases, Paget's disease, osteomalacia, healing fracture, hyperparathyroidism, hepatic disease, obstructive jaundice, hepatic metastases, pulmonary infarction, heart failure	Pernicious anemia hypoparathyroidism, hypophosphatasia
α-Fetoprotein	Hepatoma, testicular tumor, hepatitis	—
Amylase	Pancreatitis, gastrointestinal—Obstruction, mesenteric thrombosis and infarction, macroamylasemia, parotitis, renal disease, lung carcinoma, acute alcohol ingestion, after abdominal surgery	Massive pancreatic destruction

Laboratory Test	Increase	Decrease
Aspartate amino-transferase	Myocardial infarction, heart failure, myocarditis, pericarditis, myositis, trauma, hepatic disease, pancreatitis, renal infarction, neoplasia, cerebral damage, seizures, hemolysis, alcohol ingestion	Pyridoxine (vitamine B_6) deficiency, advanced stages of liver disease
Bilirubin	Hepatic disease, obstructive jaundice, hemolytic anemia, pulmonary infarction, Gilbert's disease, Dubin-Johnson syndrome	—
Calcium	Hyperparathyroidism, bone metastases, myeloma, sarcoidosis, hyperthyroidism, hypervitaminosis D, malignancy without bone metastases, milk-alkali syndrome	Hypoparathyroidism, renal failure, malabsorption, pancreatitis, hypoalbuminemia, vitamin D deficiency, overhydration
Cholesterol	Hypercholesterolemia, hypothyroidism, obstructive jaundice, nephrosis, diabetes mellitus, pancreatitis	Hyperthyroidism, infection, malnutrition, heart failure, malignancies, severe liver damage (due to chemicals, drugs, hepatitis)
High-density lipoprotein cholesterol	Vigorous exercise, increased clearance of triglyceride (very-low-density lipoprotein), moderate alcohol consumption, exogenous intake of insulin or estrogens	Malnutrition, obesity, cigarette smoking, diabetes mellitus, hypothyroidism, liver disease, nephrosis, uremia
Creatine kinase	Myocardial infarction, muscle disease or injury, burns, chest trauma, collagen-vascular disease, meningitis, drug use (e.g., lovastatin), status epilepticus, brain infarction, hyperthermia, after surgery	—
Creatinine	Renal failure, urinary obstruction, dehydration, hyperthyroidism, muscle disease	Aging (decreases creatinine clearance but not serum creatinine concentration)
Glucose	Diabetes mellitus, pheochromocytoma, hyperthyroidism, Cushing's syndrome, acromegaly, brain damage, hepatic disease, nephrosis, hemochromatosis, stress (e.g., from emotion, burns, shock, anesthesia), acute or chronic pancreatitis, Wernicke's encephalopathy (vitamin B_1 deficiency), chronic hypervitaminosis A, administration of thiazides, corticosteroids, epinephrine, estrogens, ethanol, phenytoin, propranolol, or intravenous glucose	Excess exogenous insulin, insulinoma, Addison's disease, myxedema, hepatic failure, malabsorption, pancreatitis, glucagon deficiency, extrapancreatic tumors, early diabetes mellitus, postgastrectomy, autonomic nervous system disorders, administration of oral hypoglycemic medications (factitious), malnutrition, alcoholism

Laboratory Test	Increase	Decrease
Lactate dehydrogenase	Myocardial infarction, pulmonary infarction, hemolytic anemia, pernicious anemia, leukemia, lymphoma, other malignancies, hepatic disease, renal infarction, seizures, cerebral damage, trauma, sprue	—
Lipase	Same as amylase (excluding parotitis and macroamylasemia)	—
Magnesium	Renal disease, excess exogenous magnesium	Diarrhea, malabsorption, renal tubular acidosis, acute tubular necrosis, chronic glomerulonephritis, aldosteronism, hyperthyroidism, hypercalcemia, uncontrolled diabetes, dietary deficit, administration of certain drugs (diuretics, antiboitics), alcoholism
Phosphorus	Renal failure, hypoparathyroidism, diabetic acidosis, acromegaly, hyperthyroidism, high phosphate intake (intravenous or oral), vitamin D intoxication, lactic acidosis, leukemia, volume contraction, hyperlipidemia, hyperbilirubinemia, dysproteinemia, heparin sodium contamination, spurious (prolonged refrigeration of sample)	Hyperparathyroidism, osteomalacia, hypokalemia, excess intravenous glucose, respiratory alkalosis, dietary deficit, ingestion of P-binding antacid, alcoholism, gout, hemodialysis, cirrhosis
Potassium	Hyperkalemic acidosis, diabetic acidosis, hypoadrenalism, hereditary hyperkalemia, hemolysis, myoglobulinuria, renal tubular defect, thrombocytosis, intake of potassium-retaining diuretic, angiotensin-convulsing enzyme inhibitors, or large exogenous potassium load	Cirrhosis, malnutrition, vomiting, metabolic alkalosis, diarrhea, nephrosis, hyperadrenalism, ectopic adrenocorticotropic hormone excess, β-hydroxylase deficiency, administration of diuretics
Prostate-specific antigen	Prostate cancer, benign prostatic hyperplasia, prostatic massage, prostatic abscess, prostatitis, cystoscopy	Administration of finasteride

Laboratory Test	Increase	Decrease
Sodium	Dehydration, diabetes insipidus, excessive salt ingestion, diabetes mellitus with diuresis, diuretic phase of acute tubular necrosis, hypercalcemic nephropathy with diuresis, essential hypernatremia due to hypothalamic lesions	Excess exogenous antidiuretic hormone, nephrosis, hypoadrenalism, myxedema, heart failure, diarrhea, vomiting, diabetic acidosis, adrenocortical insufficiency, hyperlipidemia, hyperglycemia, hyperproteinemia (e.g., multiple myeloma), intake of diuretics of mannitol, spurious (serum osmolality is normal or increased—avoid by using direct-reading potentiometry with ion-selective electrode)
Total protein	Multiple myeloma, myxedema, lupus, sarcoidosis, diabetes insipidus, dehydration, collagen-vascular disease	Burns, cirrhosis, malnutrition, nephrosis, malabsorption, overhydration, gastrointestinal protein loss
Triglyceride	Nephrosis, cholestatis, pancreatitis, cirrhosis, diabetes mellitus, hepatitis, familial hypertriglyceridemia	Malnutrition
Troponin	Myocardial damage	
Urea nitrogen	Renal disease, dehydration, gastrointestinal bleeding, leukemia, heart failure, shock, postrenal azotemia, obstruction of urinary tract, acute myocardial infarction	Hepatic failure, overhydration, acromegaly, dietary factors, prolonged intravenous feedings
Uric acid	Gout, renal failure, diuretic therapy, leukemia, lymphoma, polycythemia, acidosis, psoriasis, hypothyroidism, multiple myeloma, pernicious anemia, tissue necrosis, inflammation, 25% of relatives of patients with gout, cancer chemotherapy (e.g., nitrogen mustards, vincristine, mercaptopurine), hemolytic anemia, high-protein weight-reduction diet, lead poisoning, polycystic kidneys, calcinosis universalis and circumscripta, hypoparathyroidism, sarcoidosis, elevated serum triglyceride levels, use of low-dose aspirin	Administration of uricosuric drugs, allopurinol, or large doses of vitamin C; Wilson's disease

Based on material in Wallach J: *Interpretation of Diagnostic Tests,* ed 4, Little, Brown, Boston 1986, pp 41–96; used with permission.

INDEX